Intervirology

International Journal of Basic and Medical Virology

Founded 1973 by J.L. Melnick
Continued by F. Rapp (1986–1990); M.J. Buchmeier; C.R. Howard (1991–1993)
and R.W. Braun (1994–2003)

KARGER

Printed in Switzerland
on acid-free paper by
Reinhardt Druck, Basel

Appears bimonthly:
1 volume per year
(6 issues)

Guidelines for Authors

Submission

Only original papers written in English are considered and should be sent to:

Prof. U.G. Liebert
S. Karger AG
Editorial Office Intervirology
PO Box
CH–4009 Basel (Switzerland)
Tel. +41 61 306 1344
Fax +41 61 306 1434
E-Mail s.aeschbach@karger.ch

Mailing address for courier deliveries only:
Allschwilerstr. 10
CH–4055 Basel (Switzerland)

Manuscripts from Japan and South-East Asia to:
Dr. Okio Hino, MD, PhD
Professor
Department of Pathology (II)
Juntendo University School of Medicine
2-1-1, Hongo, Bunkyo-ku
Tokyo 113-8421 (Japan)
Fax +81 3 5684 1646
E-Mail ohino@med.juntendo.ac.jp

Manuscripts should be submitted threefold, i.e., one original and two copies (with three sets of illustrations of which one is an original), typewritten double-spaced on one side of the paper, with a wide margin. Please ensure that you include the entire manuscript on a disk/CD-ROM, i.e. text, tables, figures and references. The manuscript should match the file on disk exactly.

Conditions

All manuscripts are subject to editorial review. Manuscripts are received with the explicit understanding that they are not under simultaneous consideration by any other publication. Submission of an article for publication implies the transfer of the copyright from the author to the publisher upon acceptance. Accepted papers become the permanent property of 'Intervirology' and may not be reproduced by any means, in whole or in part, without the written consent of the publisher. It is the author's responsibility to obtain permission to reproduce illustrations, tables, etc. from other publications.

Arrangement

Title page: The first page of each paper should indicate the title, the authors' names, the institute where the work was conducted, and a short title for use as running head.

Full address: The exact postal address of the corresponding author complete with postal code must be given at the bottom of the title page. Please also supply phone and fax numbers, as well as e-mail address.

Key words: For indexing purposes, a list of 3–10 key words in English is essential.

Abstract: **Each paper needs an abstract of up to 200 words structured with subheadings as follows Objective(s), Methods, Results, Conclusion(s).**

Footnotes: Avoid footnotes. When essential, they are numbered consecutively and typed at the foot of the appropriate page.

Body of the paper: Manuscripts should then be divided into the following subdivisions: Introduction, Materials and Methods (as brief as possible), Results, Discussion, Acknowledgments and References.

Tables and illustrations: Tables and illustrations (both numbered in Arabic numerals) should be prepared on separate sheets. Tables require a heading and figures a legend, also prepared on a separate sheet. For the reproduction of illustrations, only good drawings and original photographs can be accepted; negatives or photocopies cannot be used. Due to technical reasons, figures with a screen background should not be submitted. When possible, group several illustrations on one block for reproduction (max. size 180 × 223 mm) or provide crop marks. On the back of each illustration, indicate its number, the author's name, and 'top' with a soft pencil. Electronically submitted b/w half-tone and color illustrations must have a final resolution of 300 dpi after scaling, line drawings one of 800–1200 dpi.

Color illustrations: Up to 6 color illustrations per page can now be integrated within the text at the special price of CHF/USD 660.00 per page. Color illustrations are reproduced at the author's expense.

References: In the text identify references by Arabic numerals [in square brackets]. Material submitted for publication but not yet accepted should be noted as 'unpublished data' and not be included in the reference list. The list of references should include only those publications which are cited in the text. Do not alphabetize; number references in the order in which they are first mentioned in the text. The surnames of the authors followed by initials should be given. There should be no punctuation other than a comma to separate the authors. Preferably, please cite all authors. Abbreviate journal names according to the Index Medicus system. (Also see International Committee of Medical Journal Editors: Uniform requirements for manuscripts submitted to biomedical journals. N Engl J Med 1997;336:309–315.)

Digital Object Identifier (DOI)
S. Karger Publishers supports DOIs as unique identifiers for articles. A DOI number will be printed on the title page of each article. DOIs can be useful in the future for identifying and citing articles published online without volume or issue information. More information can be found at www.doi.org.

Examples
(a) Papers published in periodicals: Sun J, Koto H, Chung KF: Interaction of ozone and allergen challenges on bronchial responsiveness and inflammation in sensitised guinea pigs. Int Arch Allergy Immunol 1997;112:191–195.
(b) Papers published only with DOI numbers: Theoharides TC, Boucher W, Spear K: Serum interleukin-6 reflects disease severity and osteoporosis in mastocytosis patients. Int Arch Allergy Immunol DOI: 10.1159/000063858.
(c) Monographs: Matthews DE, Farewell VT: Using and Understanding Medical Statistics, ed 3, revised. Basel, Karger, 1996.
(d) Edited books: Parren PWHI, Burton DR: Antibodies against HIV-1 from phage display libraries: Mapping of an immune response and progress towards antiviral immunotherapy; in Capra JD (ed): Antibody Engineering. Chem Immunol. Basel, Karger, 1997, vol 65, pp 18–56.

Nomenclature of viruses

Names used for viruses should be those approved by the International Committee on Taxonomy of Viruses (ICTV) and published in the fourth report of the ICTV 'Classification and Nomenclature of Viruses', Intervirology 1982;17:1–200. If desired, synonyms may be added in parentheses when the name is first mentioned. Approved generic (or group) and family names should also be used.

Short communications

In addition to regular papers, a section of the journal will publish brief communications of important findings, in which illustrative material should be limited. Such notes should include a brief summary and key words, the body of the report (without any subdivisions), brief acknowledgment, and a few selected references. The general style and submission procedures outlined above apply to the short communication.

Commentaries

Short commentaries of an editorial nature may be submitted to the journal. In these communications, usual manuscript subdivisions do not apply, and a summary statement is not needed; however, a very brief reference list may be included.

Letters to the Editor

This section provides readers with a forum in which to exchange ideas and comments on papers published in the journal. Letters should be no longer than 1–1½ double-spaced pages, including a maximum of six references, and do not require abstracts or formal section headings.

Page charges

There are no page charges for papers of 6 or fewer printed pages (including tables, illustrations and references). Each additional complete or partial page is charged to the author at CHF/USD 275.00. The allotted size of a paper is equal to approx. 16 manuscript pages (including tables, illustrations and references).

Galley proofs

Unless indicated otherwise, galley proofs are sent to the first-named author and should be returned with the least possible delay. Alterations made in galley proofs, other than the correction of printer's errors, are charged to the author. No page proofs are supplied.

Reprints

Order forms and a price list are sent to the author by the publisher after the article has been set in type. Orders submitted after the issue is printed are subject to considerably higher prices.

KARGER

Fax +41 61 306 12 34
E-Mail karger@karger.ch
www.karger.com

The Guidelines for Authors are available at:
www.karger.com/int_Guidelines

Standard forms of abbreviations: The standard abbreviations used for measurements of weight, length, volume, and time (i.e., mg, cm, ml, and min) are acceptable and may be used without definition. The abbreviations listed also require no preliminary definition. Please note that punctuation is not needed. When using other abbreviations, the name should be spelled out in full at the first mention, and followed with the abbreviation in parentheses.

°	degree centigrade (Fahrenheit will not be used)
A, C, G, T, U	adenine, cytosine, guanine, thymine, uracil
AMP	5'-monophosphates of adenosine
CMP	– cytidine
GMP	– guanosine
TMP	– thymidine
UMP	– uridine
ADP, etc.	adenosine 5'-diphosphate, etc.
ATP, etc.	adenosine 5'-triphosphate, etc.
CPE	cytopathic effect
DEAE-cellulose	diethylaminoethylcellulose
DNA	deoxyribonucleic acid
DNase	deoxyribonuclease
EDTA	ethylenediaminetetra-acetate
EOP	efficiency of plating
g	acceleration of gravity
ID_{50}	median infective dose
LD_{50}	median lethal dose
M	molar
MEM	minimum essential medium
MOI	multiplicity of infection
N	normal
ng	nanogram
nm	nanometer (10^{-9} m)
PAGE	polyacrylamide gel electrophoresis
PFU	plaque forming units
RNA	ribonucleic acid
RNase	ribonuclease
rpm	revolutions per minute
SD	standard deviation
SDS	sodium dodecyl sulfate
sp gr	specific gravity
TCD_{50}	median tissue culture infective dose
Tris	tris (hydroxymethyl) aminomethane (2-amino-2-hydroxymethylpropane-1,3-diol)
UV	ultraviolet
V	volt
W	watt

Intervirology

General Information

Publication data: 'Intervirology' is published 6 times a year. Volume 49 with 6 issues appears in 2006.

Subscription rates: Subscriptions run for a full calendar year. Prices are given per year.

Personal subscription:

Print or Online	Print/Online combined
CHF 476.35	CHF 521.35
EUR 352.80	EUR 385.80
USD 432.95	USD 473.95
postage and handling	(added to print and print/online)
CHF 33.60 Europe,	CHF 49.80 Overseas
EUR 24.30	
USD 45.60	

Institutional subscription:

Print or Online	Print/Online combined
CHF 1361.–	CHF 1470.–
EUR 1008.–	EUR 1089.–
USD 1237.00	USD 1336.00
postage and handling	(added to print and print/online)
CHF 42.– Europe,	CHF 62.40 Overseas
EUR 30.30	
USD 57.00	

Airmail surcharge: CHF 42.– / USD 38.10

Discount subscription prices: International Union of Microbiological Societies, American Society for Virology.

Microforms: Please direct all enquiries and orders to:
University Microfilms Inc.
300 North Zeeb Road, P.O. Box 1346
Ann Arbor, MI 48106-1346 (USA)

Subscription orders: Orders can be placed at agencies, bookstores, directly with the Publisher
S. Karger AG, P.O. Box
CH–4009 Basel (Switzerland)
or with any of the following distributors:
Deutschland: S. Karger GmbH, Postfach
D–79095 Freiburg
France: Librairie Luginbühl
36, bd de Latour-Maubourg
F–75007 Paris
Great Britain, Ireland: S. Karger AG
4 Rickett Street
London SW6 1RU, UK
USA: S. Karger Publishers, Inc.
26 West Avon Road, P.O. Box 529
Farmington, CT 06085, USA
India, Bangladesh, Sri Lanka:
Panther Publishers Private Ltd.
33, First Main
Koramangala First Block
Bangalore 560 034, India
Japan: Karger Japan, Inc.
Yushima S Bld. 3F
4-2-3, Yushima, Bunkyo-ku
Tokyo 113-0034, Japan

Change of address: Both old and new address should be sent to the subscription source.

Single issues and back volumes: Information can be obtained through the Publisher.

Advertising: Correspondence and rate requests should be addressed to the Publisher.

Bibliographic indices: This journal is regularly listed in bibliographic services, including *Current Contents®* and Index Medicus/MEDLINE.

Copying: This journal has been registered with the Copyright Clearance Center (CCC), as indicated by the code appearing on the first page of each article. For readers in the US, this code signals consent for copying of articles for personal or internal use, or for the personal or internal use of specific clients, provided that the stated fee is paid per copy directly to
Copyright Clearance Center Inc.
222 Rosewood Drive
Danvers, MA 01923 (USA)
A copy of the first page of the article must accompany payment. Consent does not extend to copying for general distribution, for promotion, for creating new works, or for resale. In these cases, specific written permission must be obtained from the copyright owner,
S. Karger AG,
P.O. Box, CH–4009 Basel (Switzerland).

KARGER

Fax +41 61 306 12 34
E-Mail karger@karger.ch
www.karger.com

The Journal Home Page is available at:
www.karger.com/int

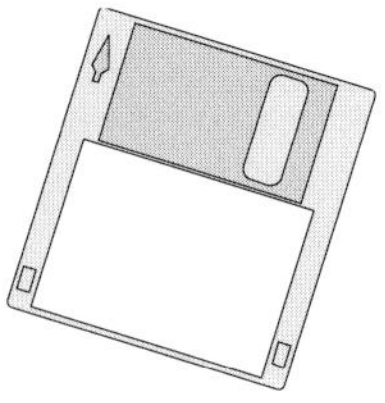

Disk Submission

A **comprehensive version** of these guidelines for the **submission of manuscripts and illustrations on disk** can be accessed online under **www.karger.com/disksubmission** or requested as a leaflet from the editorial department.

Please follow the general rules on style and arrangement in the **'Guidelines for Authors'** of the journal. Submit a **double-spaced printout** of your manuscript matching the file on disk exactly.

Technical Information
Store only data pertinent to this manuscript. Include your fonts (screen and printer fonts for Macintosh). For a **text only** manuscript, use a 3.5-inch disk. For **text and illustrations,** use 3.5 or 5.25 Magneto Optical Disc; CD-ROM (DOS or hybrid); iomega Zip/DOS (100 MB), or 44 MB, 88 MB or 200 MB SyQuest. Compress extensive data using ZIP format.

Data Description
Label your disk with the **title of the journal or book** for which it is submitted; a **short version** of the paper's title; your **name,** postal and e-mail address, fax and phone number; **hard- and software** used, including the version; and the **complete list of the file names.** File names consist of eight characters before the dot identifying the file and three characters after the dot identifying the application.

Text and Format
The **preferred word-processing package is MS-Word.** Other commonly used PC text programs and ASCII formats are accepted.
Update your data when you revise subsequent to the reviewer's or editor's decision and mark revisions clearly. Manuscripts accepted for publication are subject to **copy editing:** changes and/or questions will be marked in the manuscript, which will be returned to you with your disk and the galley proofs for checking.
Enter your text continuously flush left. Do not use any layout functions. Do not split words at the end of a line. **Do not use indentations.** Use a blank line before and a hard return at the end of paragraphs.
Arrange headings flush left. Insert only **one space after punctuation marks.** Insert Greek letters, mathematical symbols etc. with your word-processing program. Use **boldface and italics** as well as sub- and superscript where appropriate.
Tables are part of the text and should be placed at the end of the text file. Separate the individual parts of a table by lines. Use the tabulator instead of spaces. Format operation data on one line in the same column.

Legends to illustrations are part of the text and should also be listed at the end of the text file.

Illustrations
Store illustrations as separate files: do not integrate them in your text. Export **line drawings/vector graphics** as TIF, EPS or WMF format. Use Photoshop for processing and retouching **scanned half-tone images.** Save the original scan and the processed version. Export **black and white or color images** as TIF or EPS format in their anticipated size in print. **For detailed information** on how to submit illustration data on disk please consult the leaflet or **www.karger.com/disksubmission.**

KI 02 DISK

KARGER

Fax +41 61 306 12 34
E-Mail karger@karger.ch
www.karger.com

The Journal Home Page is available at:
www.karger.com/int

Intervirology

Chronic Hepatitis C in Asia: Epidemiology, Pathophysiology, Hepatocellular Carcinoma and Treatment

Proceedings of the 2nd MMRF Meeting
on Viral Hepatitis in Asia
May 15, 2004, Tokyo, Japan

Guest Editors
Hiromitsu Kumada, Tokyo
Yuzo Miyakawa, Tokyo
Shiro Iino, Tokyo

56 figures, 4 in color, and 30 tables, 2006

KARGER

Basel · Freiburg · Paris · London · New York ·
Bangalore · Bangkok · Singapore · Tokyo · Sydney

S. Karger
Medical and Scientific Publishers
Basel • Freiburg • Paris • London
New York • Bangalore • Bangkok
Singapore • Tokyo • Sydney

Disclaimer
The statements, options and data contained in this publication are solely those of the individual authors and contributors and not of the publisher and the editor(s). The appearance of advertisements in the journal is not a warranty, endorsement, or approval of the products or services advertised or of their effectiveness, quality or safety. The publisher and the editor(s) disclaim responsibility for any injury to persons or property resulting from any ideas, methods, instructions or products referred to in the content or advertisements.

Drug Dosage
The authors and the publisher have exerted every effort to ensure that drug selection and dosage set forth in this text are in accord with current recommendations and practice at the time of publication. However, in view of ongoing research, changes in government regulations, and the constant flow of information relating to drug therapy and drug reactions, the reader is urged to check the package insert for each drug for any change in indications and dosage and for added warnings and precautions. This is particularly important when the recommended agent is a new and/or infrequently employed drug.

P.O. Box, CH–4009 Basel (Switzerland)
Printed in Switzerland on acid-free paper by
Reinhardt Druck, Basel
ISBN 3–8055–8017–7

KARGER

Fax +41 61 306 12 34
E-Mail karger@karger.ch
www.karger.com

Vol. 49, No. 1–2, 2006

Intervirology

Contents

KARGER

Fax +41 61 306 12 34
E-Mail karger@karger.ch
www.karger.com

Access to full text and tables of contents, including tentative ones for forthcoming issues: www.karger.com/int_issues

Intervirology

Intervirology 2006;49:4–6

Preface

Hiroshi Suzuki

Miyakawa Memorial Research Foundation, Tokyo, and Yamanashi University, Yamanashi, Japan

On behalf of the Miyakawa Memorial Research Foundation (MMRF), I am extremely pleased and deeply honored to make the opening remarks and to start the Second MMRF Meeting on Viral Hepatitis in Asia held on May 15, 2004, here in Tokyo. The carrier rate of hepatitis B virus (HBV) in Asian countries is high at 5–10% and is responsible for a high incidence of hepatocellular carcinoma (HCC), 90% of which is induced by the persistent HBV infection. Hence, there has been a pressing need to cope with this serious situation in Asia. It has become evident that, for the establishment of the HBV carrier state, not only maternal transmission, but also horizontal transmission in the infancy plays a major role. Therefore, to prevent HBV infection, all newborns receive universal vaccination by the recommendation of the World Health Organization. The vaccination has been very effective and reduced the carrier rate to less than 1% in hyperendemic countries in Asia, represented by China and Taiwan. However, this is not enough, leaving room for future improvement.

The carrier rate of HBV in Japan was 1% in the 1970s, which is much lower than that in other Asian countries. Nevertheless, the annual incidence of HCC was high during these years at 10 per 100,000 population. Of all cases of HCC, 40% were induced by HBV infection, which urged us to cope with HCC associated with HBV. As a first step, we studied how HBV spread, because prevention of de novo infection is most effective in dealing with any diseases induced by bacteria and viruses. Regarding the results, it became evident that the vast majority of HBV carrier state in Japan is established by perinatal transmission from mothers with hepatitis B e antigen (HBeAg) in serum. In 1986, immunoprophylaxis was started as a national program on the babies born to carrier mothers with HBeAg, not only with hepatitis B vaccine but also with high-titered hepatitis B immune globulin; this is unique to Japan. The program has proven to be very effective in containing HBV infection in Japan, and the carrier rate in the Japanese younger than 15 years has become 0.03%.

As for the infection with hepatitis C virus (HCV), it spread widely all over the country during turmoil surrounding the termination of World War II through intravenous stimulants (e.g., methamphetamine) and transfusion with blood from commercial donors. The wide spread of HCV infection during these years manifests itself most vividly in the profile of HCV infection in the general population in Japan nowadays. The age-specific prevalence of HCV in Japan was surveyed during 1995–2000 on approximately 3.5 million first-time blood donors, conducted at the eight jurisdictions of the Japanese Red Cross Blood Center. The results of this large-scale survey are summarized in figure 1. Although the HCV carrier rate in the age group younger than 19 years is low at 0.1%, it increases sharply with age to 1.3% in the forties and jumps to 3.4% in the sixties. This profile differs

KARGER

Fax +41 61 306 12 34
E-Mail karger@karger.ch
www.karger.com

0300–5526/06/0492–0004$23.50/0

Accessible online at:
www.karger.com/int

Hiroshi Suzuki, MD
Miyakawa Memorial Research Foundation
Tokyo, Minami-Aoyama 2-19-8
Minato-ku, Tokyo 107-0062 (Japan)
Tel. +81 3 5414 8581, Fax +81 3 3408 3388, E-Mail drsuzuki@po.iijnet.or.jp

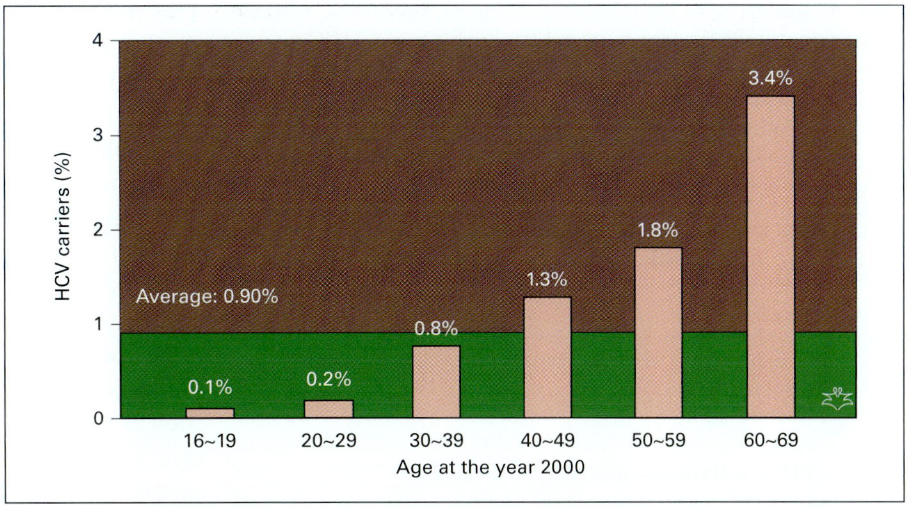

Fig. 1. Profile of HCV infection in the general population of Japan represented by the first-time blood donors. Modified from the results by Tanaka et al. [1].

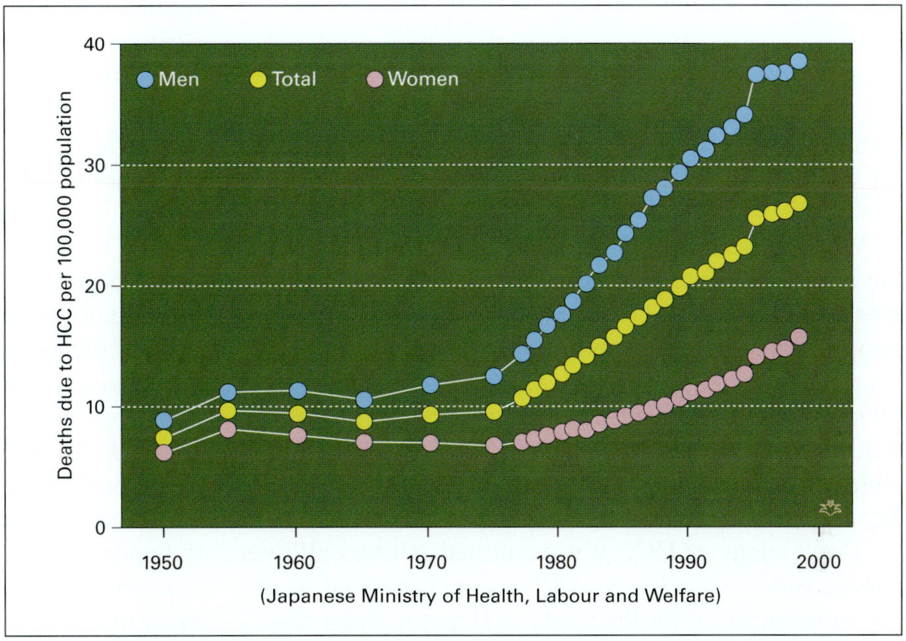

Fig. 2. Deaths due to HCC increasing with time during the past 30 years in Japan. Modified from the results by Yoshizawa et al. [2].

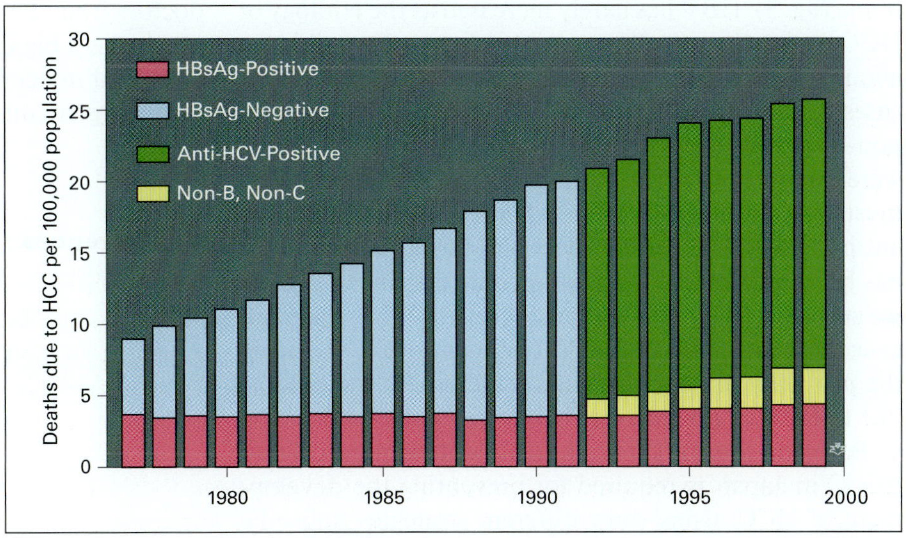

Fig. 3. The etiology of HCC changing with time in Japan. Based on data by the Japan Association for the Study of Hepatocellular Carcinoma.

Table 1. Strategies for the treatment of chronic hepatitis C toward suppression of the development of liver cirrhosis and HCC

1	Complete clearance of HCV (sustained virological response) IFN: human lymphoblast, recombinant IFN-α_{2a}, rIFN-α_{2b}, consensus, IFN-β rIFN-α_{2b} plus ribavirin (since 2001)
2	Normalization of ALT (biochemical response) Glycyrrhizin (SNMC) Ursodeoxycholic acid Phlebotomy
3	Early diagnosis of HCC (screening every 3 or 6 months) Ultrasonography Tumor markers AFP PIVKA-II (des-γ-carboxyl prothrombin)

significantly from that in the United States reported by Dr. Miriam Alter, where the carrier rate peaks in the thirties.

We have been deeply worried that deaths due to HCC have kept increasing during the last 3 decades (fig. 2). Yearly deaths due to HCC per 100,000 population in Japan started to increase rapidly since 1975 and multiplied fourfold to reach 35 per 100,000 population in the year 1995 for men. A similar increase has occurred in women, but not to such a high extent as in men. What is responsible for such a steady increase in deaths due to HCC in Japan?

The etiology of HCC was examined in cases all over Japan, and the results since 1977 were compiled by the Japan Association for the Study of Hepatocellular Carcinoma (fig. 3). HBV has barely increased as the etiology of HCC during the past 30 years; it has been responsible for about 4 deaths per 100,000 population-year. Evidently, cases without HBV infection, which were categorized in non-A, non-B etiology, started to increase after 1975 and were responsible for the rapid gain in HCC in Japan. The mystery was solved in 1991, when a serological test for antibody to HCV became possible. In retrospect, HCV has been responsible for most increments since 1975, as we suspected without solid evidence. HCV has taken an ever increasing role in the development of HCC during the past 30 years and accounts for about 75% of deaths due to HCC at present.

Based on this background, treatment of chronic hepatitis C in Japan is required for preventing the development of HCC, using three different strategies (table 1). The first option is the clearance of HCV infection by means of interferon (IFN) combined with ribavirin. Nonresponders to this treatment and patients without indication to it are treated with Stronger Neo-Minophagen C (Minophagen Pharmaceutical Company, Ltd., Tokyo, Japan) and ursodeoxycholic acid as well as phlebotomy; they are performed to normalize serum levels of alanine aminotransferase (ALT) in patients with chronic hepatitis C with or without cirrhosis. Lastly, patients with chronic hepatitis C with or without liver cirrhosis need to be examined for HCC by ultrasonography at appropriate intervals and screened for tumor markers in serum, such as α-fetoprotein (AFP) and protein induced by vitamin K absence or antagonist-II (PIVKA-II; also known as des-γ-carboxyl prothrombin). By virtue of such close follow-ups for an early detection of tumors, the 5-year survival rate of patients who are diagnosed with HCC less than 20 mm in diameter has nowadays reached more than 70%.

Fortunately, the prevalence of HCV in most Asian countries is still much lower than that in Japan. For instance, in a study performed in collaboration with the West China University in 1996, we have not found a single person with HCV RNA in serum amongst 3,000 inhabitants of farming villages in the Chendu area of Suchen. However, occasional cases of chronic hepatitis C were found among patients who visited hospitals. Looking at countries other than China, increases in transmission of HCV through intravenous drug abuse are creating much problem in Indonesia at present.

It would be very significant and fruitful for you to take the opportunity of this meeting and discuss in depth the epidemiology, pathophysiology and as well as HCC treatment of chronic hepatitis C with the many distinguished doctors from developed countries in Asia. Let me expect to witness a big development today. Finally, I would like to extend my cordial gratitude to Schering-Plough K.K. for their generous sponsorship in holding this meeting.

References

1 Tanaka J, Kumagai J, Katayama K, Komiya Y, Mizui M, Yamanaka R, Suzuki K, Miyakawa Y, Yoshizawa H: Sex- and age-specific carriers of hepatitis B and C viruses in Japan estimated by the prevalence in the 3,485,648 first-time blood donors during 1995–2000. Intervirology 2004;47:32–40.
2 Yoshizawa H: Hepatocellular carcinoma associated with hepatitis C virus infection in Japan: Projection to other countries in the foreseeable future. Oncology 2002;62:S8–S17.

Epidemiology

Intervirology

Intervirology 2006;49:7–17
DOI: 10.1159/000087257

National Prevention of Hepatocellular Carcinoma in Japan Based on Epidemiology of Hepatitis C Virus Infection in the General Population

Hiroshi Yoshizawa[a] Junko Tanaka[a] Yuzo Miyakawa[b]

[a]Department of Epidemiology, Infectious Disease Control and Prevention, Graduate School of Biomedical Sciences, Hiroshima University, Hiroshima, and [b]Miyakawa Memorial Research Foundation, Tokyo, Japan

Key Words

Chronic hepatitis · Cirrhosis · Epidemiology · Hepatitis C virus · Hepatocellular carcinoma · Prevention · Transfusion

Abstract

During the past 30 years, hepatocellular carcinoma (HCC) in Japan has kept linearly increasing from 10 to 30 per 100,000 population per year and is expected to grow further. The increment is attributed to infection with hepatitis C virus (HCV). Hence, there is a pressing need to find subjects with persistent HCV infection in the general population of Japan and take necessary measures to prevent HCC developing in them. As a first approach toward this goal, the sex- and age-specific prevalence of ongoing HCV infection was surveyed in 3,485,648 first-time blood donors during 1995–2000. Taking into account the size of subpopulations with different sex and age in Japan registered at the Census 2000, there are an estimated 884,954 HCV carriers aged from 16 to 69 years, and 759,316 (86%) of them are older than 40 years, with an increased risk for HCC; they are hidden in the society, without overt liver disease. The national 5-year project searching for HCV carriers in the general population was started in April 2002. Subjects are examinees of health check-ups, which they receive every 5 years when reaching the age of 40, as well as those at increased risk for HCV infection. The project detected HCV RNA in 14,672 of the 1,298,746 (1.1%) health check examinees and in 16,721 of the 624,734 (2.7%) high-risk individuals during the first fiscal year. Subjects found with HCV RNA have been referred to clinics and hospitals with expert hepatologists. Hopefully, this project will decrease HCC development in HCV carriers in Japan and be considered in other countries where increases in HCC are predicted from the current age-specific prevalence of anti-HCV.

Introduction

Hepatocellular carcinoma (HCC) ranks as the fourth most frequent cause of death due to malignancy in the world. HCC in men is the third most frequent malignancy in Japan, only next to lung and stomach cancers, while it is the fourth in women, following stomach, colon and lung cancers. The vast majority of patients with HCC are persistently infected with hepatitis B virus (HBV) or hepatitis C virus (HCV). The roles of HBV and HCV in the development of HCC vary widely in different countries and have changed with time. On the global scale, HBV

KARGER

Fax +41 61 306 12 34
E-Mail karger@karger.ch
www.karger.com

0300–5526/06/0492–0007$23.50/0

Accessible online at:
www.karger.com/int

Hiroshi Yoshizawa, MD
Department of Epidemiology, Infectious Disease Control and Prevention
Graduate School of Biomedical Sciences, Hiroshima University
Kasumi 1-2-3, Minami-ku, Hiroshima 734-8551 (Japan)
Tel. +81 82 257 5162, Fax +81 82 257 5164, E-Mail juntan@hiroshima-u.ac.jp

induces HCC much more frequently than HCV. There are an estimated 350 million HBV carriers (corresponding to 6% of the world population) [1], which is twice as many as 190 million who are presumed with persistent HCV infection [2].

However, several lines of epidemiological and clinical evidence predict that the role of HCV will increase and exceed that of HBV in the future. First and foremost, there is no means of preventing HCV infection with vaccines, unlike the infection with HBV that has been prevented since 1980 by hepatitis B vaccine [3]; it is proven to have a long-term effect in suppressing HCC associated with HBV infection [4]. Secondly, HCV infection can persist in 80% of adults parenterally exposed to it [5], in contrast to only a few percent of HBV infection in the adulthood that becomes chronic [6]. Thirdly, HCV infection prevails globally and keeps spreading, in remarkable contrast to HBV infection that is restricted to Asia and Africa. Finally, new HBV infections have been prevented by the global mass vaccination campaign advocated by the World Health Organization.

Hence, there is every reason to believe that HCV will have an ever increasing role in the development of HCC anywhere in the world where HCV prevails. However, it is not easy to foresee with a reasonable precision when and how often HCC develops in persistently infected individuals. The natural history of HCV infection is poorly defined [7, 8]. It varies widely according to the influence of diverse host and virus factors, of which the time factor is most important. It is presumed that 30 years elapse before HCC develops in the recipients of transfusion contaminated with HCV [9, 10]. However, the incubation time for HCC may not be constant in view of the velocity of fibrosis that differs widely by many factors, including the age at infection and gender [11–13].

Despite these differences in the development of HCC after HCV infection, a tendency would emerge if many HCV carriers are observed macroscopically en masse, in a national scale for instance. Furthermore, observing trends in HCV infection and associated HCC would help predict what will happen in the future and allow taking measures to prevent HCC arising in HCV carriers. Considering the Japanese as a whole, there has been a unique tendency for HCC during the past 50 years. Remarkably, the yearly incidence of HCC started to increase abruptly in 1975, and the role of HCV has kept increasing; now, it surpasses that of HBV by a margin of fourfold [14].

Driven by the need to comprehend how many people are at risk of developing HCC, we surveyed persistent infections with HBV and HCC in 3,485,648 first-time blood donors during 1995–2000 in the 8 jurisdictions of the Japanese Red Cross Blood Centers [15]. Based on the sex- and age-specific prevalence of infection, there are an estimated 759,316 HCV carriers in Japan who are older than 40 years and at increased risk of developing HCC. These trains of evidence have strongly indicated that HCC deaths in Japan will keep increasing at least until 2010, then flatten out and decline. This instigated doctors, as well as the personnel in the Ministry of Health, Labour and Welfare of Japan, to launch a 5-year project (which started in April 2002) to spot HCV carriers older than 40 years in Japan, urging them to take medical examination and receive treatment as required.

Geographical Distribution of Deaths due to HCC in Japan Shifting from 1975–1980 through 1991–1995 toward 1996–2000

Figure 1 pictures the distribution of deaths due to HCC examined over three 5-year ranges. Japan consists of four major islands, with Hokkaido situated up in the north, the mainland lying from northeast to southwest, accompanied by Shikoku down in the south and Kyushu in the west. There are 48 jurisdictions which are further broken down into many cities and villages. The standardized mortality rate (SMR) due to HCC in each of the 3,212 municipalities was determined by the Bay's method. The mortality rate of each municipality was classified as follows: highest (SMR >140, red), higher (SMR 140–120, orange), medium (SMR 120–80, yellow), lower (SMR 80–60, green) and lowest (SMR <60, blue). During 1971–1975, the annual incidence of HCC was pretty much the same all over Japan with most municipalities colored in yellow with the average frequency, although some areas in the southern Kyushu were in red with the highest incidence. During 1991–1995, the coloring became uneven, with areas in red or orange increasing all over Japan. The trend for this uneven distribution is further intensified on the last survey during 1996–2000. Although municipalities in green or blue increased in number, this by no means represents the incidence of decreased HCC. On the contrary, yearly incidence of HCC as well as the average total deaths due to HCC more than tripled during the three surveys covering 30 years from 1971 to 2000. Overall, the coloring highlights the incidence of HCC in Japan that decreases from Kyushu in the southwest, along the axis of Honshu toward Hokkaido in the northeast.

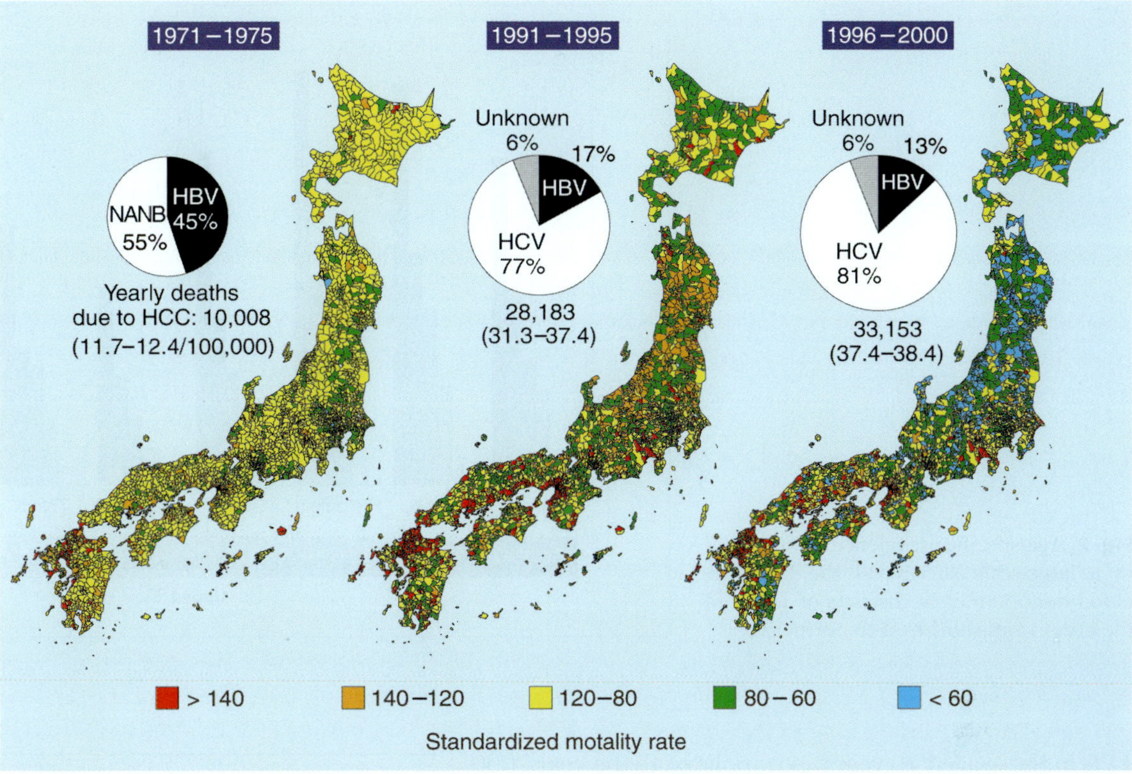

Fig. 1. Changes in the geographical distribution of deaths due to HCC in men during the past 30 years in 3,212 municipalities in Japan. Etiology of HCC is shown in a pie graph in size reflecting the yearly HCC during the survey period, with the average yearly deaths during the 5 years below and deaths due to HCC in 100,000 population per year in parentheses. Maps were produced by Dr. Yoshihiko Mirua of Saitama Prefectural University.

The center of Honshu over the skirt of Mount Fuji is an exception to this gradient. The incidence of HCC in Yamanashi prefecture stands out in red. This is due to the endemic *Schistosoma japonicum* along the Fuji River running through Yamanashi. Intravenous injection with antimony sodium tartar, performed during 1923–1980, spread HCV among patients infected with this parasite through repeated intravenous injections with insufficiently sterilized needles and syringes [16]. Similar endemic *S. japonicum* and iatrogenic diffusion of HCV happened in Saga and Fukuoka (both in northern Kyushu) and Hiroshima (in the western tail of Honshu) [17]. This was also the case along the riverside of the Nile in Egypt where *Schistosoma mansoni* once prevailed [18]. In Japan, parenteral antischistosomal treatment started to locally create small cores of HCV infection since the 1920s, and a more robust outbreak of HCV infection occurred since the end of World War II in 1945, through the 1960s to the 1970s [14].

Uneven geographical distribution of HCC in Japan, increasing with time (fig. 1), reflects the prevalence of HCV infection that differs regionally. Age-specific prevalence of HCV infection in the 3,485,648 first-time blood donors during 1995–2000 is shown in figure 2, individually for the 8 jurisdictions of the Japanese Red Cross Blood Center [15]. The frequency of HCV infection is higher in the four jurisdictions in the southwest than the other four in the northeast; there is a trend in the frequency of HCV infection, showing a decreasing gradient through the axis of Honshu from Hiroshima to Tohoku. The pattern matches the distribution of HCC in Japan at the last survey during 1995–2000, depicted in figure 1.

There are marked differences in the age-specific prevalence of HCV infection in every district (fig. 2). HCV is least prevalent in the age group of 16–19 years, gradually increases in the age group of 50–59 years and is highest in the 60–69-year-olds. Looked at more closely, in blood donors divided by a 1-year notch, the increase of HCV infection with age is even more conspicuous and reaches

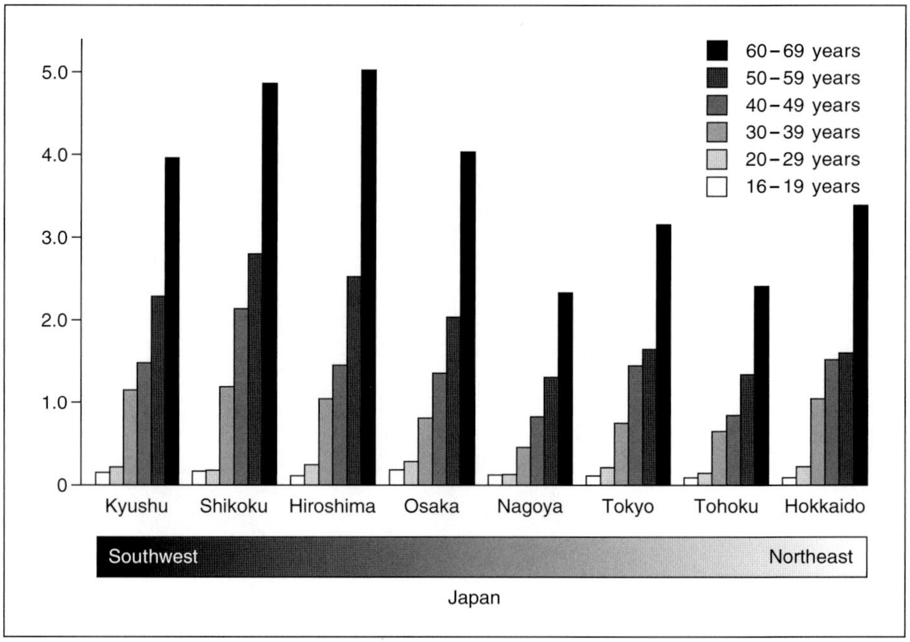

Fig. 2. Age-specific prevalence of anti-HCV in a large-scale survey on the first-time blood donors in eight districts of Japan in the order from southwest to northeast.

11% in those aged 70 years, extrapolated to the year 2000 (fig. 3). In Japan, in the year 2000, the number of total HCV carriers aged from 16 to 64 years who were eligible for blood donation was estimated at 884,954, 95% confidence interval (95% CI) 725,082–1,044,826, among 93,325,570 (0.95%) individuals aged 15–69 years [15]. They comprised 464,363 (95% CI 377,927–550,799) of the 46,638,636 (1.00%) men and 420,591 (95% CI 347,156–494,027) of the 46,686,934 (0.95%) women of the same ages. They were calculated as the sum of sex- and age-specific prevalence of HCV infection multiplied by the subpopulation with the corresponding sex and age. Thus, there are at least 759,316 HCV carriers older than 40 years who would be at increased risk of developing HCC.

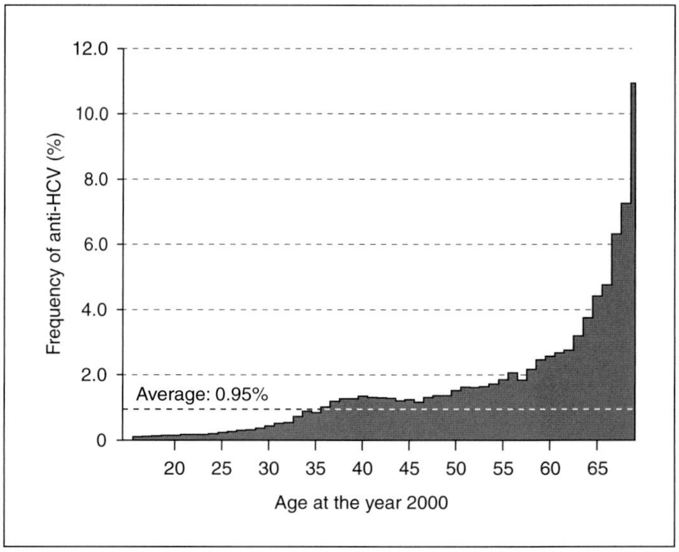

Fig. 3. Age-specific distributions in the 884,954 first-time blood donors with anti-HCV in Japan [modified from ref. 15].

Liver Disease in Blood Donors Found with Ongoing HCV Infection at the Screening

Liver disease induced by persistent HCV infection is insidious and progresses slowly at the speed differing according to various factors. Therefore, patients with HCV-associated liver disease are not aware of it before they develop signs and symptoms of cirrhosis or HCC, which even then can be missed for years due to ample reserve in the life-maintaining capacity of the liver. Hence, most HCV carriers are asymptomatic, as those typically identified among blood donors. During 10 years, from 1991 to 2000, 912 apparently healthy individuals were found to be persistently infected with HCV at a screening for blood donation at the Japanese Red Cross Blood Center in Hiroshima. They consulted doctors and were clinically examined [19]. It does strike us as a surprise that chronic

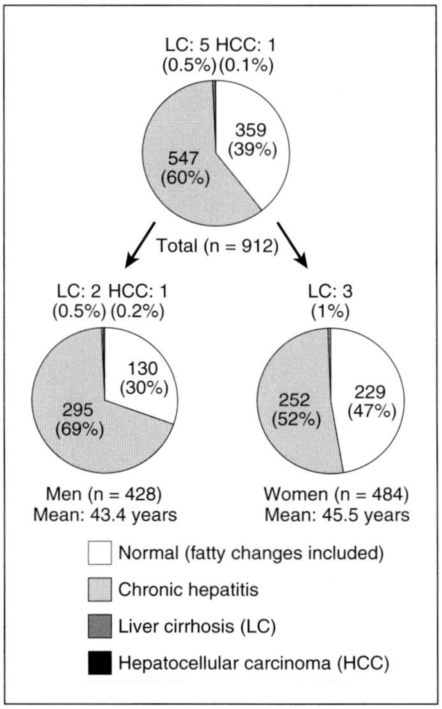

Fig. 4. Distribution of liver disease in 912 blood donors in Hiroshima who were found with HCV infection.

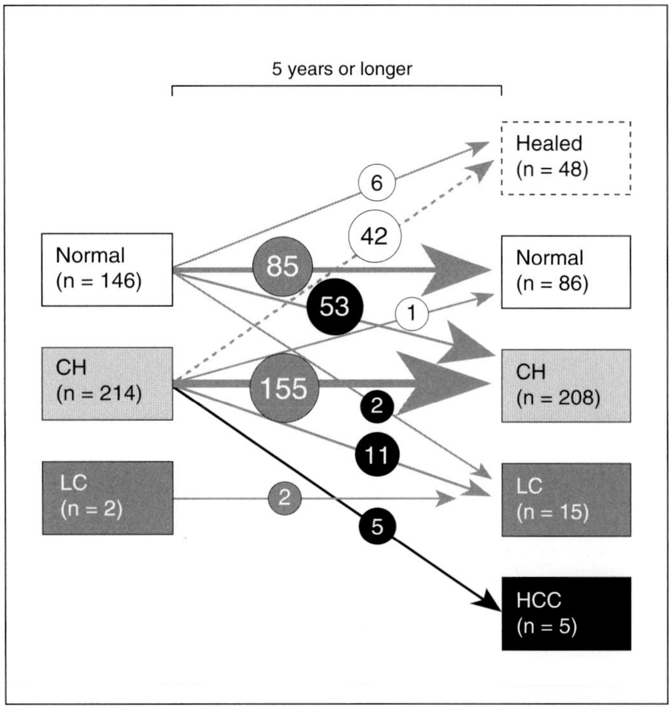

Fig. 5. Evolution of liver disease in 362 blood donors with anti-HCV in Hiroshima during follow-ups for 5 years or longer. CH = Chronic hepatitis; LC = liver cirrhosis.

hepatitis C with elevated serum levels of alanine aminotransferase was diagnosed in 60% of the subjects who had felt healthy enough to donate blood (fig. 4). Furthermore, cirrhosis had developed in 5 (0.5%) patients and HCC already in 1 (0.1%). Men had chronic hepatitis more frequently than women – 252/428 (69%) versus 252/486 (52%), $p < 0.01$ – despite the mean age which was comparable between them.

At least 5 years later (average 8.2 years, range 5.0–10.3 years), 362 (39.7%) subjects again received medical examination [19]. Clinical diagnoses remained unchanged in the majority of asymptomatic carriers and in those found with chronic hepatitis at the time of blood donation (fig. 5). However, 5 patients with chronic hepatitis had developed HCC, including 4 men at the ages of 53, 62, 64 and 68 years and 1 woman at the age of 67 years. In addition, liver cirrhosis had elicited in 11 of the 214 (5.1%) blood donors who were found with chronic hepatitis and in 2 of the 146 (1.4%) who were asymptomatic carriers at the first examination. As a positive result, HCV infection had resolved by interferon (IFN) therapy in 42 blood donors with chronic hepatitis C; they would never have received IFN, if the HCV infection had not been found at the time when they wished to donate blood. In addition, 6 of the 146 (4%) asymptomatic carriers cleared HCV infection during 5 years or longer. Five subjects resolved the infection by IFN, and the remaining one spontaneously; he might have been acutely infected with HCV and clearing it when he visited the blood center for donation.

Simulating the Natural History of HCV Infection in Asymptomatic Carriers by the Markov Model

The prospective study on blood donors who were found with HCV has unfolded liver disease advancing in some of them [19]. In order to plan the strategy to deal with inapparent HCV infection, it is necessary to foresee when and what will happen how frequently in asymptomatic carriers. However, the natural history of HCV infection is hard to define. As is evident in their wish to donate blood, subjects found with HCV infection were utterly unaware of it. The time when HCV infection was contracted is unknown in most carriers, except in those with

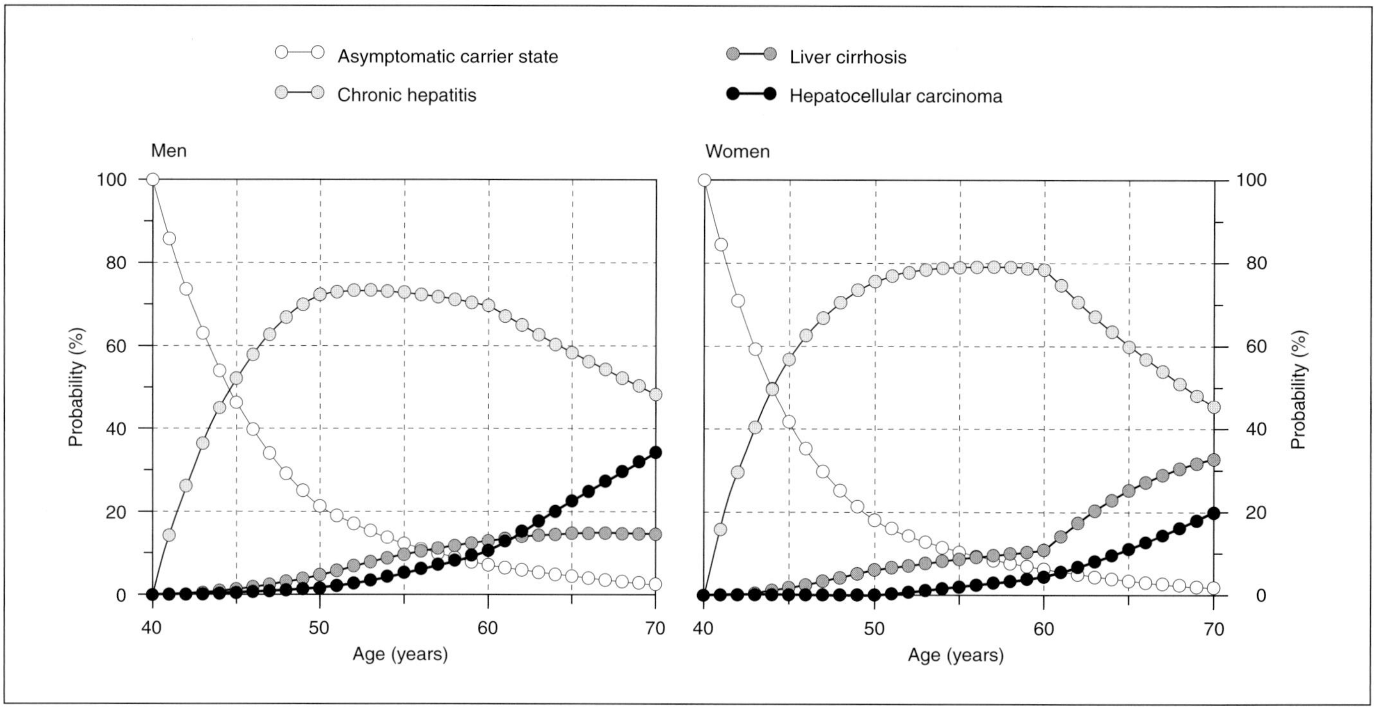

Fig. 6. Simulation of clinical courses of imaginary cohorts of 40-year-old male and female asymptomatic HCV carriers during 30 years by the Markov model [modified from ref. 21].

a history of transfusion or blood products by which they may have been infected. Since it takes decades until cirrhosis and HCC develop after HCV infection, doctors can hardly see through the entire history of their patients. Furthermore, it is unethical and not permitted to observe patients without any treatment at present.

The Markov model is powerful for simulating the natural history of chronic disease [20]. First, probabilities of transitions between any two clinical states within a cycle (usually a year) are assessed by the observation of a limited number of patients who have been followed regularly and rigorously for only a few to several years. Then, the natural history through many years is simulated in imaginary cohorts by integrating all probabilities for each transition per year that are multiplied successively for years elapsed. We have simulated the natural history of HCV infection in men and women by the Markov model [21]. Probabilities for transition per year between any of four clinical states (the asymptomatic carrier state, chronic hepatitis, cirrhosis and HCC) were calculated on 2,251 person-years from 942 patients with HCV infection who had been rigorously examined at least every year. HCC or death was defined as the absorbing state from where no transitions occur.

Based on the transition matrix constructed, the cumulative probability for developing chronic hepatitis, cirrhosis and HCC during 30 years was simulated on a hypothetical cohort of men and women who are found to be asymptomatic HCV carriers at the age of 40 (fig. 6). Of male asymptomatic carriers who enter their fifties, chronic hepatitis is estimated to develop in 72.4%, cirrhosis in 4.6% and HCC in 1.5%; 10.6% are expected to have HCC when they become 60 years old. In contrast, of female asymptomatic carriers who enter their fifties, chronic hepatitis is estimated to develop in 75.9% and liver cirrhosis in 6.2%, but HCC in none. HCC is expected to elicit only in 4.5% of female asymptomatic carriers at the age of 60, with a probability much less than 10.6% in male asymptomatic carriers. There is a steep rise in the cumulative probability for developing HCC in males in their sixties, and it reaches 34.4% at the age of 70, which is higher than that for liver cirrhosis at 14.6%. Although the cumulative probability for developing HCC increases in females reaching 70 years of age, it remains 20.0% and is much lower than that for liver cirrhosis at 32.8%.

The ability of this Markov model in predicting the clinical outcome of HCV infection was evaluated by comparing the results of 5-year follow-ups in 70 men and 83 women with those simulated by it [21]. The results were in good agreement, thereby attesting to the reliability of this model in predicting the natural history of HCV infection in asymptomatic carriers and patients with chronic hepatitis.

Efficient Screening of Individuals with Persistent HCV Infection in the General Population

There are two groups of individuals who test positive for anti-HCV. Subjects in the first group have ongoing infection with HCV RNA in serum, while those in the second group already have cleared infection without serum HCV RNA. Hence, nucleic acids need to be extracted from sera of subjects with anti-HCV, amplified by polymerase chain reaction, also known as nucleic acid amplification test (NAT), with primers deduced from the nucleotide sequence commonly expressed by HCV isolates of any genotypes, and examined for amplification products. However, this is by no means easy, demanding high cost, labor and equipment. Hence, polymerase chain reaction for detecting HCV RNA is not suitable for mass screening of ongoing HCV infection on a national scale.

We have invented a method to efficiently and sensitively screen ongoing HCV infections at low costs. The method takes advantage of the titer of anti-HCV that is higher in individuals with ongoing infection than in those who have cleared HCV infection. The bottom of anti-HCV titers over which HCV RNA can coexist and the ceiling below which HCV RNA is absent can be determined on the panel of anti-HCV-positive sera with or without HCV RNA; however, there is an inevitable grey zone in between. The flow chart depicted in figure 7 retains the benefit of this method, compensates for uncertainties given rise to by the grey zone and avoids missing rare sera with low-titered anti-HCV accompanied by HCV RNA.

First, sera of examinees are tested for anti-HCV, and those which are negative are regarded without HCV RNA and not tested further. The anti-HCV immunoassay has been calibrated for three categories of positive results: (1) high titers for the presence of HCV RNA, (2) low titers that can be very rarely accompanied by HCV RNA and (3) medium titers in the grey zone that may or may not co-occur with HCV RNA. Sera with high-titered anti-HCV are deemed to contain HCV RNA and are not examined any further. Although extremely exceptional sera with high-titered anti-HCV do not contain HCV RNA,

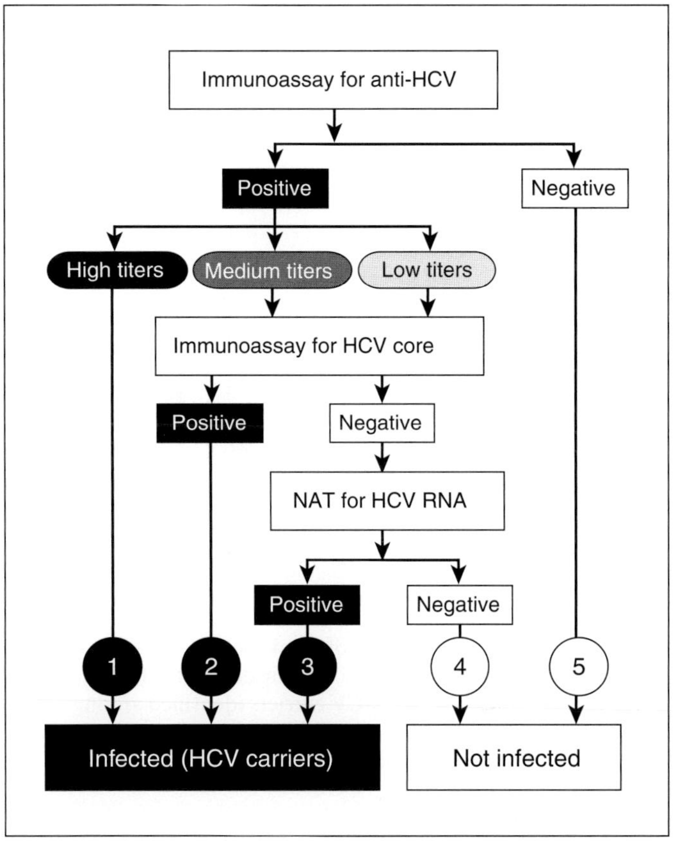

Fig. 7. Strategy for the national screening for persistent HCV infection in Japan with immunoassays for anti-HCV as well as HCV core protein combined with NAT.

we consider false-positive results far more acceptable than false-negative results in judging HCV infection and staying on the safe side. Sera with medium-titered or low-titered anti-HCV are then screened by immunoassay for HCV core antigen; it is easier and less costly than NAT for HCV RNA. If HCV core antigen is detected in the test serum, it indicates ongoing HCV infection, which is theoretically justifiable, and is not tested by NAT. Finally, NAT is performed on all sera with low- and medium-titered anti-HCV, including those that are negative for HCV core antigen. All sera fall into one of the five categories at the bottom of figure 7, of which three (1–3) indicate the presence of ongoing HCV infection and the remaining two (4 and 5) the lack of it. Examinees receive this chart with a mark on one of the categories 1–5 to let them know where they stand.

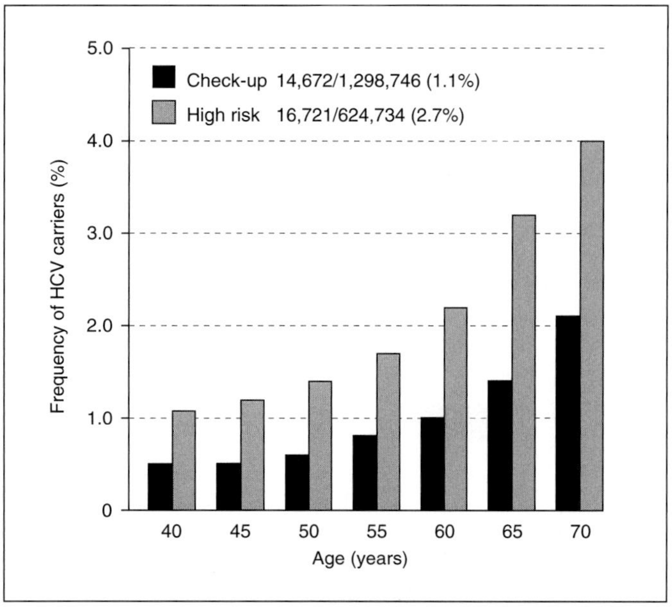

Fig. 8. Age-specific distribution of persistent HCV infection in Japan determined by the national screening during the first fiscal year (April 2002 to March 2003). HCV carriers identified among examinees at regular health check-ups and individuals at high risk, who were stratified by age, are shown separately.

A Nation-Wide Project to Spot HCV Carriers Older than 40 Years in Japan

A 5-year project for screening the Japanese for ongoing HCV and HBV infections on a national scale was launched in April 2002 [19]. It has been performed on two distinct populations. Health check-ups are offered to the Japanese every 5 years when they become 40 years old until they reach 70 years of age. Therefore, by screening health check examinees for 5 years, all carriers of hepatitis viruses who are aged 40 years or older can be identified by March 2007. Thereafter, each year, only individuals who reach 40 years of age need to be screened. This project is based on an extremely low incidence of de novo infection with HCV or HBV in Japan [14], which makes it sufficient to screen for these hepatitis viruses only once in the lifetime.

Subjects who cannot wait for the screening for HCV infection at regular health check-ups, because of an urgent requirement for it, are provided with a chance to receive it at least once. They include individuals at high risk for HCV infection: (1) those who were found with abnormal liver function in the past; (2) those who may have received transfusion with blood or its products before 1992 at a major operation or because of massive hemorrhage at delivery, which had not been screened for anti-HCV by the second-generation immunoassay, and who are not regularly monitored for their liver function; and (3) those in whom liver function tests gave abnormal results at regular examination which they receive in clinics of their companies and institutions. Individuals older than 70 years and off regular health check-ups are tested for virus markers if they wish.

The Ministry of Health, Labour and Welfare of Japan has reported results of the national screening project in the first fiscal year from April 2002 to March 2003. Of the 3,212 municipalities in Japan, 2,997 (93.3%) started this project with a good compliance. The Department of Welfare for the Aged compiled results in the first fiscal year and registered 1,923,480 examinees, of whom 31,393 (1.6%) were found with ongoing HCV infection. There were 1,298,746 examinees at regular health check-ups and 14,672 (1.1%) were found to be HCV carriers. In comparison, of 624,734 high-risk subjects who received tests on other occasions, 16,721 (2.7%) were found with ongoing HCV infection, at a frequency twice as high as that in health check examinees. The results are shown for both groups, stratified by age (fig. 8). HCV carriers were found in 3.2 and 1.3% of the individuals aged 65 at high risk and those examined at check-ups and more often in those aged 70 years, at 4.0 and 2.1%, respectively.

Figure 9 illustrates the results of persistent HCV infection in examinees of regular health check-ups and individuals at high risk from the 48 jurisdictions in Japan. Without exception, the prevalence of persistent HCV infection is higher in individuals at high risk than in health check examinees. Additionally, there is an apparent gradient in the persistent HCV infection from the southwest to the northeast of Japan; the gradient mirrors that of blood donors in the 8 jurisdictions of the Japanese Red Cross Blood Center (fig. 2).

Projection of HCC in Japan to Other Countries toward the Future

The age-specific prevalence of HCV infection in the year 2000 is compared among Japan, Ukraine and the United States (fig. 10a). It is based on 275,868 blood donors in Hiroshima for Japan, 41,021 blood donors in Kiev for Ukraine and data reported by the Center for Disease Control and Prevention for the United States. The age with the highest prevalence of anti-HCV is markedly different among the three countries. The prevalence

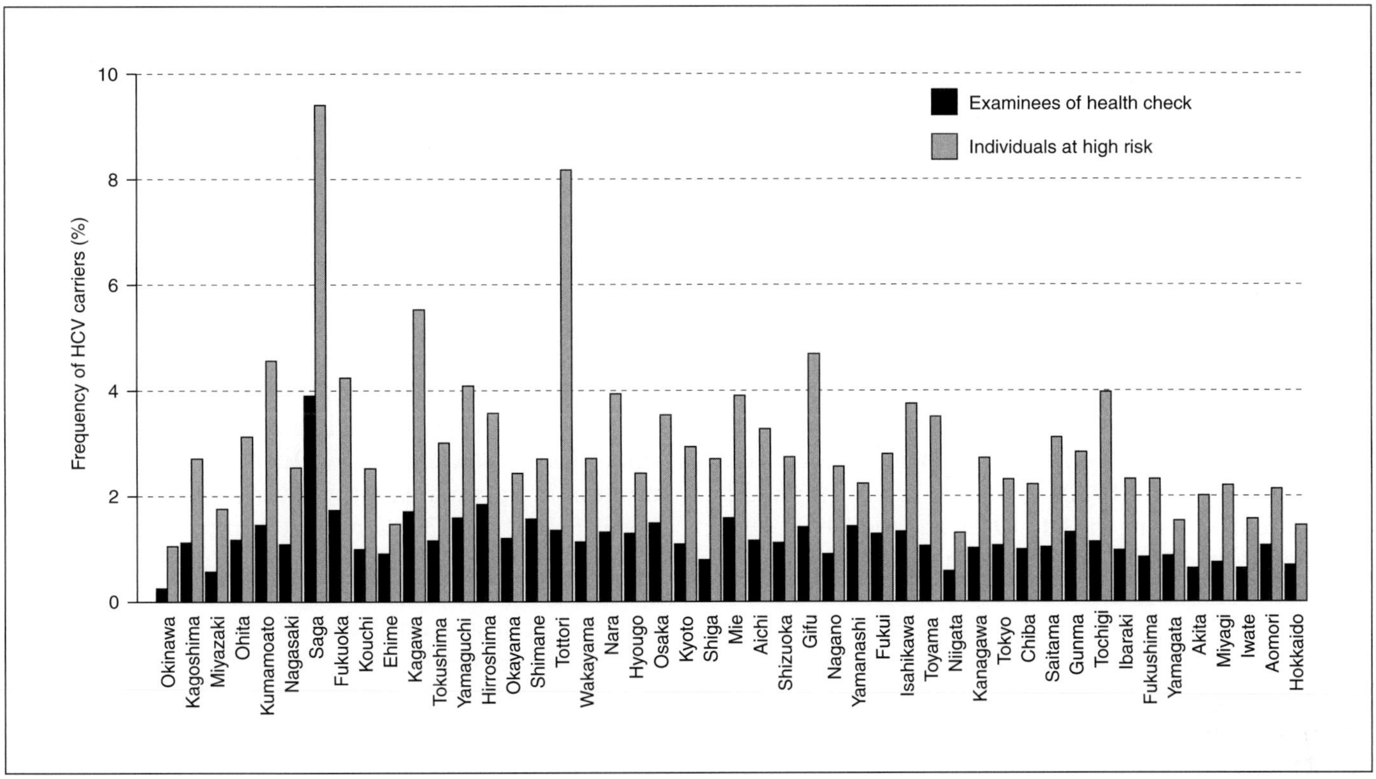

Fig. 9. Distribution of persistent HCV infection in examinees at regular health check-ups and individuals at high risk from the 48 jurisdictions in Japan detected by the national screening during the first fiscal year. The 48 jurisdictions are ordered from southeast on the left to northeast on the right.

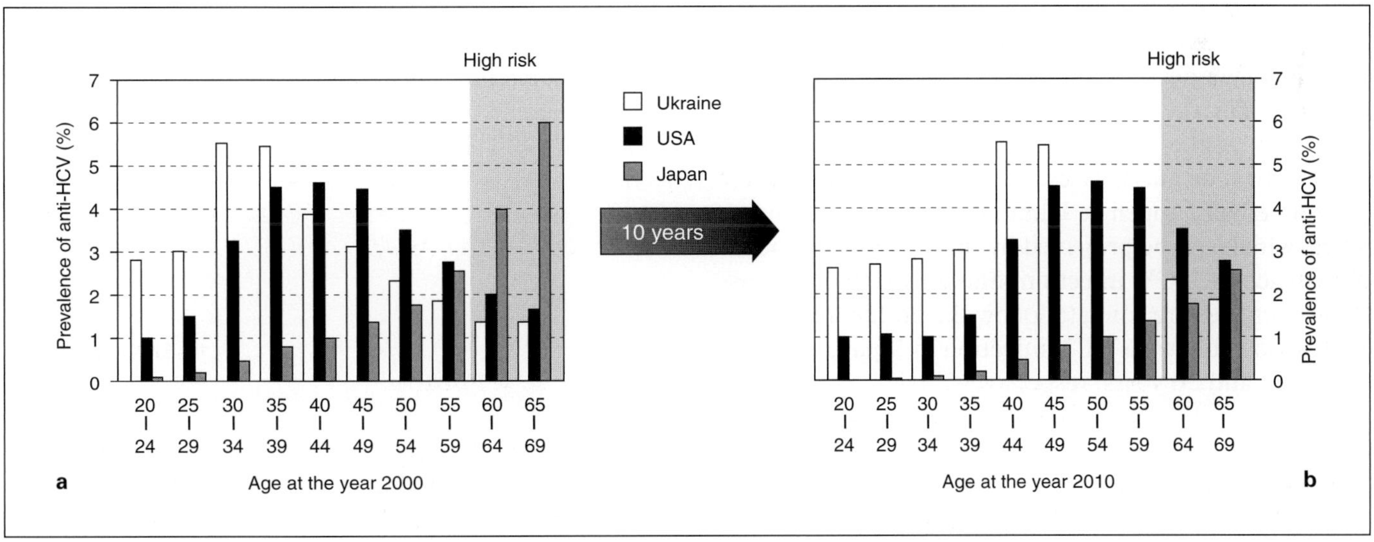

Fig. 10. Age-specific profiles of HCV infection in Japan, the United States and Ukraine. Distributions in the year 2000 (**a**) and those expected in the year 2010 (**b**) are shown.

of anti-HCV steeply increases with age in Japan; the highest is expected in the elderly who scale out of the figure. In contrast, the highest prevalence of anti-HCV is positioned at 40–44 years in the United States, and even younger at 30–35 years in Ukraine.

These wide differences in the age at which anti-HCV peaks among the three countries are attributed to distinct time points when HCV spread extensively among each population. In Japan, HCV infection infiltrated in the subpopulation of younger generations during the 1950s and 1960s in a vicious cycle, but almost completely ceased to occur since 1990 [14]. About two decades later, from the 1970s to the early 1980s, HCV infection widely diffused in the United States; the yearly incidence decreased from 230,000 in the 1980s to 38,000 in the 1990s [22]. More recently, during the late 1980s and the 1990s, HCV infection started to spread in Ukraine and has continued to invade younger generations.

It is of note that the national diffusion of HCV infection is triggered and accelerated by defeats in wars in all the three countries. They are the World War II in Japan, the Vietnam War in the United States and the Afghan War in Ukraine, all of which created a national turmoil and stimulated desperation predominantly in younger generations. What we find in the age-specific distribution of anti-HCV in the three countries at present are long-term sequelae of the wide spread of HCV infection around a major war that are shifting with time.

Age-specific distribution of anti-HCV expected in the year 2010 is depicted by shifting the present profile 10 years toward the future (fig. 10b). In Japan, with essentially no new infections, HCV carriers in their sixties will decrease. On the contrary, many individuals infected with HCV in the United States will go into their sixties along with substantial cases of HCC developing in them. The same will happen in Ukraine after an additional 10 years, which can be projected by the current age-specific prevalence of HCV infection. Should that be the case, these countries are going to follow the profile we have for HCC associated with HCV infection in Japan, with time lags of 10 and 20 years, respectively.

Conclusion

HCC is a rare cancer that is easily preventable. Individuals at high risk for developing HCC are infected with HCV or HBV, of which HCV is more universal, and they are readily identified by viral markers. It is imperative that carriers realize that they are infected with HCV, since the majority are unaware of it. Then, they can consult their present status with hepatologists and receive antiviral treatment for terminating the infection as indicated. HCV carriers who cannot clear infection are regularly followed for liver disease, and those with chronic hepatitis or cirrhosis are screened for HCC at appropriate intervals by noninvasive methods, such as ultrasonography and computed tomography, as well as tumor markers like α-fetoprotein and protein induced by vitamin K absence or antagonist-II. They need to be advised to abstain from alcohol in order to decrease the development of HCC. Antiviral and anti-inflammatory therapies are found effective in decreasing the incidence of HCC, even in patients who fail to clear HCV. Due to an extremely wide variation in the progression of liver disease and the incidence of HCC in HCV carriers, it is imperative to handle the situation on a national basis, as we are conducting in Japan. Efforts will be rewarding, with much less morbidity and mortality caused by HCV infection, and will immensely lessen the economical burden on the nation. Hopefully, interim results of our 5-year national project for spotting HCV carriers in Japan will encourage similar efforts elsewhere in the world where HCV-associated HCC is reasonably expected to increase.

Acknowledgements

We thank the Japanese Red Cross Blood Center for collecting data of the first-time blood donors and their analysis, and the members of the Hiroshima Hepatitis Study Group for follow-up and diagnosis of liver disease in blood donors found with HCV infection at the screening. This study was supported in part by Health and Labour Science Research Grants for Research on Hepatitis and BSE from the Ministry of Health, Labour and Welfare of Japan.

References

1 Lee WM: Hepatitis B virus infection. N Engl J Med 1997;337:1733–1745.
2 Cohen J: The scientific challenge of hepatitis C. Science 1999;285:26–30.
3 Szmuness W, Stevens CE, Harley EJ, Zang EA, Oleszko WR, William DC, Sadovsky R, Morrison JM, Kellner A: Hepatitis B vaccine: Demonstration of efficacy in a controlled clinical trial in a high-risk population in the United States. N Engl J Med 1980;303:833–841.
4 Chang MH, Chen CJ, Lai MS, Hsu HM, Wu TC, Kong MS, Liang DC, Shau WY, Chen DS: Universal hepatitis B vaccination in Taiwan and the incidence of hepatocellular carcinoma in children. N Engl J Med 1997;336:1855–1859.
5 Hoofnagle JH: Course and outcome of hepatitis C. Hepatology 2002;36:S21–S29.
6 Hoofnagle JH: Chronic hepatitis B. N Engl J Med 1990;323:337–339.
7 Alter HJ, Seeff LB: Recovery, persistence, and sequelae in hepatitis C virus infection: A perspective on long-term outcome. Semin Liver Dis 2000;20:17–35.
8 Seeff LB: Natural history of chronic hepatitis C. Hepatology 2002;36:S35–S46.
9 Kiyosawa K, Sodeyama T, Tanaka E, Gibo Y, Yoshizawa K, Nakano Y, Furuta S, Akahane Y, Nishioka K, Purcell RH, Alter HJ: Interrelationship of blood transfusion, non-A, non-B hepatitis and hepatocellular carcinoma: Analysis by detection of antibody to hepatitis C virus. Hepatology 1990;12:671–675.
10 Tong MJ, el-Farra NS, Reikes AR, Co RL: Clinical outcomes after transfusion-associated hepatitis C. N Engl J Med 1995;332:1463–1466.
11 Kenny-Walsh E: Clinical outcomes after hepatitis C infection from contaminated anti-D immune globulin. N Engl J Med 1999;340:1228–1233.
12 Vogt M, Lang T, Frosner G, Klingler C, Sendl AF, Zeller A, Wiebecke B, Langer B, Meisner H, Hess J: Prevalence and clinical outcome of hepatitis C infection in children who underwent cardiac surgery before the implementation of blood-donor screening. N Engl J Med 1999;341:866–870.
13 Hamada H, Yatsuhashi H, Yano K, Daikoku M, Arisawa K, Inoue O, Koga M, Nakata K, Eguchi K, Yano M: Impact of aging on the development of hepatocellular carcinoma in patients with posttransfusion chronic hepatitis C. Cancer 2002;95:331–339.
14 Yoshizawa H: Hepatocellular carcinoma associated with hepatitis C virus infection in Japan: Projection to other countries in the foreseeable future. Oncology 2002;62:S8–S17.
15 Tanaka J, Kumagai J, Katayama K, Komiya Y, Mizui M, Yamanaka R, Suzuki K, Miyakawa Y, Yoshizawa H: Sex- and age-specific carriers of hepatitis B and C viruses in Japan estimated by the prevalence in the 3,485,648 first-time blood donors during 1995–2000. Intervirology 2004;47:32–40.
16 Iida F, Iida R, Kamijo H, Takaso K, Miyazaki Y, Funabashi W, Tsuchiya K, Matsumoto Y: Chronic Japanese schistosomiasis and hepatocellular carcinoma: Ten years of follow-up in Yamanashi Prefecture, Japan. Bull World Health Organ 1999;77:573–581.
17 Tanaka Y, Hanada K, Orito E, Akahane Y, Chayama K, Yoshizawa H, Sata M, Ohta N, Miyakawa Y, Gojobori T, Mizokami M: Molecular evolutionary analyses implicate injection treatment for schistosomiasis in the initial hepatitis C endemics of Japan. J Hepatol 2005;42:47–53.
18 Frank C, Mohamed MK, Strickland GT, Lavanchy D, Arthur RR, Magder LS, El Khoby T, Abdel-Wahab Y, Aly Ohn ES, Anwar W, Sallam I: The role of parenteral antischistosomal therapy in the spread of hepatitis C virus in Egypt. Lancet 2000;355:887–891.
19 Yoshizawa H, Tanaka J: A national project for the management of viral hepatitis toward prevention of hepatocellular carcinoma in Japan; in Morrissey RF (ed): International Kilmer Conference Proceedings. Laval, Polyscience Publications, 2004, vol 8, pp 247–264.
20 Beck JR: Markov models of natural history. J Clin Epidemiol 1988;41:619–621.
21 Tanaka J, Kumada H, Ikeda K, Chayama K, Mizui M, Hino K, Katayama K, Kumagai J, Komiya Y, Miyakawa Y, Yoshizawa H: Natural histories of hepatitis C virus infection in men and women simulated by the Markov model. J Med Virol 2003;70:378–386.
22 Williams I: Epidemiology of hepatitis C in the United States. Am J Med 1999;107:S2–S9.

Epidemiology

Intervirology

Intervirology 2006;49:18–22
DOI: 10.1159/000087258

Epidemiology of Hepatitis C Virus in Korea

Hai-Rim Shin

Division of Cancer Control and Epidemiology, National Cancer Center, Goyang, Korea

Key Words
Epidemiology · Genotypes · Hepatitis C virus · Korea · Transfusion

Abstract
Mortality due to liver cancer in Korea ranks as one of the highest in the world. Both hepatitis B virus (HBV) and hepatitis C virus (HCV) infections are high-risk factors for liver cancer. Although HBV is by far the more important risk factor for the development of hepatocellular carcinoma (HCC) in Korea, HCV infection is more closely associated with HCC in elderly patients. Therefore, the evaluation of risk factors for HCV infection, including blood transfusion, is important. This study reviews the literature on HCV prevalence and risk factors among the general population, as well as the distribution of HCV genotypes in Korea. An overall estimate of the prevalence of anti-HCV among Koreans older than 40 years was 1.29% (95% confidence interval 1.12–1.48) during 1995–2000. Blood transfusion was the strongest risk factor for transmission of HCV infection. Risk factors for HCV infection in Korea other than blood transfusion and history of acupuncture have not been proven. The most prevalent HCV genotype is 1b followed by 2a. Even though the prevalence of anti-HCV in Korea has been reduced and the risk of HCV transmission through blood transfusion has markedly decreased, public-health programs to prevent de novo infections should be developed. Moreover, most people infected with HCV in Korea are older than 40 years, and therefore, the surveillance of adults (≥40 years) for HCV infection will be helpful in early detection of HCC developing in them.

Introduction

As in other countries, infections with both hepatitis B virus (HBV) and hepatitis C virus (HCV) are factors for high risk of developing hepatocellular carcinoma (HCC) in Korea [1]. Of these two, HBV is by far the more important risk factor for HCC in Korea. However, HCV infection is more closely associated with HCC in elderly patients [2]. Since the introduction of screening for anti-HCV of blood donors in Korea in April 1991, the risk of exposure to HCV in blood recipients has remarkably decreased [3]. Therefore, behavioral risk factors rather than blood transfusion influence the epidemiology of HCV infection nowadays. In this study, the literature on HCV prevalence and risk factors among the general population including health examinees in Korea has been reviewed, and the distribution of HCV genotypes in Korea is discussed.

KARGER

Fax +41 61 306 12 34
E-Mail karger@karger.ch
www.karger.com

0300–5526/06/0492–0018$23.50/0

Accessible online at:
www.karger.com/int

Hai-Rim Shin, MD
Research Institute for National Cancer & Evaluation, National Cancer Center
809 Madu-dong, Ilsan-gu, Goyang
Gyeonggi-do 411-769 (Korea)
Tel. +82 31 920 2050, Fax +82 31 920 2051, E-Mail hrshin@ncc.re.kr

Table 1. The prevalence of anti-HCV among health examinees in Korea during 1995–2000

Study year and area	Subjects n	Anti-HCV	Anti-HCV test method	Study subjects (age group)	Reference
1995–1998 Seoul	86,384	353 (0.41)	radioimmunoassay NANBDINE ^{125}C Kit (General Biologicals Corp., Hsin Chu, Taiwan)	health check-up examinees in a general hospital (≥20 years)	Seo WT et al. [9]
1997 Ulsan	10,140	133 (1.31)	3rd EIA, Cobas® Core Anti-HCV (Roche Diagnostics, Ind., USA)	examinees for health check-up at University Hospital in Ulsan (≥20 years)	Jeong TH et al. [8]
1998–2000 Cheonnam	6,790	142 (2.1)	recombinant HCr43, C200, N55 (Abbott Laboratories, Ill., USA)	examinees for health check-up at Cheonnam University Hospital (≥30 years)	Na HY et al. [10]
1997–2001 Daegu	21,291	190 (0.89)	AxSYM (Abbott Laboratories, Ill., USA)	examinees for health check-up at the health promotion center of Dongsan Hospital (≥20 years)	Park KS et al. [11]

Figures in parentheses are percentages.

Table 2. The prevalence (%) of anti-HCV among Koreans from four published data during 1995–2000[a]

	Prevalence (95% CI)
Age group	
40–49 years	0.57 (0.50–0.66)
50–59 years	1.38 (1.23–1.56)
60 years and older	2.16 (1.86–2.52)
Age-standardized prevalence (≥40 years)[b]	1.29 (1.12–1.48)
Estimated number of subjects with anti-HCV	193,000 (168,000–222,000)

[a] Data from four publications on health check-ups of middle-aged examinees [8–11].
[b] Based on the mean number of population during 1995–2002 and an age-specific estimate of anti-HCV in pooled individuals of 40 years or older.

Seroprevalence of Anti-HCV in Korea

In the 1990s, the overall prevalence of anti-HCV in Korea ranged from 0.7 to 3.5% among middle-aged and older examinees (≥40 years) at health check-ups and from 0.4 to 1.5% among healthy individuals with normal levels of alanine aminotransferase [4–9]. During 1995–2000, an overall estimate of HCV prevalence among Koreans older than 40 years was 1.29%, 95% confidence interval (CI) 1.12–1.48; it was estimated on four published data of HCV prevalence in more than 5,000 study subjects (tables 1, 2) [8–11].

Most published data indicate that the prevalence of anti-HCV increases with age. However, few studies examined children and young adults. In Seoul in the year 1995, the prevalence of anti-HCV among children aged 6–11 years was 0.81% (17/2,080) [12] and 0.4% (5/1,350) among young adults of 16–24 years [13]. In Korea, most people infected with HCV are elderly. However, future attention should be paid to the occurrence of de novo HCV infections in age groups other than the elderly.

While some published data show the prevalence of anti-HCV in men similar to that in women, three reports indicate a higher prevalence of anti-HCV in women than in men [6, 14, 15]. The reason for this discrepancy needs to be clarified in future studies.

Risk Factors for HCV Infection

Data published in eight reports unanimously name blood transfusion as the strongest risk of transmission of HCV infection in Korea, with an odds ratio ranging from 1.1 to 25.0 (table 3) [4–8, 14–17]. The average odds ratio of blood transfusion estimated on the eight data sets is 2.64 (95% CI 1.99–3.50). Since less than 1% of the general population receive blood transfusion, the risk attributed to blood transfusion is not very significant among the Korean population today. Comparison of the risk of blood transfusion before and after 1992 has revealed no risk of HCV infection among blood recipients after 1992 [15].

Among the other risk factors reported, histories of surgical operation [14] and acupuncture [15] were significant

Table 3. Odds ratios and 95% CI (in parentheses) of risk factors for HCV infection in nine published data complied

Risk factors	Seoul 1992 [4]	Seoul 1994 [5]	Seoul 1996 [16]	Pusan 1995 [6]	Three areas 1997 [7]	Ulsan 1997 [8]	Haman 1993 [14]	Haman 1999 [15]	Seoul 1994–1998 [17] (type 1b)	Seoul 1994–1998 [17] (type 2a)
Cases/controls:	72/4,239	36/105	64/128	53/1,753	57/1,624	33/99	63/253	77/623	70/97	63/97
History of hepatitis		NA	3.9 (1.4–10.7)[a]	3.4 (1.5–7.9)		2.1 (NS)				
Family history of liver disease		1.3 (0.5–3.1)			1 (0.3–3.3)	4.4 NS)				
Blood transfusion										
Yes/no	1.1 (0.5–2.4)[b]	6.7 (2.06–21.9)	2.4 (1.1–5.2)[a]	25.4 (13.8–46.9)	1.5 (0.6–4.1)	6.1 (1.7–22.5)[a]	1.1 (0.2–6.0)	1.8 (0.7–4.4)[a]	3.2 (1.3–7.8)[a]	4.6 (2.0–10.4)[b]
1992 and after								0 (0–1.3)		
Before 1992								5.5 (1.6–19.3)		
Acupuncture history										
Yes/no		0.8 (0.4–1.9)	0.7	NA	NA	0.9 (NS)		1.9 (1.0–3.6)[a]		
1992 and after							1.2 (0.6–2.4)[c]	2.4 (1.2–4.5)		
Before 1992							1.7 (0.7–4.1)[d]	3 (1.4–6.7)		
Repeated								2.1 (1.1–4.0)		
Surgical operation		0.95 (0.4–2.1)	1.8 (NS)	NA	NA	2.3 (0.8–6.7)[a]	2 (1.0–4.1)		1.63 (0.7–3.6)[a]	
Needle sharing		NS	1.8 (NS)		NA				4.08 (0.4–41.2)[b]	
Endoscopy experience					NA	2.1 (0.7–6.5)[a]			2.06 (0.9–4.5)[a]	2.16 (1.0–4.7)[a]
Tattooing		2.7 (0.8–9.3)								

NA = Nonapplicable; NS = nonsignificant.
[a] Odds ratio adjusted by multiple logistic regression. [b] Sex adjusted. [c] Less than 10 acupuncture sessions. [d] More than 10 acupuncture sessions.

risk factors among the population in the same rural area. In this area, 34.1% of men and 62.9% of women reported having had acupuncture sessions more than once; the risk of HCV infection attributable to acupuncture was 38.0% (95% CI 8.0–69.5) in total, 9.4% (95% CI 0.5–67.3) in men and 54.5% (95% CI 21.2–87.8) in women [15]. Further studies are needed to survey HCV prevalence and evaluate the role of acupuncture in other populations.

Many studies performed in Western countries have demonstrated that injection drug use is the single most important risk factor for HCV infection [18–21]. In Korea, the use of methamphetamine (Philopon) spread suddenly since the 1980s and became a serious social problem. The overall seropositivity for anti-HCV was 79.2% among 202 drug abusers [22]. The history of injection drug use has not been ascertained in most epidemiologic studies on HCV infection in Korea. According to a study investigating risk factors for HCV infection with reference to HCV genotypes, only 5.0% of the 139 anti-HCV-positive subjects studied during 1994–1998 confided having been sharing needles [17]. Hence, needle sharing was not a significant risk factor for HCV infection in Korea.

Since the incidence of transfusion-associated hepatitis C declined after the introduction of anti-HCV screening of blood donors, the overall prevalence of hepatitis C has changed in recent years. However, in Korea, the proportion of hepatitis C patients among intravenous drug abusers or individuals with risky sexual behavior is not yet definitively determined.

Intraspousal or intrafamilial infection is suggested as a route of HCV transmission. However, published data in Korea on intrafamilial [23] or intraspousal transmission [14, 15, 24] are very few, with inconsistent results.

Overall, transmission by risk factors other than blood transfusion is very rare. However, subjects at high risk of HCV infection should be monitored, including those with chronic disease related to sexual behaviors. As of now, there are virtually no data on the sexual transmission of HCV infection in Korea.

Distribution of HCV Genotypes in Korea

There have been few data on the distribution of HCV genotypes among the general population in Korea [14, 15, 17]. In a study on the distribution of HCV genotypes among 178 health examinees with anti-HCV and HCV RNA, 1b (39.9%) and 2a (38.2%) were the two most common types, followed by unclassified types (20.2%) and genotype 3 (1.1%) [17]. In another study, 1b was the pre-

Table 4. Distribution of HCV genotypes in nine studies

Reference	Number and subjects with HCV RNA studied	Study year	Method for HCV genotyping	Genotypes			
				1b	2a	others	unclassified
Shin HR et al. [14]	35; general rural population	1993–1995	RT-nested PCR	12 (37.5)	20 (62.5)	type 1a: 2 type 2a+2b: 1	
Kim CJ et al. [30]	75; patients with liver disease	before 1995	PCR for the NS5 region	45 (60.0)	25 (33.0)		5 (7.0)
Lee DS et al. [25]	138; 30 blood donors, 30 HCC patients, 33 chronic hepatitis, 15 liver cirrhosis and 30 hemodialysis patients	before 1996	method of Okamoto and the reverse hybridization method (INNO-LiPA)	98 (71.0)	33 (23.9)	type 2b: 2	2
Ohno O et al. [26]	53; HCV-infected Koreans	before 1996	a new genotyping system based on PCR with genotype-specific core region primers	35 (66.0)	9 (17.0)	type 1a: 1 type 2b: 4 type 1b+2b: 1	3
Han CJ et al. [27]	166; patients with type C chronic liver disease	before 1997	nested RT-PCR with genotype-specific primers	75 (45.2)	85 (51.2)	type 1a: 2 type 2b: 2 type 3a: 2	
Park YS et al. [28]	169; patients with HCV infections	before 1998	PCR-RFLP with four restriction endonucleases (BstUI, HaeIII, NciI, RsaI) on the 5′-untranslated region of HCV	80 (47.3)	72 (42.6)		17 (10.1)
Son HC et al. [29]	29; patients with HCV hepatitis	before 2002	standardized RT-PCR hybridization	15 (51.7)		type 2a+2c: 8 type 2b: 2	4
Kim YS et al. [17]	178; subjects with HCV-PCR in health check-up examinees	1994–1998	RT-PCR	71 (39.9)	68 (38.2)	type 1a: 1 type 3: 2	36
Shin HR et al. [15]	51; subjects with HCV RNA	1999	RT-PCR	21 (41.2)	28 (54.9)	type 1b+2a: 1	1

Figures in parentheses are percentages.

vailing type (71%), followed by 2a (23.9%), 1a (2.1%), 2b (1.5%) and unclassified types (1.5%) among 138 individuals with HCV RNA (30 blood donors, 33 patients with chronic hepatitis, 15 with liver cirrhosis, 30 with HCC and 30 on maintenance hemodialysis) [25]. In the population of the aforementioned rural area where HCV prevails [15], HCV RNA was detected in 66.2% of inhabitants with anti-HCV (51/77). The most prevalent HCV genotype was 2a (54.9% among subjects with HCV RNA), followed by 1b (41.2%), 1b+2a (2.0%) and unclassified types (2.0%). A higher prevalence of HCV genotype 2a in this rural area may be due to frequent acupunctures carried out there. However, the most prevalent HCV genotype among hepatitis patients in Korea was 1b. Estimated on nine data sets, frequencies of HCV genotypes in hepatitis patients were the highest for 1b at 50.6% (95% CI 47.2–53.9), followed by 2a at 38.0% (95% CI 34.8–41.3) (table 4) [6, 14, 15, 17, 25–29].

Discussion

There is no population-based serological study to estimate the prevalence of HCV infection in Korea. A total of 193,000 individuals (95% CI 168,000–222,000) are estimated to be positive for anti-HCV based on the age-specific prevalence compiled from four published data sets by the meta-analysis. There are no data to estimate the role of each route of HCV transmission, although high prevalence of HCV infection among older people may be due to blood transfusion before the 1990s. The risk of HCV exposure among blood recipients has decreased. In Korea, HCV has rarely been transmitted by blood transfusion after the introduction of anti-HCV screening of blood donors, which started in April 1991. The high prevalence of anti-HCV among older people is most likely due to a cohort effect caused by the higher risk of acquiring HCV infection in the distant than in the recent past.

Even though the prevalence of HCV infection in Korea has decreased and the risk of HCV transmission through blood transfusion has been markedly reduced, public health programs to prevent new infections should be developed. Moreover, in Korea, most people infected with HCV are older than 40 years, and therefore, the surveillance of HCV infection in adults (≥ 40 years) will help to efficiently detect HCC arising in them.

References

1 Shin HR, Lee CU, Park HJ, Seol SY, Chung JM, Choi HC, Ahn YO, Shigemastu T: Hepatitis B and C virus, Clonorchis sinensis for the risk of liver cancer: A case-control study in Pusan, Korea. Int J Epidemiol 1996;25:933–940.

2 Lee HS, Han CJ, Kim CY: Predominant etiologic association of hepatitis C virus with hepatocellular carcinoma compared with hepatitis B virus in elderly patients in a hepatitis B-endemic area. Cancer 1993;72:2564–2567.

3 Kim O, Kim SS, Park MS, Suh SD, Lee MW, Kim KS, Yoon JD, Lee JS: Seroprevalence of sexually transmitted viruses in Korean populations including HIV-seropositive individuals. Int J STD AIDS 2003;14:46–49.

4 Kim YS, Pai CH, Chi HS, Kim DW, Min YI, Ahn YO: Prevalence of hepatitis C virus antibody among Korean adults. J Korean Med Sci 1992;7:333–336.

5 Yoon DK, Cho KW, Hong MH, Kwon SY, Byun KS, Lee CH: Prevalence of antibody to hepatitis C virus in Korean adults (in Korean). Korean J Infect Dis 1994;26:237–247.

6 Kim WS, Dam DO, Shin HR, Jung KY, Kim JY: Epidemiologic study of hepatitis B and C among adults in Pusan (in Korean). J Pusan Med Assoc 1995;31:18–28.

7 Shin HR, Kim JY, Jung KY, Kim WS, Hong YS, Kim BK, Kim SR, Lee BO, Park TS, Lee YH, Ok ID, Ryan MK, Taniguchi M, Kim MM, Kim KI: Prevalence of hepatitis B and C virus infection among adults in Korea. Hepatol Res 1997;7:213–225.

8 Jeong TH, Jeon TH: PCR prevalence and risk factors of hepatitis C virus infection in the adult population of Ulsan (in Korean). J Korean Acad Fam Med 1998;19:364–373.

9 Seo WT, Lee SS: A study on positive rate of HBsAg, HBsAb and anti-HCV in Korean adults (in Korean). Korean J Blood Transfus 1998;9:259–272.

10 Na HY, Park MH, Park KS, Sohn YH, Joo YE, Kim SJ: Geographic characteristics of positive anti-HCV and hepatitis B surface antigen in Kwangju and Chonnam Province: Survey data of 6,790 health screenees (in Korean). Korean J Gastroenterol 2001;38:177–184.

11 Park KS, Lee YS, Lee SG, Hwang JY, Chung WJ, Cho KB, Hwang JS, Ahn SH, Park SK: A study on markers of viral hepatitis in adults living in Daegu and Gyungbuk area (in Korean). Korean J Gastroenterol 2003;41:473–479.

12 Lee JM, Lee JM, Yoo HS, Jang UK, Kim DJ, Kim YB, Kim HY, Park CK, Yoo JY: The prevalence of anti-HCV positivity in healthy Korean children (in Korean). Korean J Hepatol 1996;2:160–165.

13 Ju YH, Shin HR, Oh JK, Kim DI, Lee DH, Kim BK, Kim JI, Jung KY: Seroepidemiologic study of hepatitis B virus (HBV) and hepatitis C virus (HCV) infection in young population in parts of Busan, Korea (in Korean). Korean J Prev Med 2004, in press.

14 Shin HR, Kim JY, Ohno T, Cao K, Mizokami M, Risch H, Kim SR: Prevalence and risk factors of hepatitis C virus infection among Koreans in rural area of Korea. Hepatol Res 2000; 17:185–196.

15 Shin HR, Kim JY, Kim JI, Lee DH, Yoo KY, Lee DS, Franceschi S: Hepatitis B and C virus prevalence in a rural area of South Korea: The role of acupuncture. Br J Cancer 2002;87:314–318.

16 Kim YS, Ahn YO, Kim DW: A case-control study on the risk factors of hepatitis C virus infection among Koreans. J Korean Med Sci 1996;11:38–43.

17 Kim YS, Ahn YO, Lee HS: Risk factors for hepatitis C virus infection among Koreans according to the hepatitis C virus genotype. J Korean Med Sci 2002;17:187–192.

18 Alter MJ: Epidemiology of hepatitis C. Hepatology 1997;26:S62–S65.

19 Sladden TJ, Hickey AR, Dunn TM, Beard JR: Hepatitis C transmission on the north coast of New South Wales: Explaining the unexplained. Med J Aust 1997;166:290–293.

20 Kemp R, Miller J, Lungley S, Baker M: Injecting behaviours and prevalence of hepatitis B, C and D markers in New Zealand injecting drug user populations. N Z Med J 1998;111: 50–53.

21 Backmund M, Meyer K, Wachtler M, Eichenlaub D: Hepatitis C virus infection in injection drug users in Bavaria: Risk factors for seropositivity. Eur J Epidemiol 2003;18:563–568.

22 Kim SY, Kim JK, Lee SH: Seropositivity of anti-HCV in intravenous drug abusers (in Korean). J Korean Acad Fam Med 1997;18: 1508–1518.

23 Kim YS, Ahn YO, Kim DW: Familial clustering of hepatitis B and C viruses in Korea. J Korean Med Sci 1994;9:444–449.

24 Lee CG, Kim JS, Choi ES, Jeun MR, Chu SU, Hur C, Lee JK: Spousal transmission of hepatitis C virus (in Korean). Korean J Gastroenterol 1997;29:207–213.

25 Lee DS, Sung YC, Whang YS: Distribution of HCV genotypes among blood donors, patients with chronic liver disease, hepatocellular carcinoma, and patients on maintenance hemodialysis in Korea. J Med Virol 1996;49:55–60.

26 Ohno O, Mizokami M, Wu RR, Saleh MG, Ohba K, Orito E, Mukaide M, Williams R, Lau JY: New hepatitis C virus (HCV) genotyping system that allows for identification of HCV genotypes 1a, 1b, 2a, 2b, 3a, 3b, 4, 5a, and 6a. J Clin Microbiol 1997;35:201–207.

27 Han CJ, Lee HS, Kim HS, Choe JH, Kim CY: Hepatitis C virus genotypes in Korea and their relationship to clinical outcome in type C chronic liver diseases (in Korean). Korean J Intern Med 1997;12:21–27.

28 Park YS, Lee KO, Oh MJ, Chai YG: Distribution of genotypes in the 5′ untranslated region of hepatitis C virus in Korea. J Med Microbiol 1998;47:643–647.

29 Son HC, Yoon MS, Kim YJ, Kim IH, Kim YS: Type-specific antibody for hepatitis C virus detected by use of NS-4 peptide and hepatitis C virus genome in Korea. Rinsho Byori 2002;50: 533–540.

30 Kim CJ, Shin KS, Kim WY, Lim DS, Yoon SK, Park YM, Kim BS, Jang SK, Cho MJ: Genotype distribution and comparison of the putative envelope region of hepatitis C virus from Korean patients. J Med Virol 1995;46:380–386.

Epidemiology

Intervirology

Intervirology 2006;49:23–27
DOI: 10.1159/000087259

Viral Hepatitis C in Hong Kong

Nancy Leung[a] Carol Chu BNurs[b] John S. Tam[c]

[a]Alice Ho Miu Ling Nethersole Hospital, [b]Postgraduate Medical School, and [c]Department of Microbiology, Chinese University of Hong Kong, Hong Kong, SAR, China

Key Words
Chronic hepatitis · Epidemiology · Genotype · Hepatitis B virus · Hepatitis C virus · Hepatocellular carcinoma

Abstract
Objective: Hepatitis C virus (HCV) infection can lead to serious liver disease. Its medico-socio-economic burden on society can be immense. This study investigates the epidemiology of HCV infection in Hong Kong. ***Methods:*** Data from the Department of Health, relevant publications from Medline search and data from two acute hospitals were reviewed. ***Results:*** The prevalence of anti-HCV among voluntary blood donors is stable, remaining at approximately 0.035–0.099% over the past 10 years, and is higher in the older age group. Among the high-risk groups, the anti-HCV prevalence is as follows: (1) hospital patients 0.8%, (2) intravenous drug users 46.0%, (3) patients infected with HIV 7.9%, (4) children with transfusion-dependent hematologic disease 16.3%, (5) patients on continuous ambulatory peritoneal dialysis 1.8%, patients on hemodialysis 16.4%, recipients of kidney transplants 6.2% and (6) patients with hepatocellular carcinoma 7.3%. Among blood donors, 58.8% were infected with HCV genotype 1b and 27.0% with genotype 6a. Genotype 6a is particularly common among intravenous drug users. ***Conclusion:*** Hong Kong has a low prevalence of HCV infection. Patients are mostly infected through transfusion with blood or products prior to the introduction of anti-HCV screening to the blood transfusion service. Illicit drug use constitutes another significant risk. Since 1997, there has been a great increase in population movement between China and Hong Kong which might affect the epidemiology of HCV infection.

Introduction

Hong Kong is a region endemic for hepatitis A virus and hepatitis B virus (HBV), where viral hepatitis A accounts for most acute hepatitis, while viral hepatitis B accounts for the majority of chronic liver disease. Around 10% of the adult population are seropositive for hepatitis B surface antigen (HBsAg). In the early 1980s, posttransfusion non-A, non-B (NANB) hepatitis was recognized. With the identification of hepatitis C virus (HCV) in 1989 and the development of serological tests that followed, most of the posttransfusion NANB hepatitis was found to be HCV-related. The epidemiology of HCV infection is gradually emerging as studies were conducted. With highly sensitive and specific methodologies becoming more widely available, the clinical impact of HCV is increasingly coming to the fore. Although there is no region-wide population-based survey of HCV infection in Hong Kong, data from various studies on population subgroups are useful in identifying possible routes of HCV transmission. Public education and an improved healthcare system in Hong Kong have helped identify asymptomatic patients during medical check-ups. Hong Kong is a dy-

KARGER

Fax +41 61 306 12 34
E-Mail karger@karger.ch
www.karger.com

0300–5526/06/0492–0023$23.50/0

Accessible online at:
www.karger.com/int

Nancy Leung, MD
Department of Medicine, Alice Ho Miu Ling Nethersole Hospital
11 Chuen On Road
Taipo, NT, Hong Kong, SAR (China)
Tel./Fax +85 2 2689 3623, E-Mail leungwyn@ha.org.hk

namic cosmopolitan city hosting millions of visitors and tourists. Furthermore, after 1997, there has been a great increase in population movement between Hong Kong and the Mainland China. This is likely to have certain effects on the epidemiology of infectious diseases including HCV infection. Strategies for prevention and control of HCV infection should be planned accordingly.

Acute Hepatitis C

Acute viral hepatitis is a notifiable disease in Hong Kong. Most cases of acute hepatitis are acute hepatitis A, with occasional acute hepatitis B. Each year, a few cases fall into the category of NANB hepatitis which might include cases of acute hepatitis C. However, there is a technical difficulty in diagnosing acute hepatitis C in Hong Kong, since an assay for serum HCV RNA is not readily available in most healthcare settings. Clinicians can attend patients who are in the window period when anti-HCV antibody is not yet detectable, thus missing the diagnosis.

Clinical Impact of HCV Infection – Prevalence of Anti-HCV among Patients with Chronic Liver Disease and Hepatocellular Carcinoma

Lok et al. [1] reported high prevalence of anti-HCV among patients with posttransfusion NANB hepatitis and hepatocellular carcinoma (HCC), 87 and 37.3%, respectively, using the first-generation enzyme immunoassays on stored serum samples. On retesting with the second-generation enzyme immunoassays and neutralization assays, only 70 and 56% were confirmed positive. Another retrospective study using the first-generation recombinant assay verified by the second-generation assay also detected anti-HCV in 70% of posttransfusion NANB hepatitis, 20% of cryptogenic cirrhosis, 3% of alcoholic liver disease and 20% of autoimmune chronic active hepatitis. Only 1 of the 157 (0.6%) controls was positive for anti-HCV [2]. Among 424 consecutive patients with HCC attending the Hepatoma Clinic in a single center, 80% tested positive for HBsAg and 7.3% for anti-HCV, of whom 3.8% were positive for anti-HCV alone and 3.5% both for HBsAg and anti-HCV. The mean age of patients with anti-HCV was older than that of patients with HBsAg at 60 and 53 years, respectively [3]. Among 155 liver transplantations performed in Hong Kong, 7 (4.5%) were due to cirrhosis related to hepatitis C [4].

Coinfection with HCV and HBV

In Hong Kong, 10% of the adult population is seropositive for HBsAg. Most of them were infected at birth through mother-to-child transmission or horizontal transmission in early childhood. There has been a declining trend in HBsAg prevalence during the past two decades. Although the frequency of HCV infection in the general population remains low, 3.5% of HCC patients in Hong Kong had serological evidence for coinfection with HBV and HCV [3]. Coinfection with HBV and HCV has been shown to increase the risk of HCC. In a separate study on 571 patients with chronic hepatitis B, 4 (0.7%) were found to be anti-HCV positive; all 4 were positive for serum HCV RNA. Liver histology revealed lymphoid aggregates and bile duct changes in 3 of them. None had detectable HBV core antigen and HBV DNA was negative, while 3 had HCV RNA detected by in situ reverse transcription polymerase chain reaction (RT-PCR). Therefore, it appears that coinfection with HBV and HCV is uncommon in Hong Kong; there was no active replication of HBV in the few coinfected cases [5].

Blood Donors

Posttransfusion hepatitis C accounts for a significant proportion of chronic hepatitis C in Hong Kong. In 1991, the Hong Kong Red Cross Blood Transfusion Service introduced anti-HCV testing for all blood donors. Prior to this, HBsAg and serum alanine aminotransferase levels were screened to minimize posttransfusion viral hepatitis. Blood donation has been on voluntary basis. Potential donors are requested to complete a very comprehensive Blood Donation Registration Form to ensure his/her suitability. Inquiry includes immediate and past health (history of parenteral exposures such as surgical interventions, blood or organ transplantation, tattoo, acupuncture, body piercing and needlestick injury) and lifestyle issues (sexual activities and history of drug abuse). In an update report from the Department of Health published in December 2003, entitled 'Surveillance of viral hepatitis in Hong Kong' [6], the prevalence of anti-HCV among an average of 4,000 donors each year has remained at 0.035–0.099% since 1991; most blood donors are young adults. In the age group of 16–19 years, the prevalence of anti-HCV is 0.01–0.02%, increases to 0.1–0.2% in those aged 20–40 years and remains 0.1–0.3% in the age group over 40 years. Men tend to have a higher anti-HCV prevalence than women (table 1). The route of transmission

Table 1. Prevalence of anti-HCV in Hong Kong

Population subgroups	Anti-HCV positive	
Blood donors[a]:	men	women
All	21/20,563 (0.10)	13/21,750 (0.06)
Age groups		
16–19 years	2/12,856 (0.02)	1/13,483 (0.01)
20–29 years	7/ 4,901 (0.14)	5/4,620 (0.11)
30–39 years	5/1,716 (0.29)	3/2,115 (0.14)
40–49 years	4/841 (0.48)	3/1,213 (0.25)
>49 years	3/249 (1.20)	1/319 (0.31)
Patients on peritoneal dialysis	(1.8)	
Patients on hemodialysis	(16.4)	
IDUs[a]	97/210 (46.2)	
Patients with HIV/AIDS[a]	11/140 (7.9)	
Selected hospital-based patients	1,848/23,729 (7.8)	
Patients with chronic hepatitis B	4/571 (0.7)	
Patients with HCC	31/424 (7.1)	

Figures in parentheses are percentages.
[a] Data during 2002 from the Department of Health, Hong Kong.

among these anti-HCV-positive blood donors deserves further detailed studies.

In 1998, a review program for viral hepatitis C was launched by the Hong Kong Hospital Authority in collaboration with the Hong Kong Red Cross Blood Transfusion Service. Press releases have been made to promote checks for anti-HCV in order to identify individuals who might have been infected with HCV from a blood transfusion they received before anti-HCV screening of blood donors. Therapy was offered when indicated. This program instigated public awareness of HCV infection and encouraged individuals with a possible risk to come forward for anti-HCV testing.

Patients with End-Stage Renal Disease

The prevalence of HCV infection among patients with end-stage renal disease (ESRD) is 1.8% among those on peritoneal dialysis, 16.4% among those on hemodialysis and 6.2% among kidney transplant recipients [1, 7]. The high prevalence may be due to transfusion requirements especially for more than 5 units and parenteral exposures to HCV in their clinical courses. However, this may be an overestimation, because in these studies, the first-generation assay was performed on stored sera. On the other hand, there might be patients not diagnosed with HCV infection, because those with ESRD may not have had raised detectable anti-HCV since they are immunocompromised. HCV RNA should also be checked for the accurate diagnosis of HCV infection.

Among the 51 patients undergoing hemodialysis, 8 (16%) were positive for anti-HCV and 1 (2%) for HCV RNA alone, giving an overall HCV infection rate of 18%. Follow-up for 19 months identified an incidence of HCV infection at 5% per patient-year [7]. Patients tolerated the standard interferon (IFN)-α_{2b} well, and 27% achieved sustained virological response. Special attention must be paid to prevent aggravation of anemia resistant to erythropoietin as well as malnutrition induced during IFN therapy [8].

Recipients of renal allografts from donors seropositive for HCV RNA may have HCV-related liver disease. However, histological examinations showed lower activity scores than nonimmunosuppressed subjects, but more severe disease than patients on dialysis [9, 10].

Patients with Hematological Disorders

The thalassemia gene is common among the ethnic Chinese. Despite genetic counseling and screening of potential parents, transfusion-dependent thalassemia is not uncommon among young children. Of the 57 thalassemic children aged from 2 to 16 years, 8 (14%) were positive for anti-HCV (unpublished observation). The clinical efficacy of combination therapy with IFN-α 3 million units/m^2 three times per week and oral ribavirin 16 mg/kg daily for 12 months was evaluated in 18 treatment-naive patients with thalassemia. The median age at baseline was 16 years (range 7–29). Of those, 14 were infected with HCV genotype 1b and 4 with genotype 6a. The sustained biochemical and virological response 6 months after treatment was high at 72%. Requirement for blood transfusion was temporarily increased by 30% due to hemolysis associated with ribavirin [11].

Intravenous Drug Users

Injection drug users (IDUs) in Hong Kong have been encouraged to undergo detoxification through government-run programs including methadone clinics. These clinics supervise oral methadone administration to wean off the intravenous drug addiction. There are also inpatient drug rehabilitation centers. Surveillance for makers of HBV and HCV infections indicates a declining trend in the prevalence of anti-HCV. Of the 134 samples tested, 74% were positive during 1991–1992. Ten years later, in

2000/2001, the prevalence dropped to 46% among the 210 samples tested. Genotyping of HCV showed a high prevalence of genotype 6a among drug users. Cross-infection due to sharing syringes is common and may explain this genotype profile [6].

HIV and AIDS Patients

Hong Kong has a relatively low prevalence of HIV infection. Since 1984, a total of 2,311 HIV-infected individuals and 676 AIDS patients have been reported [6]. About 70% are ethnic Chinese, 80% have been infected through sexual contacts, of whom 70% were heterosexuals; only 5% are IDUs. They are encouraged to attend the HIV specialist services of the Department of Health or the hospital authority. In the year 2001, 75 male and 26 female patients from the Integrated Treatment Center of the Department of Health were screened. The overall anti-HCV prevalence was 7.9% (9.3% in men and 3.8% in women). Similar results were observed in the following year.

Sex Workers

There are no published data or reports on this population subgroup.

Hospital-Based Patients

The Prince of Wales Hospital and the Alice Ho Miu Ling Nethersole Hospital are two district hospitals which serve a catchment area with around 2 million inhabitants. A survey for HCV infection was performed there. Between 1993 and 2002, 23,729 tests were performed for anti-HCV. The reasons for requests were hepatitis with abnormal liver function tests, hepatitis with history of blood transfusion, previously diagnosed NANB hepatitis or current/past IDU. Using the second- and third-generation immunoassays, 1,848 (7.8%) subjects were found positive for anti-HCV, of whom two thirds were men. Anti-HCV-positive rates were 5.1, 7.1, 8.5, 7.8 and 5.2% in age groups ≤ 20, 21–40, 41–60, 61–80 and ≥ 81 years, respectively. The reason for HCV infection in 140 youngsters less than 20 years old is not entirely clear. It is postulated that they may have had blood transfusions repeatedly before the introduction of anti-HCV screening of blood donors, since most of them had suffered from hematological disorder or oncological disease. The review on case notes of 401 patients revealed a median age of 42 years (range 3–78) with a male-to-female ratio of 7:3. The possible route of transmission was IDU (44.9%), followed by history of blood transfusion including ESRD requiring dialysis and/or blood transfusion (19.5%), surgical or dental intervention (7.5%) and renal transplantation (3.7%). The possible route of transmission in the remaining 24% of the patients was not documented in the case note, although 2 might have been infected through acupuncture. Despite the HCV lookback program in 1998 to promote check-ups for anti-HCV in those with a history of blood transfusion, many patients still present with a late complication of cirrhosis [unpubl. observations].

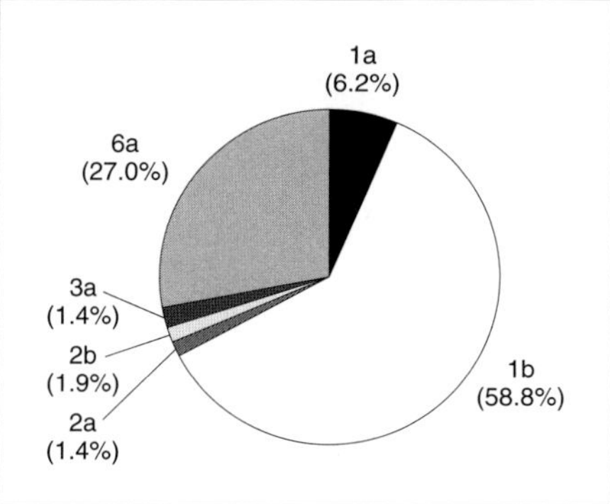

Fig. 1. Genotypes of HCV among blood donors in Hong Kong [data adapted from ref. 12].

HCV Genotypes

Among 212 blood donors, 58.5% were infected with HCV genotype 1b and 27.0% with genotype 6a. Other genotypes included 1a (6.2%), 2a (1.4%), 2b (1.4%) and 3a (1.9%) (fig. 1) [12]. In the hospital-based study at the Prince of Wales Hospital and the Alice Ho Miu Ling Nethersole Hospital, 82.4% of all patients with anti-HCV were positive for HCV RNA by PCR. In these 294 HCV RNA-positive samples, the genotype profile was similar to 1b (60.6%), 6a (28.6%) and 2a/2b/3a (10.8%) [unpubl. observations]. Among IDUs, 70% were PCR-positive for HCV RNA, and a high prevalence of genotype 6a was confirmed with 1b (33.9%), 2a/3a (7.2%) and 6a (58.9%). The rate of therapeutic response among the Chinese has not been formally assessed or compared with that in the Caucasians. Pilot studies have shown that genotype 6 behaves much the same as non-1 genotypes in the therapeutic response [pers. commun.].

Discussion

Hong Kong has a relatively low prevalence of anti-HCV in the general population. Chronic HCV infection is mainly the result of transfusion with unscreened blood or blood products in the past. The introduction of a detailed questionnaire and screening of potential blood donors for anti-HCV should have minimized the risk of infection to a negligible level; Hong Kong does not accept paid blood donation and the majority of donors are young volunteers. The fact that 0.01–0.2% of those aged between 16 and 19 years were anti-HCV-positive needs to be further investigated.

Hong Kong is undergoing great sociopolitical changes, including for example a relatively free movement of populations across the border separating Hong Kong and China. Certain regions in China have an exceedingly high prevalence of HBV, as well as HCV and HIV, largely due to failure in stemming out paid blood and organ donations. This may affect profiles of disease epidemiology in Hong Kong, including that of HCV infection.

IDU is not a major problem in Hong Kong. Young people tend to use oral drugs for recreational activities. However, for IDUs, there is no syringe change program to minimize cross-infection among the inmates. The methadone clinics were often abused by IDUs as a trafficking point. Concerted effort by the government and police department to stem out drug trafficking across the border and in the community is important. Many non-governmental organizations also provide support for IDUs to rehabilitate them in the society.

Body piercing and tattoos are back in fashion. Nail manicure is also popular. The hygienic standard of facilities providing these services is variable. Acupuncture has been and still is popular among Chinese for diverse ailments. Disposable acupuncture needles are available and acupuncturists must promote their usage. In the hospital-based study, 23.9% of the patients with anti-HCV were found to have no documented risk factors. This may be due to poor documentation or some other risk factors yet to be identified.

Therapy for chronic hepatitis C is expensive. The main focus of the healthcare system should be on the prevention of HCV infection. Public education is vital in the prevention of viral hepatitis. The awareness of risks and ways to avoid them must be promulgated.

References

1 Lok AS, Ma OC, Chan TM, Lai CL, Chung HT, Ng CP, Lam JS: Overestimation of the prevalence of antibody to hepatitis C virus in retrospective studies on stored sera. Hepatology 1991;14:756–762.

2 Lai JY, Tam JS, Lam LY, Leung NW: Prevalence of antibody to hepatitis C virus in HBsAg-negative chronic liver disease in Hong Kong using different assays. J Med Virol 1992; 37:158–160.

3 Leung NW, Tam JS, Lai JY, Leung TW, Lau WY, Shiu W, Li AK: Does hepatitis C virus infection contribute to hepatocellular carcinoma in Hong Kong? Cancer 1992;70:40–44.

4 Lo CM, Fan ST, Liu CL, Yong BH, Lai CL, Lau GK, Wei WI, Tam PK, Tsoi NS, Ng IO, Young K, Chan JK, Tso WK, Yuen KY, Wong J: Ten-year experience with liver transplantation at Queen Mary Hospital: Retrospective study. Hong Kong Med J 2002;8:240–244.

5 Lau GK, Wu PC, Lo CK, Lau V, Lam SK: Histological changes of concurrent hepatitis C virus infection in asymptomatic hepatitis B virus patients. J Gastroenterol Hepatol 1998;13:52–56.

6 'Surveillance of Viral Hepatitis in Hong Kong' – 2002 Update Report. Hong Kong, Department of Health, www.hepatitis.gov.hk.

7 Chan TM, Lok AS, Cheng IK, Chan RT: Prevalence of hepatitis C virus infection in hemodialysis patients: A longitudinal study comparing the results of RNA and antibody assays. Hepatology 1993;17:5–8.

8 Chan TM, Wu PC, Lau JY, Lok AS, Lai CL, Cheng IK: Interferon treatment for hepatitis C virus infection in patients on haemodialysis. Nephrol Dial Transplant 1997;12:1414–1419.

9 Chan TM, Wu PC, Lau JY, Lai CL, Lok AS, Cheng IK: Clinicopathologic features of hepatitis C virus infection in renal allograft recipients. Transplantation 1994;58:996–1000.

10 Chan TM, Lau JY, Wu PC, Lai CL, Lok AS, Cheng IK: Hepatitis C virus genotypes in patients on renal replacement therapy. Nephrol Dial Transplant 1998;13:731–734.

11 Li CK, Chan PK, Ling SC, Ha SY: Interferon and ribavirin as frontline treatment for chronic hepatitis C infection in thalassaemia major. Br J Haematol 2002;117:755–758.

12 Prescott LE, Simmonds P, Lai CL, Chan NK, Pike I, Yap PL, Lin CK: Detection and clinical features of hepatitis C virus type 6 infections in blood donors from Hong Kong. J Med Virol 1996;50:168–175.

Epidemiology

Intervirology

Intervirology 2006;49:28–36
DOI: 10.1159/000087260

Spread Times of Hepatitis C Virus Estimated by the Molecular Clock Differ among Japan, the United States and Egypt in Reflection of Their Distinct Socioeconomic Backgrounds

Masashi Mizokami[a] Yasuhito Tanaka[a] Yuzo Miyakawa[b]

[a]Department of Clinical Molecular Informative Medicine, Nagoya City University Graduate School of Medical Sciences, Nagoya, and [b]Miyakawa Memorial Research Foundation, Tokyo, Japan

Key Words
Evolution · Hepatitis C virus · Intravenous drugs · Molecular clock · Schistosomiasis · Transfusion

Abstract
Infection with hepatitis C virus (HCV) is taking an ever increasing role in the development of hepatocellular carcinoma (HCC) over the world. Dynamics of HCV infection were determined by the molecular clock, estimating the dissemination time when HCV entered the country and the 'spread time' when it started to grow exponentially on a national scale. A comparison of HCV dynamics in Japan, the United States and Egypt has disclosed different dissemination and spread times among the three countries. Furthermore, they faithfully mirror socioeconomic as well as medical and paramedical events inherent to each country responsible for the wide spread of HCV infection during the past. Epidemic histories of HCV would enable us to predict what is going to happen in the future for HCV infection, in special reference to HCC associated with it. Population dynamics of HCV need to be determined in other countries where HCV prevails and compared with those in the three countries described. These studies should help foresee what will happen in the near future for HCV infection in a given country, time the future development of HCC and take measures for preventing it.

Introduction

Of the total population in the world, 190 million people (3%) are infected with hepatitis C virus (HCV) [1], which is half as many as the 400 million people persistently infected with hepatitis B virus (HBV), accounting for 6% of the world population [2]. The most severe consequence of persistent infections with HBV and HCV is hepatocellular carcinoma (HCC) that now ranks fourth in yearly deaths due to malignancies worldwide. In contrast to HBV, the presence of which has been known since 1964, and which enabled serological diagnosis in the early 1970s [3], the history of HCV is much younger. For a long time, the diagnosis of HCV has been made by excluding infection with HBV or hepatitis A virus (thus called non-A, non-B), until a subgenomic sequence of the HCV genome was discovered by Choo et al. [4] in 1989 and instantaneously applied to enzyme immunoassay for anti-HCV [5].

Although much information on HCV has been gained during the past 15 years since its discovery, there remains plenty to investigate. First and foremost, the natural history of HCV infection is hard to define due to the insidious nature of the liver disease it induces and a long incubation time before serious complications develop, such as decompensated cirrhosis and HCC. Necroinflammatory changes that keep wax and wane in the liver of patients with chronic hepatitis C are healed and replaced by

KARGER
Fax +41 61 306 12 34
E-Mail karger@karger.ch
www.karger.com

0300–5526/06/0492–0028$23.50/0

Accessible online at:
www.karger.com/int

Masashi Mizokami, MD
Department of Clinical Molecular Informative Medicine
Nagoya City University Graduate School of Medical Sciences
Nagoya 467-8601 (Japan)
Tel. +81 52 853 8292, Fax +81 52 842 0021, E-Mail mizokami@med.nagoya-cu.ac.jp

fibrosis, and cirrhosis eventually develops; more than 90% of HCV-associated HCC occurs in cirrhotic patients. Many factors influence fibrosis of the liver and the development of HCC, including the duration of infection, ethnicity, sex, iron load, obesity, alcohol intake and HCV genotypes.

It takes a long time for HCC to develop in a person infected with HCV, although it is estimated to happen only in about 30% of those who are infected, if they live long enough. It has been reported that 30 years elapse from the time of HCV infection through transfusion until recipients come down with HCC [6, 7], although the age when they are infected can make much difference [8]. Hence, there is no doubt about the crucial role of the time factor in the development of HCC. The impact of time when people are infected with HCV becomes even more important when HCV-associated HCC is looked at as a social problem on a national scale. There is a pressing need to estimate dynamics of the national spread of HCV infection in a given country, which will not only determine the present situation, but may also predict what will happen in the foreseeable future. By means of the molecular clock based on the coalescent theory [9, 10], we have reproduced population dynamics of effective HCV infections in Japan, the United States and Egypt [11, 12]. Time of diffusion and spread of HCV infection were estimated to differ among these countries in reflection of socioeconomic events which happened in the remote past. Hopefully, these studies will help to predict and prevent what will happen in the future in other countries where HCV prevails and determine its population dynamics.

Differences in Present Profiles of HCC between Japan and the United States despite Comparable Prevalence of Anti-HCV

Table 1 compares the annual incidence of HCC between Japan and the United States in reference to their backgrounds. With half the population but the same prevalence of anti-HCV at 1.7% in the general population, the total cases of HCC in Japan are four times more than those in the United States; in Japan, 90% of HCC is caused by HCV infection, which stands in remarkable contrast to only about 40% in the United States. HCC is nine times commoner at face value, and after adjustment to the population size, HCC due to HCV infection is twenty times more frequent in Japan than in the United States. Why is there such a big difference? There are many factors involved, including the time after exposure (duration of HCV infection), genetic differences in distinct ethnicity (Mongoloid vs. Caucasian), 1b as the most frequent HCV genotype at 70% in Japan against 1a at 60% in the United States, coinfection with or past exposure to HBV (which is far more common in Japan than in the United States), environmental factors like eating habits accelerating the obesity, and probably many more.

Table 1. Differences in yearly incidence of HCC between Japan and the United States despite the same prevalence of anti-HCV in the general population

	Japan	United States
Total population	125 million	250 million
Subjects with anti-HCV	2 million (1.7%)	4 million (1.7%)
Yearly deaths due to HCC	40,000	10,000
HCC due to HCV infection	36,000 (90%)	4,000 (40%)
Ratio of HCV-related HCC	9	1
Population-adjusted ratio		
HCC associated with HCV	20	1

We envisage that the most important difference between Japan and the United States is the duration of infection, in terms of years that have elapsed after exposure of the general population to HCV. How then do we know the time of mass HCV infection in the Japanese and Americans?

Evolutionary Analysis with the Molecular Clock

The molecular clock was invented more than 40 years ago [9, 10]. It has been very instrumental in analyzing the dynamics of evolution and has been extended to studies on the epidemic behavior of HCV [13]. We have employed it to calculate the time when HCV infection entered and started to spread and found much difference between Japan and the United States [11]. Scientific evolutionism was first reported by Charles Darwin in 1858. In his famous book *The Origin of Species,* he proposed that evolution occurs by mutations and a natural selection of the fittest. However, we know now that most evolutions cannot be explained by mutations and the natural selection alone. In Japan in 1968, Dr. Kimura [14] came up with the neutral theory. In that theory, he states that evolution is created by mutations of nucleotides which constitute the genes. More importantly, he proposed that

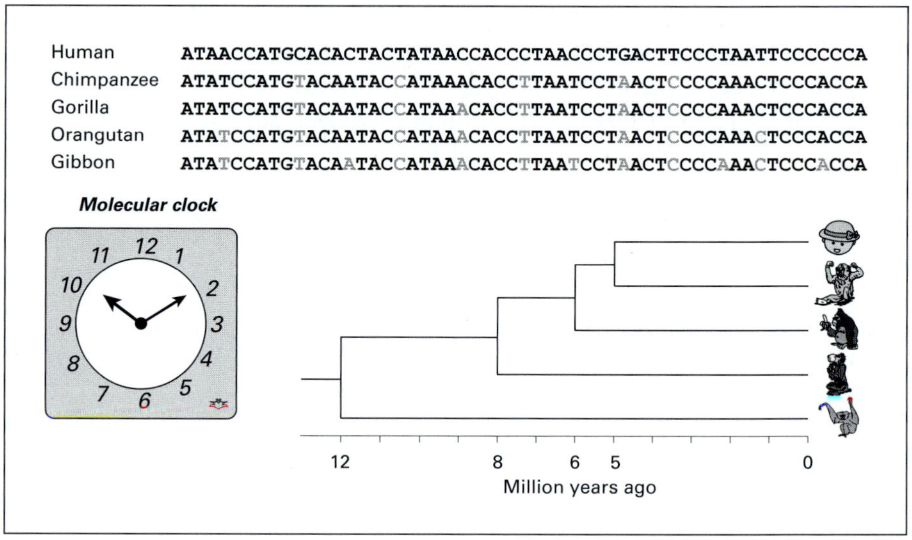

Fig. 1. From which of the four great apes did we divert how many years ago? The method is schematically explained on putative sequences of 55 nucleotides. Based on mutations in nucleotide sequences (upper half), a phylogenetic tree is constructed (lower half). The number of different nucleotides (grey letters) is divided by the known mutation rate per site per year for human DNA to estimate how long ago each primate diverted (by the molecular clock). The genetic kinship between species is determined by bifurcation on the phylogenetic tree.

nucleotide mutations should be accounted for systematically by mathematical and statistical analyses. We applied the molecular clock to HCV infection, because HCV is subject to very rapid mutations.

The most famous application of the neutral theory was performed to investigate the origin of human beings (fig. 1). We all know that humans originated in primates. However, no one knows for sure which species of the great apes, including chimpanzee, gorilla, orangutan and gibbon, is the origin of humans; they all look very similar. How then can we recognize our direct ancestor, *Homo sapiens,* in any one of them? The evolutionary analysis with the molecular clock has proven that chimpanzees are our direct ancestors and that we evolved from them about 5 million years ago, based on statistical and systematic evaluation of differences in the number of mutations in the corresponding nucleotide sequences of a mitochondria gene among humans and the four great apes.

With the use of this molecular clock method, the duration after HCV infection that may significantly influence its clinical sequelae was compared between Japan and the United States [11]. Materials were 62 sera including 36 serial serum samples from 10 patients sampled 2–7 times at intervals of 7–21 years, all of whom participated in the Transfusion-Associated Hepatitis Study started in 1972 [15]. In addition, single sera from 11 long-term (>20 years) carriers of HCV were analyzed [16]. All of them were infected with HCV genotype 1a and had not received treatment with interferon (IFN) which can modify mutation rates of the HCV genome, thereby affecting the viral evolution. For comparison, serial serum samples from 6 Japanese patients infected with HCV genotype 1b were studied; none had received IFN therapy.

HCV RNA was extracted from these sera, amplified by polymerase chain reaction, and a sequence of 1,778 nucleotides assorted from the core gene, E1 and E2 regions as well as the NS5b region was determined and subjected to molecular evolutionary analyses. Then, phylogenetic trees were constructed on these subgenomic areas, and the results were analyzed by the molecular clock to precisely determine the mutation rate per site per year of the Hutchinson strain of genotype 1a (the prototype of HCV) [4].

The ordinal pairwise comparison method is a simple way to estimate when two genomic sequences were separated from the same path into two distinct directions. More feasibly, a recently developed technique of linear regression analysis deals with the time elapsed from the origin to every diversification that is indicated by a bifurcation in phylogenetic trees. Results are displayed in two dimensions with the x-axis for years when serum samples were collected and the y-axis for length in nucleotides between any two diversifications. Thus, partial sequences of the Hutchinson strain were determined at the year of its detection in 1977, and changes in sequences were successively followed five times in 1982, 1989, 1990, 1995 and 1996 (fig. 2). They were all plotted on a straight line in a constant slope. Small deviations from the linearity arise because evolution is sometimes slower or faster. When examining these plots by the linear regression method, the results are perfectly in accord; they all stayed within the 95% confidence interval (CI). The evolution-

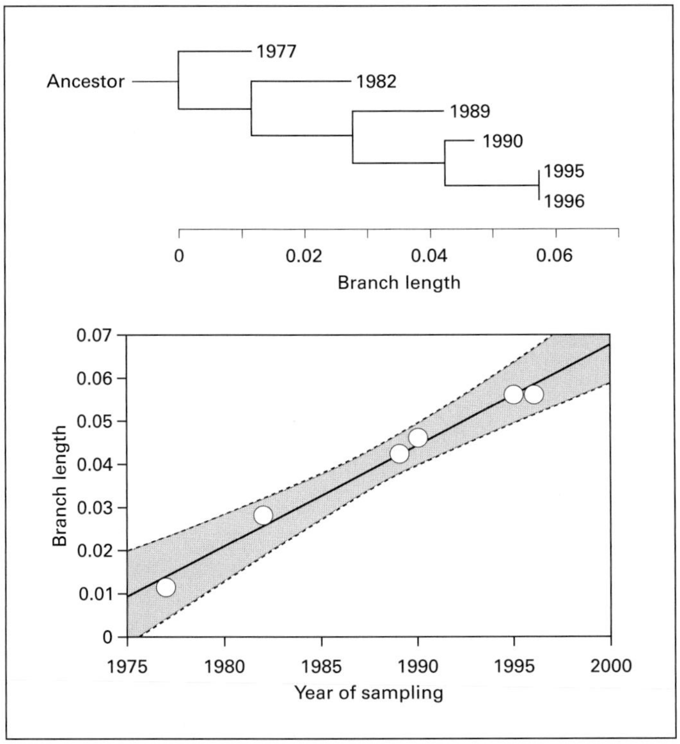

Fig. 2. Evolution of the prototype HCV (the Hutchinson strain) during 20 years. Phylogenetic trees were constructed on nucleotide sequences of the core gene as well as E1 and NS5 regions from 6 serum samples recovered from the same HCV carrier in the years indicated (upper half). They were plotted by branch lengths from the beginning of divergence (y-axis) against the time scale in years (x-axis). All plots remained on a straight line, by which the mutation rate of nucleotides in HCV was estimated at 0.58×10^{-3} per site per year.

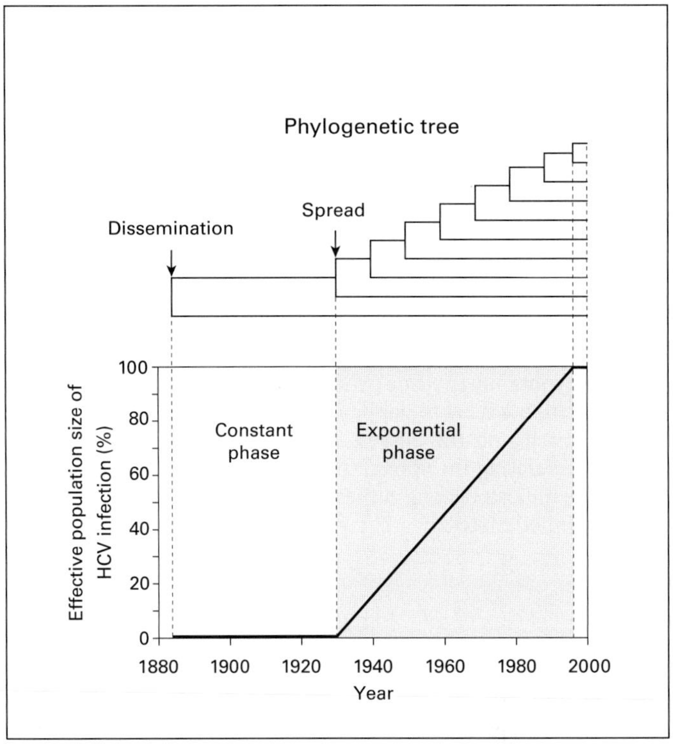

Fig. 3. The principle of the population dynamics study with the molecular clock enforced. A phylogenetic tree is constructed on the corresponding genomic area of HCV isolates available at present (the year 2000) (upper half). Thereafter, the effective population size is estimated by the molecular clock (lower half). In essence, a point on the curve at a given year represents in percent the number of genetically different HCV populations divided by that of populations at present. The dissemination time is defined by the time when HCV entered the country. The spread time is defined by the year when the exponential increase started.

ary rate of HCV calculated on five HCV isolates is 0.58×10^{-3} (95% CI $0.53–0.65 \times 10^{-3}$) per site per year, which is the most reliable figure at present. It is substantially smaller than 1.92×10^{-3} [17], 1.35×10^{-3} [18] and 1.44×10^{-3} per site per year [19], figures that have been estimated on HCV isolates in limited HCV isolates recovered from the same carriers during a short period of time.

Based on the speed of HCV evolution, we have calculated the time when HCV entered the United States and Japan [11]. From the linear regression analysis of all 47 HCV isolates of genotype 1a from the United States of which sequences in comparison are available, the most recent ancestor of HCV genotype 1a is estimated to have entered the United States around the year 1909 (95% CI 1900–1914). We extended this method to 17 serial serum samples from patients infected with HCV genotype 1b in Japan and estimated the time of its entry around 1882 [11].

Dynamics of HCV Infection Simulated by the Effective Population Size

Recently, a more sophisticated technique became available for estimating evolution with an added precision. It has been used for viral population studies based on the neutral theory [20] and was extended to HCV [13]. In general, the time scale in phylogenetic trees is converted to the genetic distance. However, in the neutral theory, this distance is converted to a time scale using the molecular clock (fig. 3). In essence, past changes in the effec-

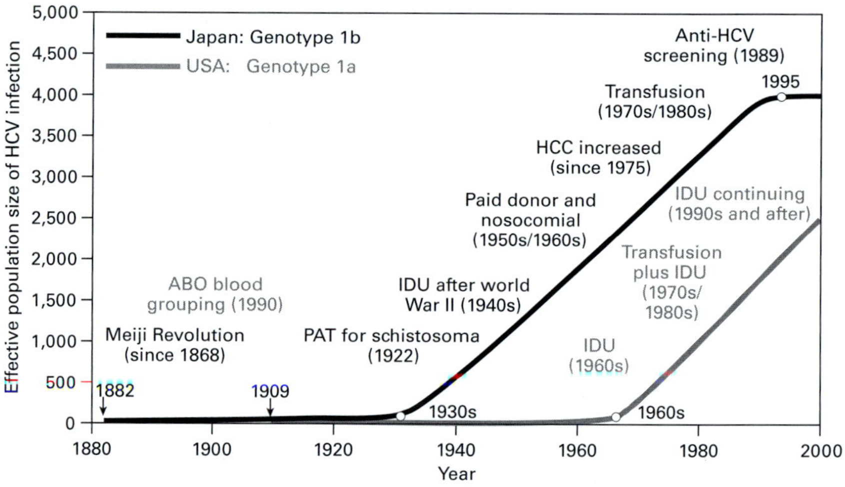

Fig. 4. Dynamics of the expansion of effective population size of HCV infections in Japan and the United States estimated by the molecular clock. Number of effective HCV infections are estimated on the basis of HCV isolates from Japan and the United States [11]. The divergence time (when the HCV infection entered each country) is indicated by an arrow, and the spread time as well as the containment time (when de novo HCV infection ceased to happen) are indicated as circles on the curves. Important events accelerating the spread of HCV infection are indicated along curves for Japan and the United States.

tive population size of infections are estimated on present viral populations in limited numbers. First, a phylogenetic tree is constructed, and then, with the application of the substitution rate obtained by the molecular clock (fig. 2), a phylogenetic tree is displayed on the x-axis for the time scale to track down when any two distinct HCV populations diverted.

For the sake of simplification, let us assume that we have 10 genetically distinct populations of HCV at the year 2000. We also had 100% of the HCV population in 1995, indicating that no new HCV infections have occurred. Only one HCV isolate existed from 1882 to 1930, when it started to spread with the exponential growth that continued until 1995. Each transition time can be estimated by the piecewise expansion model [21, 22]. Thus, by means of converting sequence divergence of limited HCV isolates available into the effective size of HCV infection at any given time during the past, this method can estimate when HCV entered the country (dissemination time) and when HCV started to spread exponentially (spread time).

We applied this technique to HCV infection in Japan, comparing it with that in the United States (fig. 4). In Japan, HCV genotype 1b was introduced in 1882 and started to spread exponentially in the 1920s and the1930s [11]. The spread was terminated in 1995, with essentially no de novo HCV infection eliciting since then [23]. From the age-specific distribution of HCV carriers in Japan [23, 24], we can foresee that the curve of the effective population size of HCV will flatten out during 2010–2015 and then decrease. In remarkable contrast, HCV genotype 1a infection entered the United States in the year 1909, with its exponential phase since the 1960s; the expansion is still going on at present, principally among intravenous drug users (IDUs). Hence, effective measures need to be taken to decrease future spread of HCV and diminish the size of the presently effective population by antiviral treatment.

These analyses are supported by epidemiological and socioeconomical backgrounds, which differ between the two countries. Based on the population dynamics of HCV in the United States that are assumed to represent those in Japan 30 years ago, one can reasonably expect that the United States will have the same population dynamics for HCV-associated HCC within the next few decades which we have in Japan nowadays, that is, if they do not take appropriate and efficient strategies to prevent it. Already, deaths due to HCC are increasing in the United States [25, 26]. There have been some studies to indicate that IFN can decrease the development of HCC in patients persistently infected with HCV, not only in those who have cleared infection [27], but also in those in whom necroinflammation is kept suppressed by IFN [28].

It is our consensus that HCV has less infectious activity than HBV. Infection with HCV occurs in 2–3% of individuals who are accidentally exposed to HCV by needlesticks breaking the integument [29, 30] and in 2.8% of sexual partners who have been infected with HCV of the same genotype [31]. In contrast, IDU is very efficient in transmitting HCV and infects about three quarters of users who share needles and syringes [32, 33]. Hence, at present, the most important factor for the spread of HCV infection in the United States is IDU.

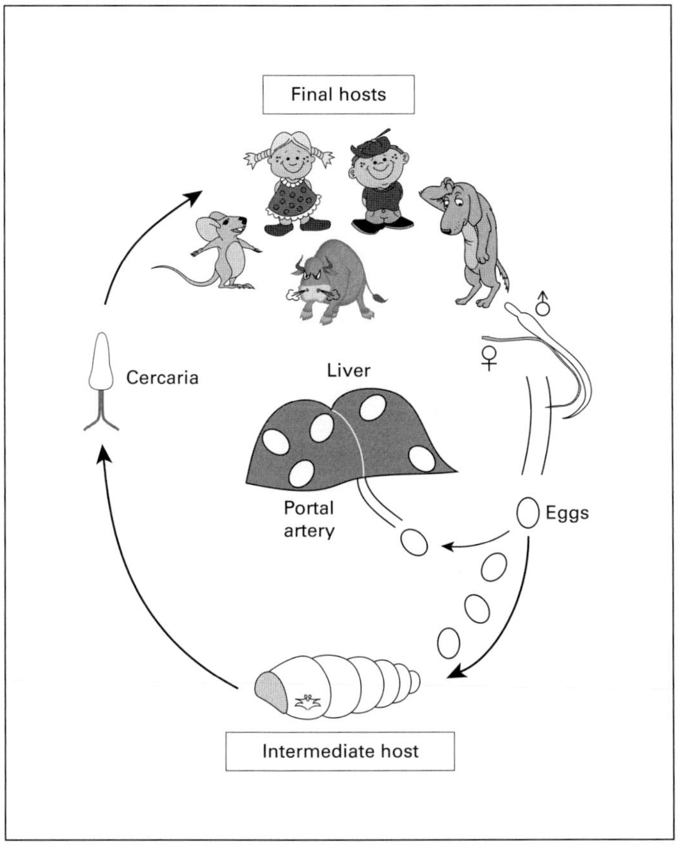

Fig. 5. The life cycle of *S. japonicum.* The final hosts are mammals paddling in the river and/or living along the riverside. The parasite (congruent male and female) hooks in the walls of the intestines and mesenteric arteries and lays tens of thousands of eggs. Some eggs are deposited in the liver and cause fibrosis, but they never hatch. Others are excreted and infect the intermediate host of small shellfish in which they proliferate, evolve into cercaria and are excreted into water. By means of proteolytic enzyme contained in filaments, cercaria penetrates the skin of mammals, hatches to parasite and infects them for life.

Next to the United States, we also investigated the factors which were responsible for the wide spread of HCV in Japan. We estimate that HCV was introduced to Japan in the era of the Meiji Revolution started in 1868. Since then, Japan imported medical techniques from the Western countries with much enthusiasm, especially surgical operation techniques. And more importantly, in 1921, intravenous antimony was introduced for treatment of schistosomiasis japonica. Since there was no sterilization of needles and syringes between injections of two or more patients, the treatment spread HCV infection very efficiently among those infected with *Schistosoma japonicum* in endemic areas [34]. During the turmoil surrounding the end of World War II, intravenous methamphetamine use was popular among soldiers to stay awake at night and stir up their fighting spirits, and thus, spread among subpopulations in Japan, especially among paid blood donors [23]. During these years, tuberculosis of the lung was rampant in Japan due to a poor socioeconomic status after the war, and surgical operations were frequently performed on patients suffering from lung tuberculosis. Through transfusions that patients received at thoracoplasty, HCV in remunerated blood was transmitted. Some 30 years later, in 1975, this dissemination of HCV among the general population in Japan started to take tolls, and the incidence of HCC started to increase [23], as has recently been the case in Scotland [35]. Lacking any means for serological diagnosis of HCV infection, diffusion of HCV by transfusion of blood or blood products continued to occur through the 1970s and the 1980s, even though paid blood donation was abolished in 1964. It was not until 1992 when posttransfusion HCV infection was completely stopped by the second-generation screening for anti-HCV [36].

In the United States, in 1900, Dr. Landsteiner discovered the ABO blood grouping, and in the following year, his pupil Dr. Castero identified the AB group for the safe blood transfusion without complication of hemolysis in recipients. It is conceivable that transfusion set HCV to spread, although, for a long time, its impact was small due to a very low population size of HCV infection in the United States. However, suddenly during the late 1960s, HCV started to diffuse among soldiers in the Vietnam War by IDU. This vice continued in veterans after they came back to the United States and spread widely among younger generations. The dissemination of HCV continued efficiently through the 1970s and the 1980s by IDU and transfusions not screened for anti-HCV. Although transmission of HCV by transfusion and blood products ceased to occur in 1990 when screening for anti-HCV was introduced to blood banks in the United States, the spread of HCV by shared needles and syringes for IDU seems to continue.

Dynamics of Effective Population Size of HCV Infections of Genotype 4a in Egypt

Once, Egypt was heavily endemic for *Schistosoma mansoni.* The parasite has a peculiar life cycle, with human beings and other mammals as the final host and small shellfish as the intermediate host (fig. 5). It is a hermaphrodite, stays in the liver as well as the intestines and

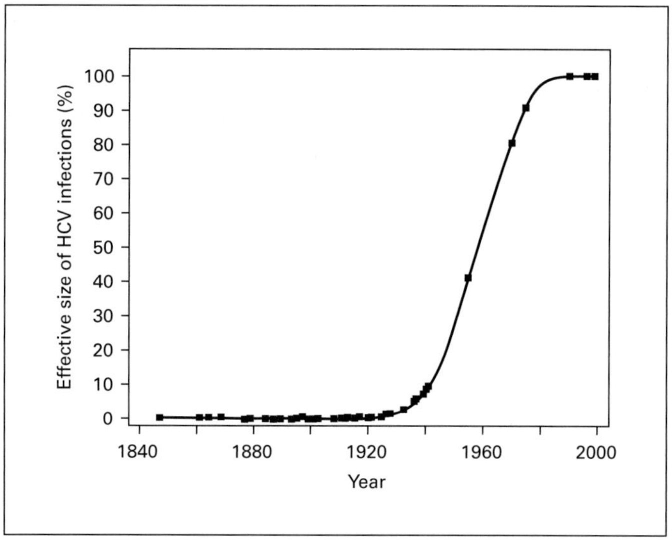

Fig. 6. Dynamics of the effective population size of infection with HCV genotype 4a in inhabitants along riversides of the Nile River in Egypt.

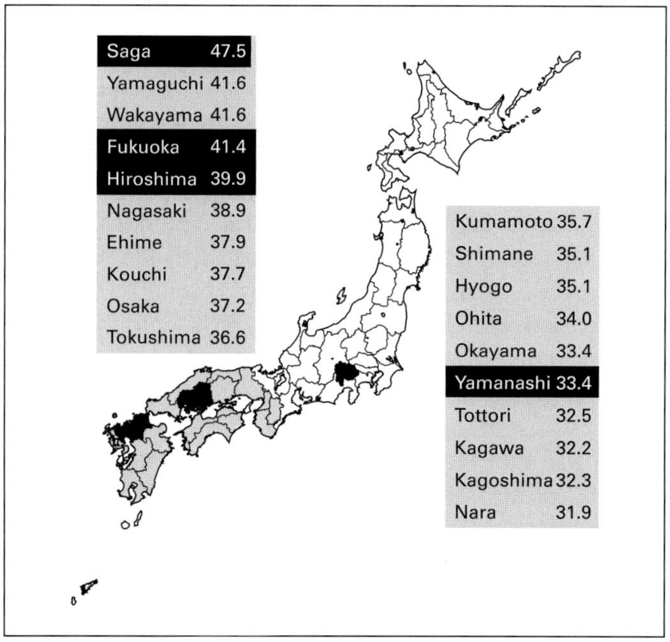

Fig. 7. The top 20 prefectures in Japan with a mortality due to HCC in excess of 30 per 100,000 population in the year 2002. The average of yearly deaths per 100,000 population in the 48 prefectures in Japan is 27.5, and those with high numbers cluster in southwestern districts including Shikoku and Kyushu, with the exception of Yamanashi situated in the center of Honshu. Four prefectures previously endemic for *S. japonica* are highlighted in white on black background, in which Yamanashi is included together with Saga, Fukuoka and Hiroshima that are within the top five for a high incidence of HCC.

continues to bear eggs, some of which are excreted. Eggs do not infect other humans horizontally, but shellfish can harbor, hatch and grow them to cercaria; it swims in the water and penetrates the skin of animals that paddle in rivers and swamps. Thus, *S. mansoni* preferentially infected inhabitants along the Nile River. To cope with schistosomiasis rampant in Egypt, nation-wide campaigns for parenteral antischistosomal therapy (PAT) were started in the 1940s, which widely and efficiently disseminated HCV among patients with this disease [37].

The prevalence of anti-HCV in Egypt is the highest in the world, with 25% of people having been exposed to it [1]. HCV infections in Egypt are very peculiar in that more than 90% are of genotype 4a, as genotype 6 is the most common in Hong Kong [38]. In collaboration with local doctors, we determined sequences of HCV isolates from Egyptians living alongside the Nile River and constructed a phylogenetic tree [12]. Based on this phylogenetic tree constructed on an NS5b sequence of 339 nucleotides from 47 HCV isolates of genotype 4a, we simulated the dynamics of HCV in Egypt by the molecular clock (fig. 6). Again, the profile mirrors social backgrounds, as it does for Japan and the United States (fig. 4). The exponential spread of HCV occurred during the national project for PAT. It was started in 1961 and continued until 1986 when oral medicine for schistosomiasis was introduced to take over the injection treatment [37]. These results stand in strong corroboration with those in a recent report of Pybus et al. [39]. Cases of HCC keep increasing in Egyptians at present [40], some of which are a long-term outcome of PAT conducted until 20 years ago.

A situation similar to this happened in districts in Japan where schistosomiasis japonica was once endemic [34]. These districts are all located along big rivers, and eggs of this parasite were detected in excrements from 60% of primary school children living there in the 1920s. The ramifications of a possible spread of HCV infection by intravenous antimony are evident in the current distribution of HCC in Japan. The mortality due to HCC in Japan during the year 2002 averages 27.5 per 100,000 population. There were 20 prefectures that exceeded 30 deaths due to HCC per 100,000 population (fig. 7). They are all situated in the southwest of Japan, including all 4 prefectures in Shikoku and all 7 in Kyusu. Yamanashi is exceptional in that it stands out with a high incidence of HCC-associated deaths despite its location in the center of Honshu and far east to the other 19 prefectures with a high incidence. Schistosomiasis once prevalent in Yamanashi is the clue to this mystery. There are an additional 3 prefectures where schistosomiasis japonica was rampant, and they all rank within the top five in the list for high incidence of HCC in Japan. We applied the effective population method with the molecular clock in patients infected with HCV genotype 1b [41], as we did in the analysis of HCV genotype 4a infection in Egypt [12], and have found the exponential growth of HCV infection during the years when PAT was conducted there. Dynamics of the effective population size of HCV genotype 1b infections in Yamanashi are much different from those in Nagoya where schistosomiasis japonica was not endemic [41].

Conclusion

In conclusion, different divergence and spread times of HCV in Japan, the United States and Egypt mirror distinct socioeconomic backgrounds and unfortunate events which each country has gone through in the remote or recent past. In the 1920s and the 1930s, HCV started to spread widely in Japan by PAT, IDU and transfusion, in the 1960s in the United States through IDU and transfusion and in the 1960s in Egypt by PAT. HCV genotypes are different among the three countries: 1b in Japan, 1a in the United States and 4a in Egypt.

Population dynamics of HCV estimated by the molecular clock predict that the burden of HCC in the United States will be increasing during the next few decades, in the wake of what has happened and is occurring in Japan for HCC. In fact, the incidence of HCC has already started to increase in the United States [25, 26]. The virtue of the molecular clock in combination with an effective population study, capable of accurately estimating the dynamics of HCV based on a limited number of isolates, has been very informative in looking back at epidemic spreads of HCV infection in Japan, the United States and Egypt. Hopefully, the method we used will be extended to any other countries in the world where HCV is prevalent and an increase in HCC is expected in the foreseeable future.

References

1 Cohen J: The scientific challenge of hepatitis C. Science 1999;285:26–30.
2 Lee WM: Hepatitis B virus infection. N Engl J Med 1997;337:1733–1745.
3 Blumberg BS: Polymorphisms of the serum proteins and the development of iso-precipitins in transfused patients. Bull NY Acad Med 1964;40:377–386.
4 Choo QL, Kuo G, Weiner AJ, Overby LR, Bradley DW, Houghton M: Isolation of a cDNA clone derived from a blood-borne non-A, non-B viral hepatitis genome. Science 1989; 244:359–362.
5 Kuo G, Choo QL, Alter HJ, Gitnick GL, Redeker AG, Purcell RH, Miyamura T, Dienstag JL, Alter MJ, Stevens CE, et al: An assay for circulating antibodies to a major etiologic virus of human non-A, non-B hepatitis. Science 1989;244:362–364.
6 Kiyosawa K, Sodeyama T, Tanaka E, Gibo Y, Yoshizawa K, Nakano Y, Furuta S, Akahane Y, Nishioka K, Purcell RH, Alter HJ: Interrelationship of blood transfusion, non-A, non-B hepatitis and hepatocellular carcinoma: Analysis by detection of antibody to hepatitis C virus. Hepatology 1990;12:671–675.
7 Tong MJ, el-Farra NS, Reikes AR, Co RL: Clinical outcomes after transfusion-associated hepatitis C. N Engl J Med 1995;332:1463–1466.
8 Hamada H, Yatsuhashi H, Yano K, Daikoku M, Arisawa K, Inoue O, Koga M, Nakata K, Eguchi K, Yano M: Impact of aging on the development of hepatocellular carcinoma in patients with posttransfusion chronic hepatitis C. Cancer 2002;95:331–339.
9 Zuckerkandel E, Pauling L: Evolutionary divergence and convergence in proteins; in Bivson V, Vogel HJ (eds): Evolving Genes and Proteins. New York, Academic Press, 1962, pp 97–166.
10 Margoliash E: Primary structure and evolution of cytochrome C. Proc Natl Acad Sci USA 1963;50:672–679.
11 Tanaka Y, Hanada K, Mizokami M, Yeo AE, Shih JW, Gojobori T, Alter HJ: A comparison of the molecular clock of hepatitis C virus in the United States and Japan predicts that hepatocellular carcinoma incidence in the United States will increase over the next two decades. Proc Natl Acad Sci USA 2002;99: 15584–15589.
12 Tanaka Y, Agha S, Saudy N, Kurbanov F, Orito E, Kato T, Abo-Zeid M, Khalaf M, Miyakawa Y, Mizokami M: Exponential spread of hepatitis C virus genotype 4a in Egypt. J Mol Evol 2004;58:191–195.
13 Pybus OG, Charleston MA, Gupta S, Rambaut A, Holmes EC, Harvey PH: The epidemic behavior of the hepatitis C virus. Science 2001; 292:2323–2325.
14 Kimura M: Evolutionary rate at the molecular level. Nature 1968;217:624–626.
15 Alter HJ, Purcell RH, Shih JW, Melpolder JC, Houghton M, Choo QL, Kuo G: Detection of antibody to hepatitis C virus in prospectively followed transfusion recipients with acute and chronic non-A, non-B hepatitis. N Engl J Med 1989;321:1494–1500.
16 Conry-Cantilena C, VanRaden M, Gibble J, Melpolder J, Shakil AO, Viladomiu L, Cheung L, DiBisceglie A, Hoofnagle J, Shih JW, et al: Routes of infection, viremia, and liver disease in blood donors found to have hepatitis C virus infection. N Engl J Med 1996;334:1691–1696.
17 Ogata N, Alter HJ, Miller RH, Purcell RH: Nucleotide sequence and mutation rate of the H strain of hepatitis C virus. Proc Natl Acad Sci USA 1991;88:3392–3396.
18 Ina Y, Mizokami M, Ohba K, Gojobori T: Reduction of synonymous substitutions in the core protein gene of hepatitis C virus. J Mol Evol 1994;38:50–56.
19 Okamoto H, Kojima M, Okada S, Yoshizawa H, Iizuka H, Tanaka T, Muchmore EE, Peterson DA, Ito Y, Mishiro S: Genetic drift of hepatitis C virus during an 8.2-year infection in a chimpanzee: Variability and stability. Virology 1992;190:894–899.

20 Stumpf MP, Pybus OG: Genetic diversity and models of viral evolution for the hepatitis C virus. FEMS Microbiol Lett 2002;214:143–152.
21 Pybus OG, Rambaut A: GENIE: Estimating demographic history from molecular phylogenies. Bioinformatics 2002;18:1404–1405.
22 Lemey P, Pybus OG, Wang B, Saksena NK, Salemi M, Vandamme AM: Tracing the origin and history of the HIV-2 epidemic. Proc Natl Acad Sci USA 2003;100:6588–6592.
23 Yoshizawa H: Hepatocellular carcinoma associated with hepatitis C virus infection in Japan: Projection to other countries in the foreseeable future. Oncology 2002;62:S8–S17.
24 Tanaka J, Kumagai J, Katayama K, Komiya Y, Mizui M, Yamanaka R, Suzuki K, Miyakawa Y, Yoshizawa H: Sex- and age-specific carriers of hepatitis B and C viruses in Japan estimated by the prevalence in the 3,485,648 first-time blood donors during 1995–2000. Intervirology 2004;47:32–40.
25 El-Serag HB: Hepatocellular carcinoma and hepatitis C in the United States. Hepatology 2002;36:S74–S83.
26 Nair S, Shiv Kumar K, Thuluvath PJ, Shivakumar KS, Shiva Kumar K: Mortality from hepatocellular and biliary cancers: Changing epidemiological trends. Am J Gastroenterol 2002;97:167–171.
27 Ikeda K, Saitoh S, Arase Y, Chayama K, Suzuki Y, Kobayashi M, Tsubota A, Nakamura I, Murashima N, Kumada H, Kawanishi M: Effect of interferon therapy on hepatocellular carcinogenesis in patients with chronic hepatitis type C: A long-term observation study of 1,643 patients using statistical bias correction with proportional hazard analysis. Hepatology 1999;29:1124–1130.
28 Yabuuchi I, Imai Y, Kawata S, Tamura S, Noda S, Inada M, Maeda Y, Shirai Y, Fukuzaki T, Kaji I, Ishikawa H, Matsuda Y, Nishikawa M, Seki K, Matsuzawa Y: Long-term responders without eradication of hepatitis C virus after interferon therapy: Characterization of clinical profiles and incidence of hepatocellular carcinoma. Liver 2000;20:290–295.
29 Sodeyama T, Kiyosawa K, Urushihara A, Matsumoto A, Tanaka E, Furuta S, Akahane Y: Detection of hepatitis C virus markers and hepatitis C virus genomic-RNA after needlestick accidents. Arch Intern Med 1993;153:1565–1572.
30 Takagi H, Uehara M, Kakizaki S, Takahashi H, Takezawa J, Kabeya K, Satoh K, Kojima A, Saito S, Matsumoto T, Hashimoto Y, Abe T, Yamada T, Konaka K, Shimoda R, Takayama H, Takehara K, Nagamine T, Mori M: Accidental transmission of HCV and treatment with interferon. J Gastroenterol Hepatol 1998;13:238–243.
31 Terrault NA: Sexual activity as a risk factor for hepatitis C. Hepatology 2002;36:S99–S105.
32 van den Hoek JA, van Haastrecht HJ, Goudsmit J, de Wolf F, Coutinho RA: Prevalence, incidence, and risk factors of hepatitis C virus infection among drug users in Amsterdam. J Infect Dis 1990;162:823–-826.
33 Galeazzi B, Tufano A, Barbierato E, Bortolotti F: Hepatitis C virus infection in Italian intravenous drug users: Epidemiological and clinical aspects. Liver 1995;15:209–212.
34 Iida F, Iida R, Kamijo H, Takaso K, Miyazaki Y, Funabashi W, Tsuchiya K, Matsumoto Y: Chronic Japanese schistosomiasis and hepatocellular carcinoma: Ten years of follow-up in Yamanashi Prefecture, Japan. Bull World Health Organ 1999;77:573–581.
35 De Vos Irvine H, Goldberg D, Hole DJ, McMenamin J: Trends in primary liver cancer. Lancet 1998;351:215–216.
36 Schreiber GB, Busch MP, Kleinman SH, Korelitz JJ: The risk of transfusion-transmitted viral infections. The Retrovirus Epidemiology Donor Study. N Engl J Med 1996;334:1685–1690.
37 Frank C, Mohamed MK, Strickland GT, Lavanchy D, Arthur RR, Magder LS, El Khoby T, Abdel-Wahab Y, Aly Ohn ES, Anwar W, Sallam I: The role of parenteral antischistosomal therapy in the spread of hepatitis C virus in Egypt. Lancet 2000;355:887–891.
38 McOmish F, Yap PL, Dow BC, Follett EA, Seed C, Keller AJ, Cobain TJ, Krusius T, Kolho E, Naukkarinen R, et al: Geographical distribution of hepatitis C virus genotypes in blood donors: An international collaborative survey. J Clin Microbiol 1994;32:884–892.
39 Pybus OG, Drummond AJ, Nakano T, Robertson BH, Rambaut A: The epidemiology and iatrogenic transmission of hepatitis C virus in Egypt: A Bayesian coalescent approach. Mol Biol Evol 2003;20:381–387.
40 Angelico M, Renganathan E, Gandin C, Fathy M, Profili MC, Refai W, De Santis A, Nagi A, Amin G, Capocaccia L, Callea F, Rapicetta M, Badr G, Rocchi G: Chronic liver disease in the Alexandria governorate, Egypt: Contribution of schistosomiasis and hepatitis virus infections. J Hepatol 1997;26:236–243.
41 Tanaka Y, Hanada K, Orito E, Akahane Y, Chayama K, Yoshizawa H, Sata M, Ohta N, Miyakawa Y, Gojobori T, Mizokami M: Molecular evolutionary analyses implicate injection treatment for schistosomiasis in the initial hepatitis C endemic of Japan. J Hepatol 2005;42:47–53.

Intervirology

Intervirology 2006;49:37–43
DOI: 10.1159/000087261

Comparison between Subgenomic Replicons of Hepatitis C Virus Genotypes 2a (JFH-1) and 1b (Con1 NK5.1)

Michiko Miyamoto[a] Takanobu Kato[a, b] Tomoko Date[a] Masashi Mizokami[b] Takaji Wakita[a]

[a]Department of Microbiology, Tokyo Metropolitan Institute for Neuroscience, Tokyo, and
[b]Department of Clinical Molecular Informative Medicine, Nagoya City University Graduate School of Medical Sciences, Nagoya, Japan

Key Words
Genotypes · Hepatitis C virus · Interferon · Replicon

Abstract
Although replicon systems for hepatitis C virus (HCV) recently developed have enabled the replication of HCV in cultured cells, limited genotypes are available for them. We have isolated HCV cDNA of genotype 2a (JFH-1 strain) from serum of a patient with fulminant hepatitis. A subgenomic replicon of JFH-1 was constructed and compared with the HCV replicon of genotype 1b (Con1 NK5.1) which possessed adaptive mutations. Huh7 cells transfected with replicon RNAs that had been transcribed in vitro were cultured in the presence of neomycin sulfate (G418), and selected colonies were isolated and expanded. Then, growth rates and replication of HCV RNA were evaluated on isolated cells hosting replicons. Saturation densities were lower for cells propagating JFH-1 than Con1 NK5.1 or untransfected Huh7 cells, and the mean doubling time was longer for JFH-1 than for Huh7 cells. Levels of HCV RNA replication in isolated clones were similar between JFH-1 and Con1 NK5.1 cells. Replication of RNA decreased reciprocally with cell densities in both JFH-1 and Con1 NK5.1 cells. The replication of HCV RNA was more resistant to interferon-α in JFH-1 than in Con1 NK5.1 cells based on the comparison of an inhibitory concentration of 50%. In conclusion, we found differences between HCV replicon clones of genotypes 1b and 2a. However, these differences may result from strain-specific characteristics, such as the source of HCV, rather than characteristics of distinct genotypes. Therefore, further investigation may be needed on more HCV isolates of diverse genotypes.

Introduction

Hepatitis C virus (HCV) is a positive-strand RNA virus categorized in a flavivirus by structural similarities. The genomic RNA of HCV comprises approximately 9,600 nucleotides encoding a single open reading frame encoding about 3,000 amino acid residues [1–4]. HCV displays marked genetic heterogeneity and is currently classified into six major genotypes which are broken down into many subgroups [5]. Some HCV genotypes have regional distribution, and of those, genotypes 1 and 2 occur worldwide. In Japan, genotype 1b is the most frequent genotype, followed by genotype 2a [6]. Differences be-

KARGER

Fax +41 61 306 12 34
E-Mail karger@karger.ch
www.karger.com

0300–5526/06/0492–0037$23.50/0

Accessible online at:
www.karger.com/int

Takaji Wakita, MD
Department of Microbiology, Tokyo Metropolitan Institute for Neuroscience
2-6 Musashidai, Fuchu-shi
Tokyo 183-8526 (Japan)
Tel. +81 42 325 3881, ext. 4605, Fax +81 42 321 8678, E-Mail wakita@tmin.ac.jp

tween these two HCV genotypes have been noted in clinical profiles, severity of liver disease, and most importantly, response to antiviral therapies [7]. These clinical differences may be due to viral characteristics, and systems to deepen the understanding of molecular mechanisms underlying such differences have been proposed.

Lohmann et al. [8] reported subgenomic replicons of HCV RNA selectable by neomycin sulfate (G418) which can autonomously replicate in Huh7 cells. This system provides a novel powerful tool for studying mechanisms of HCV replication and selecting potential antiviral agents. Despite big advantages of this system, replication-competent replicons have been engineered only from HCV isolates of genotype 1 [8–11]. Recently, we established a subgenomic HCV replicon derived from the JFH-1 clone of genotype 2a, which had been isolated from a patient with fulminant hepatitis [12]. The JFH-1 replicon system has high efficiency in colony formation and robust RNA replication not only in Huh7 cells, but also in other liver-derived cell lines such as HepG2 and IMY-N9 [13], as well as nonhepatic cell lines like HeLa and 293 cells [14]. The availability of this replicon has enabled comparison in replication between replicons of distinct genotypes in cultured cells. The aim of the present study is to compare JFH-1 (genotype 2a) and Con1 NK5.1 (genotype 1b) [8, 15] replicons with respect to cellular growth, HCV RNA titer of replicons in culture and sensitivity to interferon (IFN).

Materials and Methods

Cell Culture System and IFN

Huh7 cells were cultured and maintained in conditions described previously [12]. Recombinant human IFN-α_{2a} (Roferon-A) was obtained from Nippon Roche, Tokyo, Japan.

Constructs of Subgenomic HCV Replicons

The construct of a subgenomic HCV replicon of genotype 1b, pFK-I_{389}neo/NS3-3′/NK5.1 (pFK/Con1 NK5.1) [8, 15], was a generous gift from Dr. Ralf Bartenschlager (University of Heidelberg, Heidelberg, Germany). The construct of a subgenomic HCV clone of genotype 2a, pSGR-JFH1 (accession number AB114136), was prepared using the JFH-1 strain isolated from a patient with fulminant hepatitis [12].

RNA Synthesis

pFK/Con1 NK5.1 was linearized by treatment with *Sca*I. pSGR-JFH1 was digested with *Xba*I and then treated with a mung bean nuclease (New England Biolabs, Beverly, Mass., USA) as described elsewhere [12]. Linearized plasmid DNAs were purified and used as templates for RNA synthesis. Subgenomic HCV RNA was synthesized in vitro with the use of a MEGAscript™ T7 kit (Ambion, Austin, Tex., USA). Synthesized RNA was treated with DNase I (RQ1™ RNase-free DNase, Promega, Madison, Wisc., USA) and extracted with acid phenol to remove any remaining template DNA.

Transfection with RNA

Synthesized replicon RNAs were transfected into Huh7 cells by electroporation as described [12]. Briefly, synthesized RNA (0.1 ng to 1 μg) was mixed with suspension of trypsinized Huh7 cells (400 μl; 7.5×10^6 cells/ml). Cells were then pulsed at 260 V and 950 μF in a Gene Pulser II™ apparatus (Bio-Rad, Hercules, Calif., USA). Transfected cells were immediately transferred to culture dishes of 10 cm in diameter, each containing 8 ml of culture medium. G418 (Nacalai Tesque, Kyoto, Japan) in a concentration of 1.0 mg/ml was added to culture medium at 16–24 h after transfection. Culture medium supplemented with G418 was replaced twice weekly. Three weeks after the transfection, cells were fixed with buffered formalin and stained with crystal violet, and some grown colonies were cloned.

Isolation and Analysis of G418-Resistant Cells

G418-resistant colonies were independently isolated using a cloning cylinder (Asahi Techno Glass Co., Tokyo, Japan) and cultured until approximately 90% confluence in 10-cm dishes (Corning Inc., N.Y., USA). Total RNA was isolated from cells using the Isogen reagent (Nippon Gene, Tokyo, Japan). Isolated clones and parental Huh7 cell were seeded at 1×10^5 cells/well in 6-well plates (Corning Inc.). In some experiments, replicon cells were seeded at 2×10^5 cells/well in 6-well plates. Cells were harvested daily for determining cell growth and HCV RNA titers. At 24 h after G418 had been removed from the culture medium, serial dilutions of IFN-α (Nippon Roche) were added to wells, and cells were harvested after culture for 72 h.

Northern Blot Analysis

Isolated RNA (2.5 or 4 μg) was separated by electrophoresis on 1% (weight/vol) agarose gel containing formaldehyde, then transferred to a positively charged nylon membrane (Hybond-N+, Amersham Pharmacia, Bucks., UK) and immobilized with the use of the Stratalinker UV cross linker (Stratagene, La Jolla, Calif., USA). Hybridization was performed using a DNA probe labeled with [α-^{32}P]dCTP in Rapid-Hyb buffer (Amersham Pharmacia). The DNA probe was deduced from *neo^r* and encephalomyocarditits virus internal ribosome entry site genes and synthesized in the Megaprime DNA labeling system (Amersham Pharmacia).

Quantification of HCV RNA by Real-Time Reverse Transcrpition Polymerase Chain Reaction

Copy numbers of HCV RNA were determined by the real-time detection reverse transcription polymerase chain reaction (RTD-PCR) described previously [16] in the ABI Prisom 7700 sequence detector system (Applied Biosystems Japan, Tokyo, Japan). Data were standardized by the concentration of intracellular glyceraldehyde-3-phosphate dehydrogenase.

Statistics

Statistical analysis was performed by Student's t test, Welch's t test or the Mann-Whitney U test. Differences with a p value <0.05 were considered statistically significant.

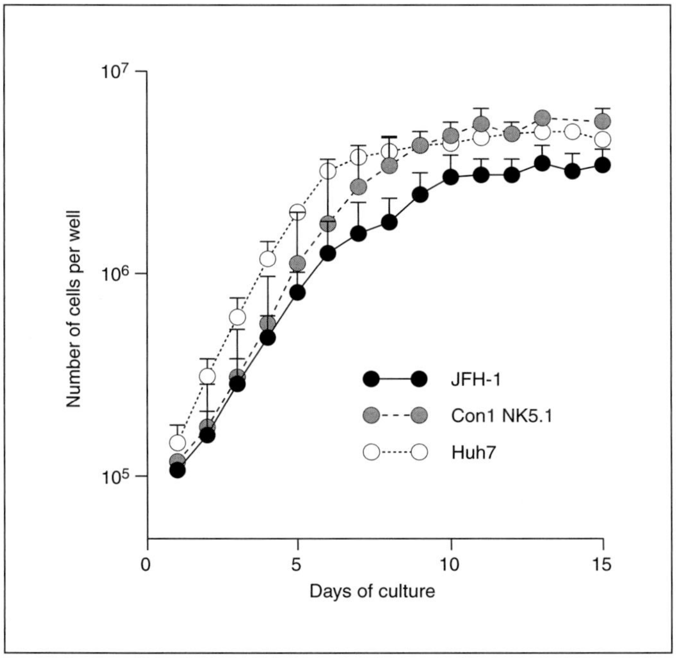

Fig. 1. Rate of cell growth. JFH-1 replicon clones, Con1 NK5.1 replicon clones and Huh7 cells were grown in 6-well culture plates and counted daily. Results are expressed by the mean ± SD cell number/well.

Table 1. HCV RNA copies detected in isolated clones carrying HCV replicon

Replicon clone	Number of isolated clones	HCV RNA copies/μg, RNA[a]
JFH-1	19	$2.73 \pm 2.16 \times 10^7$
Con1 NK5.1	6	$2.38 \pm 2.04 \times 10^7$

[a] Mean ± SD.

Table 2. Growth rates and cell densities (mean ± SD) of Huh7 and other cell lines harboring HCV replicon

Cell line	Mean doubling time, h	Saturation density $\times 10^5$ cells/cm^2
Huh7	27.4 ± 3.5[b]	5.17 ± 0.33[c]
JFH-1[a]	31.2 ± 2.7	3.41 ± 0.48
Con1 NK5.1[a]	28.9 ± 2.9	5.56 ± 0.34[c]

[a] Ten clones of the JFH-1 replicon and 4 clones of Con1 NK5.1 were used in this experiment.
[b] $p < 0.05$ versus JFH-1.
[c] $p < 0.001$ versus JFH-1.

Results

Replication of HCV RNA in Clones Transfected with JFH-1 or Con1 NK5.1 Subgenomic HCV RNA

To determine the replicative ability of the JFH-1 clone, synthetic RNA transcribed from linearized pSGR-JFH1 or pFK/Con1 NK5.1 was transfected into Huh7 cells by electroporation, as described previously [12]. Cells transfected with the Con1 NK5.1 replicon became confluent more rapidly than those transfected with the JFH-1 replicon, until they started to die because of G418; transfected cells were cultured for 3 weeks in the presence of 1 mg/ml G418. Efficiencies of colony formation were 53,200 and 909 colony forming units/μg RNA for JFH-1 and Con1 NK5.1 replicons, respectively [12].

A total of 19 clones were isolated for the JFH-1 replicon and 6 clones for the Con1 NK5.1 replicon. Each clone had been cultured until approximately 80–90% confluence was achieved on the culture dish, whereupon it was harvested. Total RNA was extracted from each replicon clone, and the replication of RNA was confirmed using Northern blot analysis (data not shown). Mean replication levels of HCV RNA determined by RTD-PCR were similar for both replicon clones, $2.73 \pm 2.16 \times 10^7$ copies/μg RNA for JFH-1 and $2.38 \pm 2.04 \times 10^7$ copies/μg RNA for Con1 NK5.1 (table 1). Expressions of HCV proteins were confirmed in all replicon clones by Western blot and immunofluorescence assay (data not shown).

Growth Curves of Replicon Cells

Rates of cellular growth were determined on parental Huh7 cells, 10 cloned cells harboring JFH-1 replicon and 4 cloned cells supporting Con1 NK5.1. Each cell line was seeded at 1.0×10^5 cells/well in 6-well plates, harvested daily and counted. Figure 1 depicts mean rates of cell growth for the JFH-1 replicon, the Con1 NK5.1 replicon and Huh7 cells. The mean doubling time during the logarithmic growing phase was 31.2 ± 2.7 h for JFH-1, 28.9 ± 2.9 h for Con1 NK5.1 and 27.4 ± 3.5 h for Huh7 (JFH-1 vs. Huh7, $p < 0.05$) (table 2). Saturation densities determined by cell counts after they had reached the confluence were $3.41 \pm 0.48 \times 10^5$ cells/cm^2 for JFH-1, 5.56 ± 0.34 010^5 cells/cm^2 for Con1 NK5.1 and $5.17 \pm 0.33 \times 10^5$ cells/cm^2 for Huh7 (JFH-1 vs. Con1 NK5.1 or Huh7, $p < 0.001$) (table 2). Thus, JFH-1 replicon cells had slower cell growth and lower cell density than parental Huh7 cells.

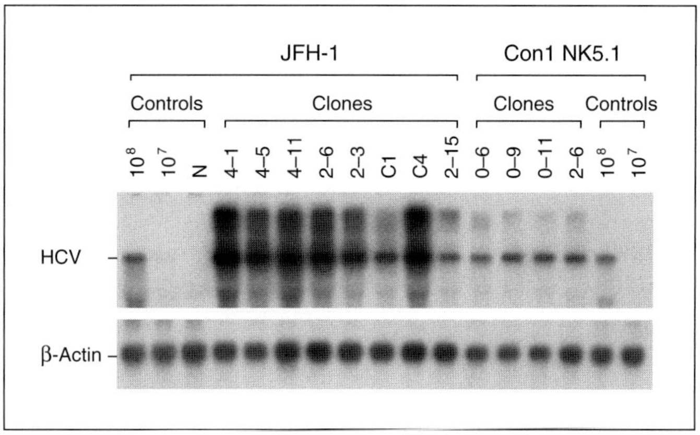

Fig. 2. Northern blot analysis of replicon RNA 1 day after the cell passage. Total cellular RNAs (2.5 μg) isolated from JFH-1 and Con1 NK5.1 replicon cells at the next day of passage were loaded onto agarose gel. After electrophoresis, RNAs of HCV or β-actin were detected by the Northern blot with random-primed DNA probes specific to encephalomyocarditits virus internal ribosome entry site and *neo*^{r} or β-actin sequences, respectively.

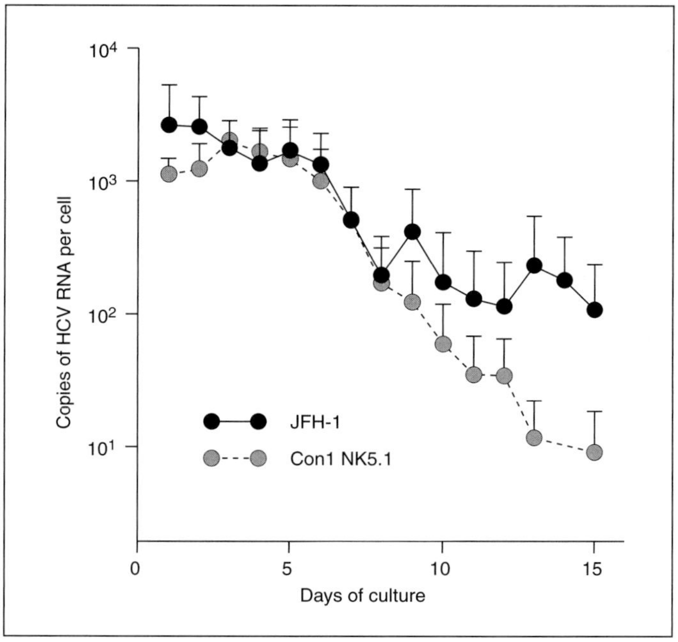

Fig. 3. Replication levels of HCV RNA during cell growth. HCV RNA replicating in JFH-1 or Con1 NK5.1 replicon cells were determined by the quantitative RTD-PCR.

Pietschmann et al. [17] reported that the replication level of the Con1 NK5.1 replicon is inversely related to cell growth. Therefore, we compared the number of HCV RNA copies determined by RTD-PCR between JFH-1 and Con1 NK5.1 replicon clones that had been examined for the cell growth. Mean titers of HCV RNA at 1 day after seeding were $2.65 \pm 2.36 \times 10^3$ copies/cell for JFH-1 and $1.14 \pm 0.28 \times 10^3$ copies/cell for Con1 NK5.1 ($p = 0.396$). However, most JFH-1 replicon clones emitted HCV RNA signals stronger than those of Con1 NK5.1 replicon clones in Northern blot analysis (fig. 2). HCV RNA levels of both JFH-1 and Con1 NK5.1 replicon cells decreased gradually and became comparable during days 3–8 (fig. 3). Both replicon cells became confluent around day 7–9. However, the mean RNA titer of JFH-1 clones remained around 100 copies/cell, while that of Con1 clones decreased to some 10 copies/cell during days 9–15. When all replicon cells were expanded after cloning, they were 80–90% confluent with HCV RNA titers comparable between JFH-1 and Con1 NK5.1 (table 1). The mean levels of replicon RNA at day 15 were $9.84 \pm 12.58 \times 10^1$ copies/cell for JFH-1 and $0.93 \pm 0.86 \times 10^1$ copies/cell for Con1 NK5.1 ($p = 0.0897$). During this experiment, culture medium was replaced on days 4, 8 and 12. The mean level of replicon RNA in JFH-1 clones increased the day after replacement of culture medium. However, RNA levels of Con1 NK5.1 clones were not affected by the replacement of culture medium.

Effects of IFN on the Replication of Subgenomic RNA

HCV replicon clones of genotype 1b are reportedly sensitive to IFN-α [10, 18]. However, in the clinical setting, HCV genotype 1b is generally considered resistant to IFN-α, in contrast to HCV genotype 2a which is more sensitive to it. To compare sensitivities of JFH-1 and Con1 NK5.1 replicons to IFN, serially diluted IFN-α was added to cultures of these replicons. After cultivation for 72 h, replicon cells were harvested and cellular RNA was extracted from each culture. RNAs isolated from cloned replicon cells, JFH-1/4–1 and Con1 NK5.1/0–11, were subjected to Northern blot analysis (fig. 4). The copy number of replicon RNA was also determined by RTD-PCR. IFN-α at a concentration of 10 U/ml clearly reduced the replication of Con1 NK5.1/0-11 replicon RNA, whereas JFH-1/4-1 replicon RNA did not decrease with 10 U/ml IFN-α (fig. 4). Copy numbers of HCV RNA were determined by RTD-PCR in 4 clones each for JFH-1 and Con1 NK5.1 replicons. Changes in the copy number of HCV RNA are expressed by the percentage of that cultured without IFN-α shown in figure 5. Inhibitory concentration of 50% (IC_{50}) thus calculated was 30.61 ± 15.19 U/ml for JFH-1 replicons and 2.94 ± 1.59 U/ml for Con1 NK5.1 replicons ($p < 0.05$). Although there is a

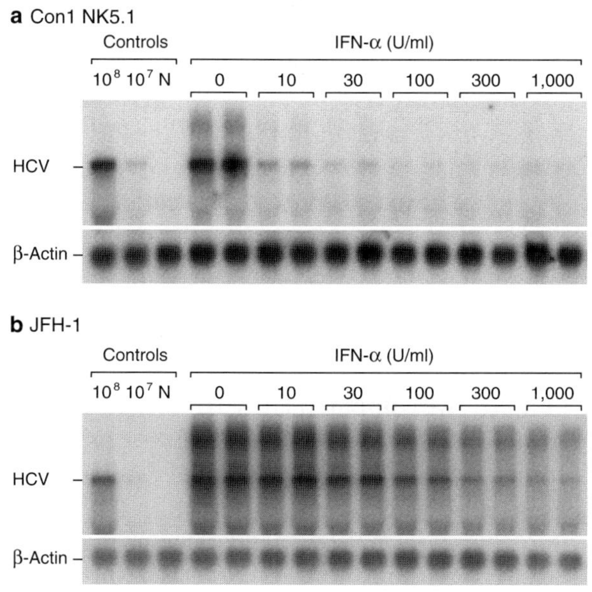

Fig. 4. Northern blot analysis of HCV RNAs in Con1 NK5.1/0-11 (**a**) and JFH-1/4-1 (**b**) replicon clones having undergone treatment with IFN-α. Cells were cultured for 72 h in the absence (lanes 4–5) or presence (lanes 6–15) of 10–1,000 U/ml IFN-α.

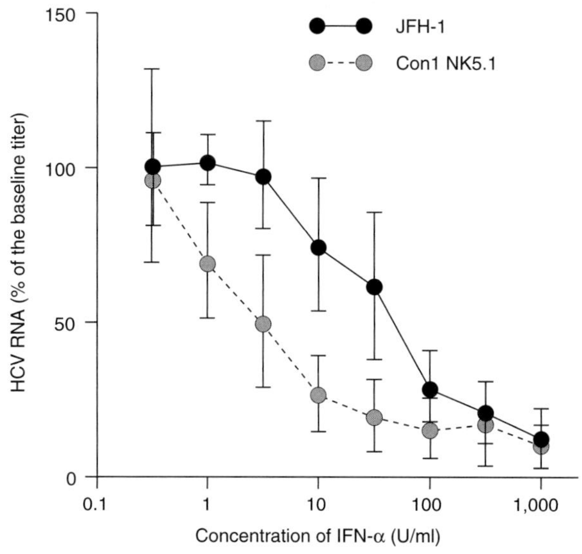

Fig. 5. Inhibition of HCV replicons by IFN-α. Four clones each of JFH-1 and Con1 NK5.1 replicons were cultured for 72 h in the absence or presence of 0.3–1,000 U/ml IFN-α. HCV RNA titers in replicon cells were determined by the quantitative RTD-PCR. HCV RNA levels from control cells (without IFN) were set at 100%. The percentage of HCV RNA levels of the JFH-1 or Con1 NK5.1 replicon was calculated and plotted against the concentration of IFN-α. Data were normalized based on the concentration of an internal control (glyceraldehyde-3-phosphate dehydrogenase).

significant difference in IC_{50} between replicons of genotypes 1b and 2a, the mean copy number of HCV RNA extracted from cells in the absence of IFN was different, namely $5.77 \pm 3.7 \times 10^7$ copies/μg RNA for JFH-1 and $5.56 \pm 6.21 \times 10^6$ copies/μg RNA for Con1 NK5.1. Thus, the difference in IC_{50} between genotypes may be due to different replication capacities of the clones tested rather than a distinct response to IFN-α.

Discussion

Since the discovery of HCV, numerous sequences of HCV isolates have been reported. Comparison of these sequences has highlighted a marked genetic heterogeneity of the HCV genome, by which HCV isolates have been classified into six genotypes. Among them, genotypes 1 and 2 are distributed worldwide [6]. Increasing lines of evidence indicate that patients infected with HCV of different genotypes may present with distinct clinical profiles, in terms of severity of liver disease and response to antiviral therapies [7]. For example, genotype 1b is known to be resistant to IFN, whereas genotype 2a is sensitive to it. However, because of its ubiquity, investigations of viral characteristics have been mostly conducted on HCV isolates of genotype 1b. The newly established subgenomic replicon of genotype 2a [12] has provided opportunities for evaluating differences in viral characteristics between genotypes 1 and 2 to improve our understanding on mechanisms of viral replication and persistence.

In this study, we compared subgenomic HCV replicons of genotype 1b with genotype 2a, using Con1 NK5.1and JFH-1 strains, respectively. As reported previously [12], the efficiency of colony formation is higher for JFH-1 than for Con1 NK5.1. However, HCV RNA titers of both replicons did not differ when harvested after cloning procedures (table 1). The efficiency in colony formation may reflect the replication capacity of the original HCV strain rather than HCV RNA titers of replicon cells, since levels of HCV RNA replication in the selected clones may have been enhanced through G418 selection and cloning procedure. However, a high replication efficiency of the JFH-1 replicon has been demonstrated in a transient replication of JFH-1 in Huh7 cells in the absence of G418 selection [12], in contrast to Con1 NK5.1 that did not efficiently replicate in conditions of transient transfection (data not shown). It would have been necessary for HCV RNA titers of replicon clones to remain at levels high enough to overcome the selection pressure of G418. In support of this view, the Con1 NK5.1 replicon has acquired adaptive mutations to maintain efficient replication in Huh7 cells [15]. However, adaptive mutations are not always necessary to maintain the replication of HCV RNA, since JFH-1 replicates in Huh7, HepG2, IMY-N9 and other cell lines as well [12–14].

The present study has shown the mean doubling time and saturation densities of JFH-1 replicon clones significantly lower than those of parent Huh7 cells. However, Con1 NK5.1 replicon clones did not show such decreases, in consistence with the original report [17]. Hence, RNA replication and protein expression of the JFH-1 replicon may suppress the cell growth. Otherwise, slower growing Huh7 subclones may have been preferentially selected for the JFH-1 replicon. Several HCV proteins are reported to suppress cell growth when expressed stably or by induction [19–21]. The core protein of HCV has a relatively weak effect on the cell growth [22], and conditional expression of structural HCV proteins (core, E1 and E2) and some nonstructural proteins (NS2 and NS3) completely suppresses it [23]. In contrast, nonstructural proteins such as NS5A may accelerate the rate of cell growth [24]. The viral protein responsible for a phenotype for slower growth of the JFH-1 replicon should therefore be sought for.

HCV titers of JFH-1 and Con1 NK5.1 replicon clones were monitored in analysis for cell growth (fig. 2). After cells reached the confluence, HCV copy numbers of JFH-1 replicon clones remained at around 100 copies/cell contrasting with those of Con1 NK5.1 that decreased to some 10 copies/cell. Furthermore, copy numbers of JFH-1 clones increased by the exchange of culture medium, whereas Con1 NK5.1 clones did not respond to it (fig. 2). This result may suggest that JFH-1 and Con1 HCV replicons replicate in Huh7 cells with the use of different cellular factors or by utilizing the same factors in distinct manners.

Clinical experiences have indicated that infection with HCV genotype 1b is resistant to IFN, while that with genotype 2a is usually sensitive to it [7]. In the present study, the JFH-1 replicon of genotype 2a exhibited a phenotype more resistant to IFN than to the Con1 NK5.1 replicon of genotype 1b. Previous reports have described efficient responses of HCV and Con1 NK5.1 replicons, both of genotype 1, to type I IFN [10, 18]. At present, it is unclear whether or not the response to IFN, which is different between these replicons of genotypes 1b and 2a, contradicts distinct characteristics of genotypes in the clinical setting. However, infections with HCV genotype 2a are not always sensitive to IFN, and the JFH-1 strain may represent a rare IFN-resistant genotype 2a clone. Certainly, more strains need to be isolated for experiments with replicons to compare the phenotype between genotypes 1b and 2a. However, a higher replicative capacity of JFH-1 may depend on IFN-resistant characteristics, especially under the experimental conditions used in this study.

In summary, we compared HCV RNA replication, cell growth and sensitivity to IFN between subgenomic replicons of genotypes 1b and 2a transfecting Huh7 cells. JFH-1, representing genotype 2a, exhibited a higher efficiency in colony formation than Con1 NK5.1 of genotype 1, even though copy numbers of replicating RNA did not significantly differ between them. Of note, JFH-1 was found to be more resistant to IFN than Con1 NK5.1, at least in experiments with subgenomic replicons.

Acknowledgments

We thank Dr. Ralf Bartenschlager for providing the pFK-I_{389}neo/NS3-3′/NK5.1. We are also grateful to Dr. Satoshi Koike and Dr. Kotaro Yasui for their helpful discussions. This work is supported in part by a Grant-in-Aid for Scientific Research from the Japan Society for the Promotion of Science, a grant from Toray Industries, Inc., the Program for Promotion of Fundamental Studies in Health Sciences of the Pharmaceuticals and Medical Devices Agency (PMDA), as well as the Research on Health Sciences focusing on Drug Innovation from the Japan Health Sciences Foundation and the Japanese Society of Gastroenterology.

References

1 Kato N, Hijikata M, Ootsuyama Y, Nakagawa M, Ohkoshi S, Sugimura T, Shimotohno K: Molecular cloning of the human hepatitis C virus genome from Japanese patients with non-A, non-B hepatitis. Proc Natl Acad Sci USA 1990;87:9524–9528.

2 Choo QL, Richman KH, Han JH, Berger K, Lee C, Dong C, Gallegos C, Coit D, Medina-Selby R, Barr PJ: Genetic organization and diversity of the hepatitis C virus. Proc Natl Acad Sci USA 1991;88:2451–2455.

3 Takamizawa A, Mori C, Fuke I, Manabe S, Murakami S, Fujita J, Onishi E, Andoh T, Yoshida I, Okayama H: Structure and organization of the hepatitis C virus genome isolated from human carriers. J Virol 1991;65:1105–1113.

4 Reed KE, Rice CM: Overview of hepatitis C virus genome structure, polyprotein processing, and protein properties. Curr Top Microbiol Immunol 2000;242:55–84.

5 Bukh J, Purcell RH, Miller RH: Sequence analysis of the core gene of 14 hepatitis C virus genotypes. Proc Natl Acad Sci USA 1994;91:8239–8243.

6 Ohno O, Mizokami M, Wu RR, Saleh MG, Ohba K, Orito E, Mukaide M, Williams R, Lau JY: New hepatitis C virus (HCV) genotyping system that allows for identification of HCV genotypes 1a, 1b, 2a, 2b, 3a, 3b, 4, 5a, and 6a. J Clin Microbiol 1997;35:201–207.

7 Yoshioka K, Kakumu S, Wakita T, Ishikawa T, Itoh Y, Takayanagi M, Higashi Y, Shibata M, Morishima T: Detection of hepatitis C virus by polymerase chain reaction and response to interferon-alpha therapy: Relationship to genotypes of hepatitis C virus. Hepatology 1992;16:293–299.

8 Lohmann V, Korner F, Koch J, Herian U, Theilmann L, Bartenschlager R: Replication of subgenomic hepatitis C virus RNAs in a hepatoma cell line. Science 1999;285:110–113.

9 Blight KJ, Kolykhalov AA, Rice CM: Efficient initiation of HCV RNA replication in cell culture. Science 2000;290:1972–1974.

10 Guo JT, Bichko VV, Seeger C: Effect of alpha interferon on the hepatitis C virus replicon. J Virol 2001;75:8516–8523.

11 Ikeda M, Yi M, Li K, Lemon SM: Selectable subgenomic and genome-length dicistronic RNAs derived from an infectious molecular clone of the HCV-N strain of hepatitis C virus replicate efficiently in cultured Huh7 cells. J Virol 2002;76:2997–3006.

12 Kato T, Date T, Miyamoto M, Furusaka A, Tokushige K, Mizokami M, Wakita T: Efficient replication of the genotype 2a hepatitis C virus subgenomic replicon. Gastroenterology 2003;125:1808–1817.

13 Date T, Kato T, Miyamoto M, Zhao Z, Yasui K, Mizokami M, Wakita T: Genotype 2a hepatitis C virus subgenomic replicon can replicate in HepG2 and IMY-N9 cells. J Biol Chem 2004;279:22371–22376.

14 Kato T, Date T, Miyamoto M, Zhao Z, Mizokami M, Wakita T: Nonhepatic cell lines HeLa and 293 cells support efficient replication of hepatitis C virus genotype 2a subgenomic replicon. J Virol 2005;79:592–596.

15 Krieger N, Lohmann V, Bartenschlager R: Enhancement of hepatitis C virus RNA replication by cell culture-adaptive mutations. J Virol 2001;75:4614–4624.

16 Takeuchi T, Katsume A, Tanaka T, Abe A, Inoue K, Tsukiyama-Kohara K, Kawaguchi R, Tanaka S, Kohara M: Real-time detection system for quantification of hepatitis C virus genome. Gastroenterology 1999;116:636–642.

17 Pietschmann T, Lohmann V, Rutter G, Kurpanek K, Bartenschlager R: Characterization of cell lines carrying self-replicating hepatitis C virus RNAs. J Virol 2001;75:1252–1264.

18 Frese M, Barth K, Kaul A, Lohmann V, Schwarzle V, Bartenschlager R: Hepatitis C virus RNA replication is resistant to tumour necrosis factor-alpha. J Gen Virol 2003;84:1253–1259.

19 Aizaki H, Harada T, Otsuka M, Seki N, Matsuda M, Li YW, Kawakami H, Matsuura Y, Miyamura T, Suzuki T: Expression profiling of liver cell lines expressing entire or parts of hepatitis C virus open reading frame. Hepatology 2002;36:1431–1438.

20 Moradpour D, Kary P, Rice CM, Blum HE: Continuous human cell lines inducibly expressing hepatitis C virus structural and nonstructural proteins. Hepatology 1998;28:192–201.

21 Arima N, Kao CY, Licht T, Padmanabhan R, Sasaguri Y: Modulation of cell growth by the hepatitis C virus nonstructural protein NS5A. J Biol Chem 2001;276:12675–12684.

22 Moradpour D, Englert C, Wakita T, Wands JR: Characterization of cell lines allowing tightly regulated expression of hepatitis C virus core protein. Virology 1996;222:51–63.

23 Moradpour D, Wakita T, Wands JR, Blum HE: Tightly regulated expression of the entire hepatitis C virus structural region in continuous human cell lines. Biochem Biophys Res Commun 1998;246:920–924.

24 Ghosh AK, Steele R, Meyer K, Ray R, Ray RB: Hepatitis C virus NS5A protein modulates cell cycle regulatory genes and promotes cell growth. J Gen Virol 1999;80:1179–1183.

Pathophysiology

Intervirology

Intervirology 2006;49:44–50
DOI: 10.1159/000087262

Use of an in vitro Model and Yeast Two-Hybrid System to Investigate the Pathogenesis of Hepatitis C

Seng Gee Lim[a, b] Yee Joo Tan[a] Phuay Yee Goh[a] Siew Pheng Lim[a] Wan Jin Hong[a]

[a]Institute of Molecular and Cell Biology, and [b]National University Hospital, Singapore, Singapore

Key Words
Chemokines · Hepatitis C virus · Mutations · Pathogenesis · Plasmid, inducible · Protein-protein interactions · Viral replication · Yeast two-hybrid system

Abstract
Fifteen years after the discovery of hepatitis C virus (HCV) in 1989, much remains to be learnt about the cell biology of this virus. Using the serum from a patient containing HCV RNA in high titer as a source, a Singapore strain of genotype 1b was recovered and characterized. This full-length HCV genome was then constructed into a tetracycline-inducible vector using the pSTAR plasmid. Transfection of hepatoma cell lines with this HCV genome under tetracycline induction indicated that chemokines (RANTES and monocyte chemoattractant protein-1) were upregulated, possibly contributing to the induction of immune responses. Using the yeast two-hybrid system to discover protein-protein interactions, nonstructural region NS3 was found to interact with itself, forming a dimer that increased helicase activity but was not essential for its activity, thereby disqualifying it as a suitable target of drug actions. The significance of the interaction between core and NS5A is unclear, and the cleavage of NS5A is related to the development of apoptosis. However, the interaction of p68 and NS56B appears to be important because the knockdown of p68 reduced the viral replication. Finally, a new cell model using chimeric CD81 linked to the cytoplasmic domain of either a low-density lipoprotein receptor or a transferrin receptor led to productive infection of HCV that had been recovered from infected serum. These studies allow us to examine the pathogenesis of HCV infection in more detail.

Introduction

Since the discovery of hepatitis C virus (HCV) in 1989 [1], there has been an exponential increase in the knowledge about HCV [2, 3], its behavior in the host [4, 5] and the mechanism of viral pathogenicity [6]. However, the investigation of viral pathogenesis is hampered by the lack of reliable cell cultures [7] and animal models. The entry of the virus into host cells results in infection by releasing viral RNA and polymerase for initiating the viral replicative process. This process depends on the ability of the virus to usurp host proteins and the machinery for its replication. In addition, unexpected or unintended interactions with host proteins may induce pathogenicity by interfering with cellular pathways.

KARGER

Fax +41 61 306 12 34
E-Mail karger@karger.ch
www.karger.com

0300–5526/06/0492–0044$23.50/0

Accessible online at:
www.karger.com/int

Seng Gee Lim, MD
Institute of Molecular and Cell Biology
Department of Medicine, National University Hospital
5 Lower Kent Ridge Road, 119074 Singapore (Singapore)
Tel. +65 67795555, ext. 4369, Fax +65 67794112, E-Mail mdclimsg@nus.edu.sg

In 1997, the Institute of Molecular and Cell Biology in Singapore launched a new research team, the Collaborative Anti-Viral Research (CAVR) Group, to perform translational research on HCV. At the outset, we identified three areas that would be our strategic foci. The first was to isolate a full-length clone of HCV and create a plasmid that can induce the replication of full-length HCV. The second was to use this model and related constructs to investigate interactions of HCV proteins, either with other viral proteins or with host proteins, particularly those critical for viral replication or responsible for host pathology. Finally, we attempted to create a novel cell model that would be permissive for entry and infection with HCV.

Isolation of a Singapore Strain of HCV and Production of an Inducible Full-Length HCV Genome

We initially identified a Singapore patient infected with HCV who had high viral titers in serum. This patient had acquired HCV through multiple transfusions for thalassemia major. Nine overlapping cDNA clones covering the entire viral genome were recovered from the serum by reverse transcription polymerase chain reaction (RT-PCR). 5′-RACE (rapid amplification of cDNA ends) was used to amplify the 5′-noncoding region. The final sequence comprised 9,609 nucleotides and a single open reading frame of 3,011 amino acids (aa). Its genotype was 1b, and phylogenetic analysis revealed it to be most closely related to the Taiwan strain (HCV-TW) and another Japanese strain (HCV-K1-R1) [8].

Next, we sought to produce a full-length HCV genome that would be inducible [9]. A full-length genome of HCV was constructed from the overlapping cDNA clones and inserted into the construct pSTAR under the control of a tetracycline-inducible cytomegalovirus promoter (fig. 1). The entire vector was transfected into HepG2 and Huh7 cells. Under tetracycline induction, transcriptions of positive and negative strands of HCV RNA were identified at 1 and 12 h by RT-PCR and confirmed by transcription products in vitro. Similarly, the translation of HCV proteins including core, E1, E2, NS3, NS4B, NS5A and NS5B was demonstrated by Western blotting. A kinetic study showed that these HCV proteins were expressed at times varying from 6–96 h after the induction. At 5 days after tetracycline induction, culture media were harvested and treated with anti-E2 beads. After treatment of beads with DNase and RNaseA, RNA was extracted and PCR products of the expected size, which were absent in uninduced cells, were obtained from it. Five days after tetracycline, when culture media were subjected to centrifugation in a sucrose density gradient and fractions examined by RT-PCR, viral RNA was detected. In addition, viral particles were visualized in the cytoplasm of tetracycline-induced cells by electron microscopy; they stained positive with anti-HCV core and anti-E2 antibodies. Culture media fractionated by centrifugation in sucrose density gradient were found to contain viral particles of 50 nm in size and stained positive with anti-E2 antibodies as well.

Media of tetracycline-induced cell culture were then layered onto stable Huh7 cells expressing CD81 (the putative receptor for HCV). Negative-strand HCV RNA was found in the cell lysate, thereby indicating productive HCV infection in these cells transmitted by tetracycline-induced culture media. The infection of CD81-expressing Huh7 cells with HCV was blocked by pretreatment with anti-E2 antibodies. These findings demonstrated that the full-length HCV inserted into a vector under tetracycline induction was able to transcribe viral RNA, translate viral proteins, produce viral particles in cytoplasm, and more importantly, secrete viral particles into the supernatant that can productively infect Huh7 cells expressing CD81, the putative HCV receptor. Such a model can be exploited not only to investigate viral pathogenesis and events in the viral lifecycle, but also to evaluate potential antiviral drugs.

There have been similar inducible systems for examining interaction and cellular localization of NS3-4A [10] and expression of structural proteins [11], but they do not employ the full-length HCV genome. Myung et al. [12] used a replication-deficient adenovirus carrying the T7 RNA polymerase gene and the full-length HCV genome. They confirmed viral replication with positive- and negative-strand RNA, presence of viral proteins by Western blotting and viral particles observed in electron microscopy. However, transfection of permissible cell lines, with these viral particles or culture supernatant, was not performed in their studies, which would have been important. There are advantages of a full-length HCV genome over reproducible replicon systems [13] in that it allows for exploring interactions between all viral proteins and examining viral assembly and secretion; it would closely reproduce in vivo events.

We continued to use this model to investigate the pathogenesis of HCV infection. The question of how HCV infection induces immune responses may be addressed by using the tetracycline-inducible model. Previ-

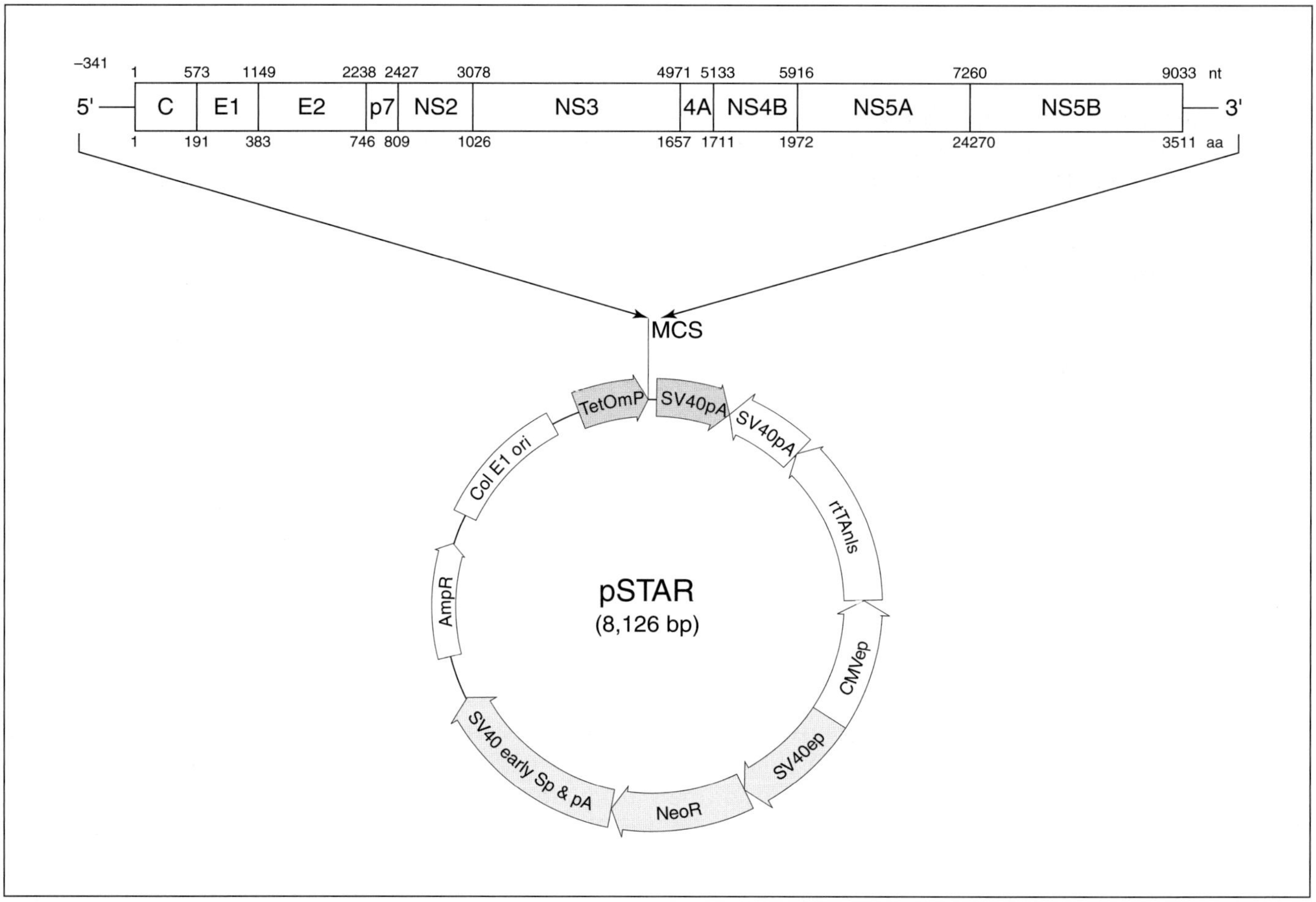

Fig. 1. Schematic diagram of the Singapore HCV isolate, HCV-S1. Predicted coding sequences for structural (C, E1, E2, p7) and nonstructural proteins (NS2, NS3, NS4A, NS4B, NS5A and NS5B) are shown with their terminal nucleotides (nt) and amino acids (aa) positions. The full-length genome was inserted into the multiple cloning site (MCS) of the pSTAR vector so that the expression of the viral proteins is under the control of a tetracycline-inducible cytomegalovirus (CMV) promoter.

ously, RANTES (regulated on activation, normal T cell expressed and secreted) and monocyte chemoattractant protein-1 (MCP-1), which are members of the CC chemokine family, were induced in a wide variety of cells during viral infection [14–16]. These chemokines recruit lymphocytes and monocytes for stimulating immune responses. Transfection with the full-length HCV under control of tetracycline promoter significantly induced the transcription of RANTES and MCP-1 in HeLa, Huh7 and HepG2 cells (fig. 2) [17]. A semi-quantitative PCR analysis of the expression of these chemokines on serial dilutions of cDNA has shown them upregulated at least 16-fold over the baseline level 3 days after induction. Electromobility shift assays and supershift assays have demonstrated the full-length HCV-enhanced promoter activities of MCP-1 and RANTES. In the case of MCP-1, the binding AP-1 to MCP-1 promoter was specifically induced by transfection with the full-length HCV. On the other hand, the expression of RANTES was upregulated by increased binding of NFκB in cultured cells transfected with the full-length HCV.

These experiments indicate that HCV infection affects the promoter activities of CC chemokines and that the resultant increase in their expression may trigger chemoattraction of lymphocytes as well as monocytes for the initiation of immunopathology in the liver. In support of our view, RANTES polymorphisms appear to be an important predictor of less severe inflammation in the liver

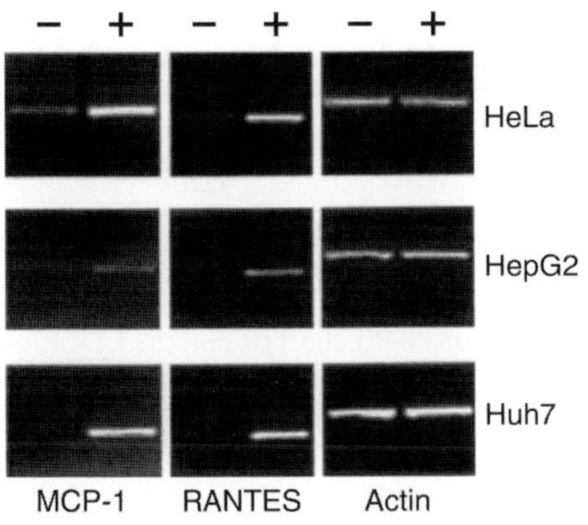

Fig. 2. RT-PCR results showing the upregulation of MCP-1 and RANTES transcripts in non-liver (HeLa) and liver-derived (HepG2 and Huh7) cell lines transfected with empty vector (–) or the plasmid-containing full-length HCV (+). Levels of endogenous actin mRNA are shown as controls.

[18], while polymorphisms of MCP-1 have been associated with more severe liver disease [19]. Exploitation of the tetracycline-inducible full-length HCV vector may yield further information about other chemokines and interactions that are relevant to viral immunopathology and replication. The alteration in chemokines or cytokines clearly plays an important role in the immunopathology of liver disease induced by HCV [20].

Protein-Protein Interactions

The replication of HCV may require interactions of viral proteins, and replication within hepatocytes occurs by viral elements usurping host proteins. In order to investigate mechanisms by which these occur, protein-protein interactions were investigated using the yeast two-hybrid system.

Each viral protein was used independently as a 'bait' in the yeast two-hybrid system (Matchmaker, Clontech Laboratories, Inc., Palo Alto, Calif., USA) with three reporters, HIS3, ADE2 and LacZ; the latter two are indicators of a stronger interaction than HIS3. When NS3 was used as the bait, we found that it interacted strongly with itself [21]. This interaction was confirmed by coimmunoprecipatation. By construction of deletions, the area of interaction was mapped to a specific subdomain of 174 aa in the N terminus of the helicase region. Random mutations were generated in this 174-aa domain to characterize mutants that failed to interact with the wild-type 174-aa fragment. A helicase assay was used which detected the proportion of double-stranded and unwound oligonucleotides utilizing the ^{32}P-labeling method. Four mutants (T266A, Y267S, M288T and AAA) induced 10–100% reduction in the helicase activity. Although the AAA mutation allowed for dimerization, it had no helicase activity, suggesting that dimer formation and helicase activity are separate but closely related. Monomeric forms of NS3 also demonstrated helicase activity albeit at reduced rates, suggesting that while dimerization enhances helicase activity, it is not critical. Hence, helicase dimerization, while important in the viral replication process, does not appear a critical target for the discovery of antiviral drugs.

Further screening of viral proteins with the yeast two-hybrid system disclosed another novel interaction between NS5A and core proteins [22]. Again, this interaction was confirmed by coimmunoprecipitation and in vitro binding assays in COS-7 cells. Overexpression of core induced apoptosis as evidenced by DNA laddering and truncation of poly(ADP-ribose) polymerase 1. Coexpression of core and NS5A resulted in the cleavage of NS5A. Both apoptosis and cleavage of NS5A were inhibited by the caspase inhibitor Z-VAD. Although the biological significance of this interaction is unclear, one may speculate that this interaction may couple viral replication to the viral assembly.

Moving onto interactions between viral and host proteins, NS5B was used as a bait in the yeast two-hybrid system for screening a human spleen cDNA library. The interaction between NS5B (RNA-dependent RNA polymerase) and p68 was noted to be strong and confirmed using coimmunoprecipitation [23]. Truncations of NS5B have shown that the C terminus is essential for this interaction. When NS5B is overexpressed, p68 relocalized from nucleus to cytoplasm as demonstrated by immunofluorescence staining on HeLa cells. Truncations in various sizes of the N terminus of NS5B altered its cytoplasmic localization. This effect of relocalization of p68, when NS5B is overexpressed, was also demonstrable with a replicon cell line (9-13). In a separate system, the full-length HCV in a mammalian vector pcDNA3.1(+) was transiently expressed in Huh7 and 293 cells that were cotransfected with p68 siRNA. A positive correlation was established between knockdown of p68 siRNA and reduction in negative-strand HCV RNA, thereby indicating that

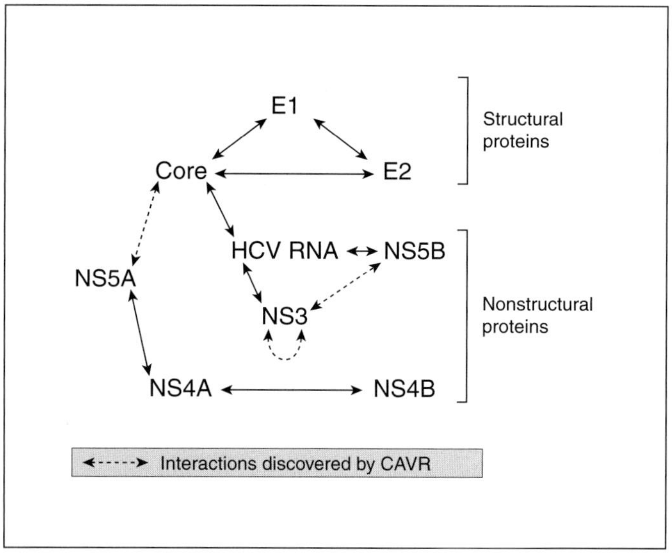

Fig. 3. Schematic diagram of viral protein interactions in the yeast two-hybrid system. Yeast two-hybrid interactions discovered by the CAVR Group at the Institute of Molecular and Cell Biology in Singapore.

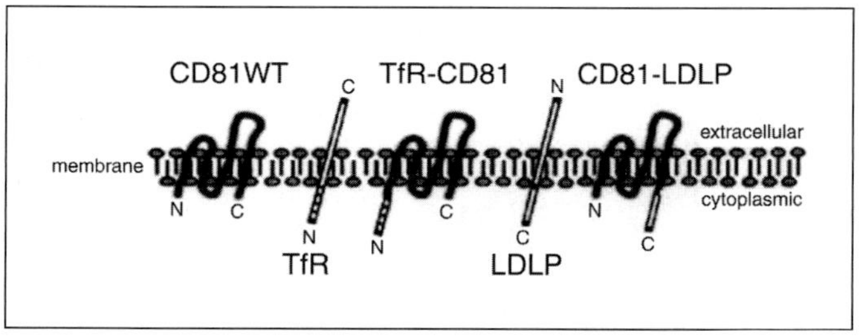

Fig. 4. Schematic diagram showing membrane topologies of the wild-type CD81 (CD81WT), the TfR and the LDLR as well as predicted topologies of CD81 chimeras (TfR-CD81 and CD81-LDLR). TfR-CD81 is obtained by linking the cytoplasmic domain of the TfR to the N terminus of CD81, and CD81-LDLR is obtained by linking the cytoplasmic domain of the LDLR to the C-terminus of CD81.

transcription was affected. It seems that p68, a cellular helicase, interacts with NS5B permitting viral transcription, possibly through the replication complex. The protein-protein interactions discovered by the CAVR Group are summarized in figure 3. These interactions demonstrated by our group only represent part of the patchwork of interactions reported by various investigators that contribute to our understanding of the cell biology of HCV, which was recently succinctly reviewed [24, 25].

A New Cell Model

A number of publications attest to the infection of liver cell lines with HCV. However, none of them have been established as a reliable and reproducible model. Consequently, the development of a new permissive cell line is of high priority. CD81 is shown to bind to the E2 protein, but its role as a putative HCV receptor is controversial. Taking advantage of its ability to bind E2, we constructed two CD81 chimeras by linking them to the cytoplasmic domains of recycling surface receptors, i.e. the low-density lipoprotein receptor (LDLR) and the transferrin receptor (TfR) (fig. 4) [26]. These chimeras also expressed CD81 in high levels. Using antibody to hCD81, binding to CD81 and subsequent internalization were evaluated by immunofluorescence. Chimeric CD81 was internalized more efficiently than wild-type CD81. Furthermore, similar results were demonstrated with recombinant E2 protein and E2-enveloped viral particles. After internalization, these viral particles could produce positive- and negative-strand HCV RNA as well as replicative intermediates, thereby attesting to productive infection. Such a cell model allows us to examine a full replicative cycle of HCV infection, unlike the truncated cycle of HCV replicons. Now, interactions with host proteins and pathogenesis of HCV infection can be dissected in more detail.

This concept is extrapolated to HIV in that antibody to HIV-gp120, expressed as an endocytotoxic transmembrane protein and similarly linked to cation-independent mannose 6-phosphate receptor or the LDLR, can internalize into HIV-1 [27]. Furthermore, using a luciferase HIV-1 reporter, viral replication is shown to occur following internalization. Both these studies indicate that linking a cytoplasmic domain of a rapidly recycling receptor to either a cellular receptor of the virus in question or an antibody to the virus acting as a receptor can be used to create a new cell model for productive viral infection. Other cell models of HCV replication have also been developed. Although models based on the replicon system are powerful tools [13], their application is limited to examination of the replication cycle of HCV in the absence of structural proteins and the viral assembly system. The full-length HCV genome, as reported by our group in an inducible system [9], can significantly advance our understanding of the cell biology. Interestingly, adaptive mutations that enable high viral replication in cell culture appear to be one way of optimizing this system [7]. However, many of the cell lines used are transformed, and therefore, the proteins expressed may or may not significantly differ from those in authentic hepatocytes [28, 29]. Hence, in vivo validation of such systems are crucial before we can accept cell culture systems as truly representative of all that is occurring in vivo.

Conclusions

A multipronged strategy to investigate HCV pathogenesis has led to creation of an inducible full-length HCV vector, which initially increased the production of CC chemokines (RANTES and MCP-1), suggesting that induction of immune responses could originate from productive HCV infection in hepatocytes. Subsequent exploration into protein-protein interactions demonstrated that NS3 existed as a dimer, which enhanced the activity of HCV helicase, but dimerization was not critical to the helicase activity. The interaction between core and NS5A was intriguing, as the cleavage of NS5A was related to the development of apoptosis, but the biological function of this interaction remains unclear. On the other hand, the interaction of p68 and NS56B resulted in the translocalization of p68 from nucleus to cytoplasm, and the knockdown of p68 reduced viral replication. Finally, to pursue the goal of productive HCV infection in hepatocytes, a new cell model of permissive HCV infection was developed with the use of chimeric CD81 linked to the cytoplasmic domain of the LDLR or TfR that led to productive HCV infection. Having established useful tools to examine the cell biology of HCV, we are now dissecting out aspects of HCV infection that will impact viral replication and pathogenesis.

References

1 Choo QL, Kuo G, Weiner AJ, Overby LR, Bradley DW, Houghton M: Isolation of a cDNA clone derived from a blood-borne non-A, non-B viral hepatitis genome. Science 1989; 244:359–362.
2 Penin F, Dubuisson J, Rey FA, Moradpour D, Pawlotsky JM: Structural biology of hepatitis C virus. Hepatology 2004;39:5–19.
3 Moradpour D, Brass V, Gosert R, Wolk B, Blum HE: Hepatitis C: Molecular virology and antiviral targets. Trends Mol Med 2002;8: 476–482.
4 Giannini C, Brechot C: Hepatitis C virus biology. Cell Death Differ 2003;10:S27–S38.
5 Dubuisson J, Penin F, Moradpour D: Interaction of hepatitis C virus proteins with host cell membranes and lipids. Trends Cell Biol 2002; 12:517–523.
6 Pavio N, Lai MM: The hepatitis C virus persistence: How to evade the immune system? J Biosci 2003;28:287–304.
7 Bartenschlager R, Kaul A, Sparacio S: Replication of the hepatitis C virus in cell culture. Antiviral Res 2003;60:91–102.
8 Lim SP, Khu YL, Hong WJ, Tay A, Ting AE, Lim SG, Tan YH: Identification and molecular characterisation of the complete genome of a Singapore isolate of hepatitis C virus: Sequence comparison with other strains and phylogenetic analysis. Virus Genes 2001;23:89–95.
9 Lim SP, Soo HM, Tan YH, Brenner S, Horstmann H, MacKenzie JM, Ng ML, Lim SG, Hong W: Inducible system in human hepatoma cell lines for hepatitis C virus production. Virology 2002;303:79–99.
10 Wolk B, Sansonno D, Krausslich HG, Dammacco F, Rice CM, Blum HE, Moradpour D: Subcellular localization, stability, and trans-cleavage competence of the hepatitis C virus NS3-NS4A complex expressed in tetracycline-regulated cell lines. J Virol 2000;74:2293–2304.
11 Moradpour D, Wakita T, Wands JR, Blum HE: Tightly regulated expression of the entire hepatitis C virus structural region in continuous human cell lines. Biochem Biophys Res Commun 1998;246:920–924.
12 Myung J, Khalap N, Kalkeri G, Garry R, Dash S: Inducible model to study negative strand RNA synthesis and assembly of hepatitis C virus from a full-length cDNA clone. J Virol Methods 2001;94:55–67.
13 Lohmann V, Korner F, Koch J, Herian U, Theilmann L, Bartenschlager R: Replication of subgenomic hepatitis C virus RNAs in a hepatoma cell line. Science 1999;285:110–113.
14 Peterson KE, Robertson SJ, Portis JL, Chesebro B: Differences in cytokine and chemokine responses during neurological disease induced by polytropic murine retroviruses Map to separate regions of the viral envelope gene. J Virol 2001;75:2848–2856.
15 Lin YL, Liu CC, Chuang JI, Lei HY, Yeh TM, Lin YS, Huang YH, Liu HS: Involvement of oxidative stress, NF-IL-6, and RANTES expression in dengue-2-virus-infected human liver cells. Virology 2000;276:114–126.
16 Matikainen S, Pirhonen J, Miettinen M, Lehtonen A, Govenius-Vintola C, Sareneva T, Julkunen I: Influenza A and sendai viruses induce differential chemokine gene expression and transcription factor activation in human macrophages. Virology 2000;276:138–147.
17 Soo HM, Garzino-Demo A, Hong W, Tan YH, Tan YJ, Goh PY, Lim SG, Lim SP: Expression of a full-length hepatitis C virus cDNA up-regulates the expression of CC chemokines MCP-1 and RANTES. Virology 2002;303:253–277.
18 Hellier S, Frodsham AJ, Hennig BJ, Klenerman P, Knapp S, Ramaley P, Satsangi J, Wright M, Zhang L, Thomas HC, Thursz M, Hill AV: Association of genetic variants of the chemokine receptor CCR5 and its ligands, RANTES and MCP-2, with outcome of HCV infection. Hepatology 2003;38:1468–1476.
19 Muhlbauer M, Bosserhoff AK, Hartmann A, Thasler WE, Weiss TS, Herfarth H, Lock G, Scholmerich J, Hellerbrand C: A novel MCP-1 gene polymorphism is associated with hepatic MCP-1 expression and severity of HCV-related liver disease. Gastroenterology 2003;125: 1085–1093.
20 Heydtmann M, Shields P, McCaughan G, Adams D: Cytokines and chemokines in the immune response to hepatitis C infection. Curr Opin Infect Dis 2001;14:279–287.
21 Khu YL, Koh E, Lim SP, Tan YH, Brenner S, Lim SG, Hong WJ, Goh PY: Mutations that affect dimer formation and helicase activity of the hepatitis C virus helicase. J Virol 2001;75: 205–214.
22 Goh PY, Tan YJ, Lim SP, Lim SG, Tan YH, Hong WJ: The hepatitis C virus core protein interacts with NS5A and activates its caspase-mediated proteolytic cleavage. Virology 2001; 290:224–236.

23 Goh PY, Tan YJ, Lim SP, Tan YH, Lim SG, Fuller-Pace F, Hong W: Cellular RNA helicase p68 relocalization and interaction with the hepatitis C virus (HCV) NS5B protein and the potential role of p68 in HCV RNA replication. J Virol 2004;78:5288–5298.
24 Tellinghuisen TL, Rice CM: Interaction between hepatitis C virus proteins and host cell factors. Curr Opin Microbiol 2002;5:419–427.
25 Dimitrova M, Imbert I, Kieny MP, Schuster C: Protein-protein interactions between hepatitis C virus nonstructural proteins. J Virol 2003; 77:5401–5414.
26 Tan YJ, Lim SP, Ng P, Goh PY, Lim SG, Tan YH, Hong W: CD81 engineered with endocytotic signals mediates HCV cell entry: Implications for receptor usage by HCV in vivo. Virology 2003;308:250–269.
27 Tan YJ, Lim SP, Ting AE, Goh PY, Tan YH, Lim SG, Hong W: An anti-HIV-1 gp120 antibody expressed as an endocytotic transmembrane protein mediates internalization of HIV-1. Virology 2003;315:80–92.
28 Wilkening S, Bader A: Influence of culture time on the expression of drug-metabolizing enzymes in primary human hepatocytes and hepatoma cell line HepG2. J Biochem Mol Toxicol 2003;17:207–213.
29 Wilkening S, Stahl F, Bader A: Comparison of primary human hepatocytes and hepatoma cell line Hepg2 with regard to their biotransformation properties. Drug Metab Dispos 2003;31: 1035–1042.

Pathophysiology

Intervirology

Intervirology 2006;49:51–57
DOI: 10.1159/000087263

Hepatitis C Virus Infection Can Present with Metabolic Disease by Inducing Insulin Resistance

Kazuhiko Koike

Department of Infectious Diseases, Internal Medicine, Graduate School of Medicine, University of Tokyo, Tokyo, Japan

Key Words
Diabetes · Hepatitis C virus · Insulin resistance · Insulin receptor substrate · Transgenic mouse

Abstract
Although hepatitis C virus (HCV) targets the liver, it has become increasingly evident that HCV can induce diseases of many organs. Recently, much attention is drawn to metabolic disorders in HCV infection. First, hepatic steatosis and derangement in lipid metabolism have been found characteristic of HCV infection, and later on, a correlation was noted between HCV infection and diabetes as well as insulin resistance. We have demonstrated that HCV by itself can induce insulin resistance through disturbing the insulin signaling pathway by HCV proteins. The fact that HCV infection induces insulin resistance by the virus itself may influence the progression of chronic liver disease and open up novel therapeutic approaches. In conclusion, towards the future, HCV infection needs to be viewed not only as a liver disease but also as a metabolic disease.

Introduction

Hepatitis C virus (HCV) infects approximately 1.8 million people in Japan alone and as many as 200 million over the world and induces liver disease ranging from chronic hepatitis through cirrhosis to hepatocellular carcinoma (HCC) [1, 2]. It has been noticed soon after the discovery that the infection with HCV does not exclusively involve the liver. In fact, type II cryoglobulinemia [3] and membranoproliferative glomerulonephritis [4] frequently occur in patients infected with HCV. Furthermore, strong associations of HCV infection with Sjogren's syndrome [5] and lichen planus [6] have been noted, which is verified in the animal model [7]. In addition, the relation between HCV infection and B cell lymphoma has attracted attention especially in Europe [8].

Recently, there have been increasing lines of evidence to indicate metabolic disturbances in HCV infection which, in turn, would influence the pathogenesis of chronic hepatitis C. The discovery of HCV in 1989 [9] enabled a comparison between chronic hepatitis C and other chronic liver diseases. As shown in the results, it has been repeatedly reported that steatosis is significantly associated with chronic hepatitis C [10, 11]. Steatosis in HCV infection is reproduced in animal models [12–14] to reinforce a pathologic role of HCV. Furthermore, patients infected with HCV have abnormalities in serum lipids, such as hypocholesterolemia and abnormal levels of apolipoproteins in serum [15, 16]; they are rectified in sustained virological responders to interferon (IFN) [16]. Thus, the association between HCV infection and a derangement in lipid metabolism has become increasingly strong, both in patients and experimental systems in animals. Finally, patients with chronic hepatitis C accompanied by severe steatosis develop hepatic fibrosis with an

KARGER

Fax +41 61 306 12 34
E-Mail karger@karger.ch
www.karger.com

0300–5526/06/0492–0051$23.50/0

Accessible online at:
www.karger.com/int

Kazuhiko Koike, MD
Department of Infectious Diseases, Internal Medicine
Graduate School of Medicine, University of Tokyo
7-3-1 Hongo, Bunkyo-ku, Tokyo 113-8655 (Japan)
Fax +81 3 5800 8799, E-Mail kkoike-tky@umin.ac.jp

increased velocity [17]. All in all, we could say that abnormal lipid metabolism in HCV infection is deeply involved in the pathogenesis of hepatitis C.

HCV Infection and Diabetes

Diabetes is suggested as another metabolic disease in association with HCV infection. In 1994, Allison et al. [18] reported an epidemiological link between diabetes and HCV infection. However, doubts were cast on the association in view of a decreased glucose tolerance in advanced chronic hepatitis as well as an increased opportunity for HCV infection in diabetics who frequently receive determination of blood sugar. Several reports from the same group and others followed along this line. The trend to accept the solid association between diabetes and HCV infection seems to have been triggered in the United States by the population study by Metha et al. [19].

However, the association between diabetes and HCV infection is blemished by factors responsible for decreased glucose tolerance, such as advanced cirrhosis, obesity and ageing common in patients with hepatitis C; they make it difficult to prove this association. Hence, there is a need to evaluate the association by basic studies in experimental systems.

HCV Infection Induces Insulin Resistance

We set out to demonstrate the association between HCV infection and diabetes using the animal model. Mice transgenic for the HCV core gene were employed to this end [12, 13]. These mice are engineered to have the HCV core gene of genotype 1b in the absence of other viral genes. They express HCV core protein of the expected size in the liver, in levels comparable with those of patients with chronic hepatitis C (fig. 1). Half of them develop HCC later during their lives [13]. These transgenic mice were fed with their normal littermates, and the glucose metabolism was compared between them [20].

Although mice transgenic for the core gene did not develop overt diabetes, they had markedly elevated serum levels of insulin. Plasma glucose levels were somewhat higher in transgenic mice than in their normal littermates, both in the fast and after ample feeding, with no significant differences between them. In remarkable contrast, serum insulin levels were significantly higher in transgenic than in normal mice in both conditions (fig. 2). Since such a combination of normal glucose levels and hyperinsulinemia points to insulin resistance, glucose and insulin tolerance tests were conducted.

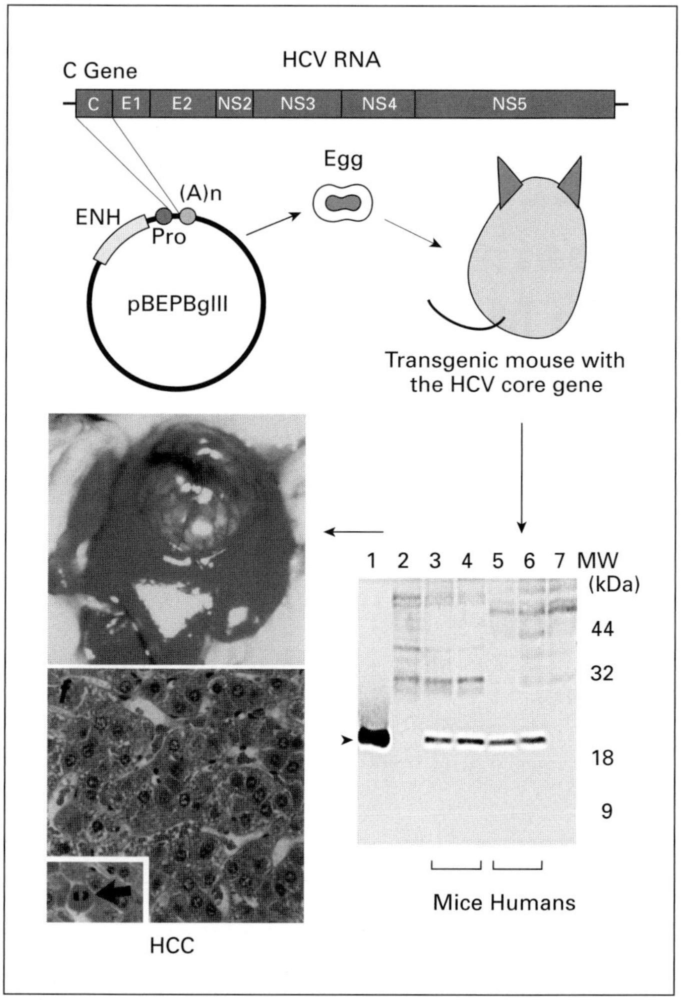

Fig. 1. Expression of HCV core gene in transgenic mouse. It carries the core gene of HCV genotype 1b alone and expresses the core protein of expected size in the liver, at levels similar to those in human patients. Mice eventually develop HCC later in their lives.

Mice transgenic for the HCV core gene exhibited glucose levels a little higher than those in normal littermates, without any significant differences between them. In insulin tolerance tests, glucose levels were significantly higher in transgenic than in normal mice, both 40 and 60 min after they were injected with insulin intraperitoneally (fig. 3). These results indicate suppression of the activity of insulin to decrease blood glucose levels for inducing insulin resistance in core-transgenic mice. Since only the HCV core gene had been incorporated into these transgenic mice, HCV core protein was able to induce insulin resistance in vivo.

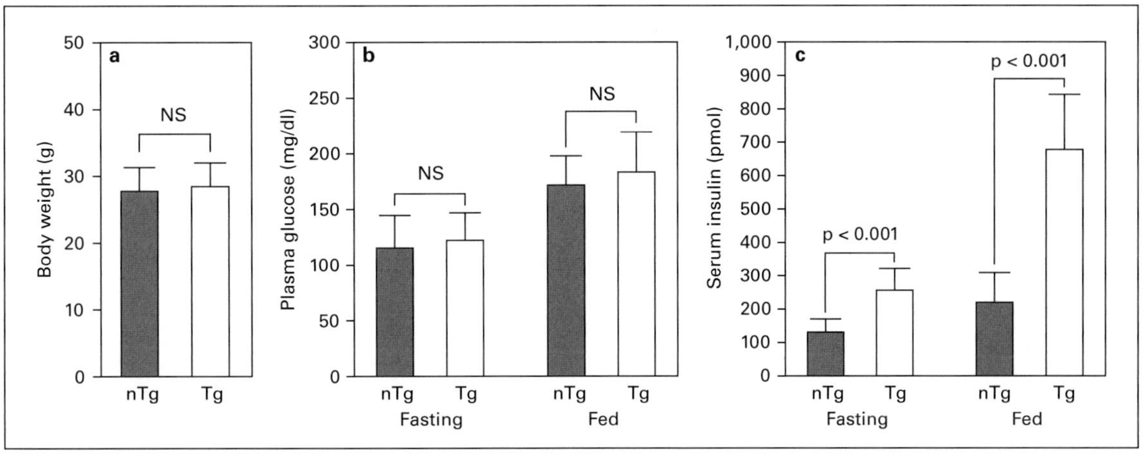

Fig. 2. Altered homeostasis of glucose in mice transgenic for the HCV core gene. Body weight of 2-month-old mice (**a**), plasma glucose levels in fasting or fed mice (**b**) and serum insulin levels in fasting or fed mice (**c**) are shown. Values represent means ± SE. NS = Not significant statistically; nTg = nontransgenic mice; Tg = transgenic mice.

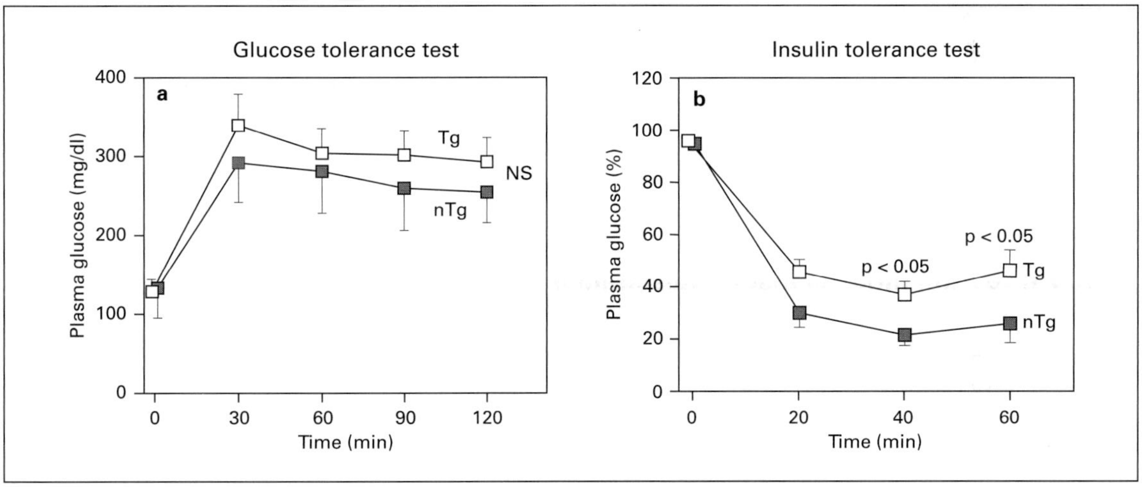

Fig. 3. Insulin resistance in transgenic mice. Glucose tolerance in mice after overnight fasting (**a**). *D*-Glucose (1 g/kg body weight) was given intraperitoneally to conscious mice, and plasma glucose levels were determined at time points indicated. **b** Insulin tolerance in mice fasted overnight. Human insulin (1 U/kg body weight) was injected intraperitoneally, and glucose concentrations were determined sequentially. Values were normalized to the baseline glucose concentration at the time of insulin administration. NS = Not significant statistically; nTg = nontransgenic mice; Tg = transgenic mice.

By what mechanism does insulin resistance arise in this animal model? The insulin resistance is considered to involve two factors, namely central and peripheral insulin resistances (table 1) [21]. The hyperinsulinemic-euglycemic clamp method was employed to differentiate between them. In this method, hepatic glucose production (HGP) is calculated on the basis of amounts of glucose required to keep plasma glucose levels within a certain range at serum insulin levels higher than physiological ones. In normal control mice, HPG was suppressed by 60% by the administration of insulin, in contrast to core-transgenic mice in which there was no appreciable suppression of HGP by insulin (fig. 4). These results indicate a hepatic (central) origin of the insulin resistance

Table 1. Two types of insulin resistance

Type	Mechanism
Peripheral	A shortage of insulin action in the muscle due to deficit in the insulin-induced uptake of glucose into muscles
Central	A shortage of insulin action in the liver due to deficit in the insulin-induced suppression of glucose production in hepatocytes

in transgenic mice. For further confirmation, an uptake of glucose into muscle was determined. There were no differences in the uptake in response to administration of insulin between normal and transgenic mice. Therefore, the insulin resistance in mice transgenic for the HCV core gene is central and hepatic.

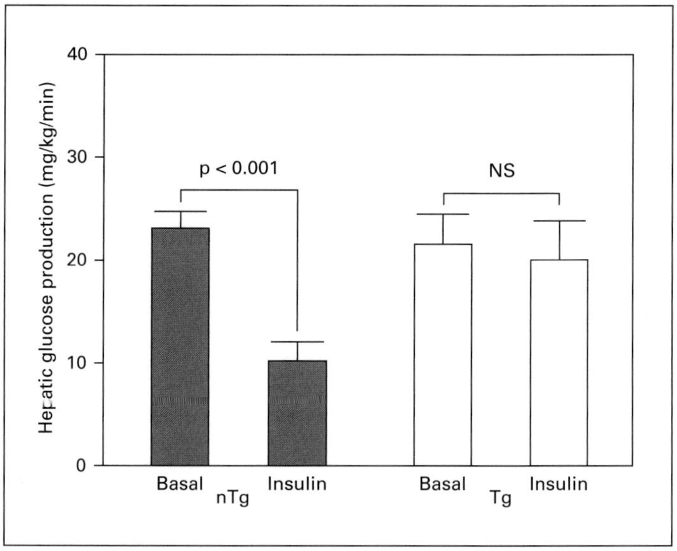

Fig. 4. Characterization of glucose metabolism in transgenic mice. Glucose production in the liver was calculated using the hyperinsulinemic-euglycemic clamp method. NS = Not significant statistically; nTg = nontransgenic mice; Tg = transgenic mice.

HCV Core Protein Suppresses the Transduction of Insulin Signaling in Hepatocytes

Next, we evaluated how insulin resistance elicits in mice transgenic for the HCV core gene. For this purpose, liver homogenate was immunoblotted with antiphosphotyrosine and antiphosphoserine antibodies after insulin receptor substrate (IRS)-1 and IRS-2 had been immunoprecipitated. Tyrosines in IRS-1 were weakly phosphorylated both in normal and transgenic mice before they received insulin, with no differences between them. However, after the administration of insulin, the phosphorylation of tyrosines in IRS-1 increased in normal but not in transgenic mice (fig. 5). Obtained results suggested disturbance in tyrosine phosphorylation as one of the factors responsible for insulin resistance in the liver. There were no differences in phosphorylation of serines in IRS-1 or tyrosines in IRS-2 between normal and transgenic mice. Combined, they provided experimental evidence for the development of insulin resistance by the presence of HCV in the liver that would occur by disturbing the transduction of insulin signaling in hepatocytes (fig. 6).

There remains a possibility for the HCV core protein to directly prohibit phosphorylation of tyrosines, or else, it might inhibit tyrosine phosphorylation via certain cytokines. In our extensive searches for the expression of cytokines in the liver of transgenic mice, only TNF-α and IL-1β have been found with an increased expression [22]. Therefore, for the purpose of evaluating the role of

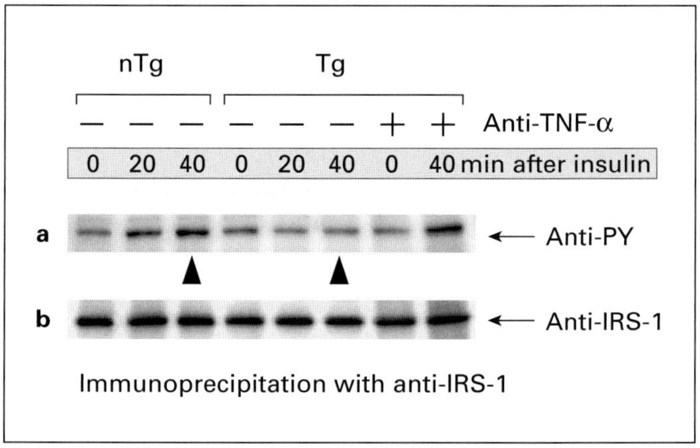

Fig. 5. Phosphorylation of tyrosine in IRS-1 in response to insulin stimulation. Liver tissues from control mice, transgenic mice with or without anti-TNF-α antibody treatment, were analyzed before and 20 as well as 40 min after administration of insulin. Samples were subjected to immunoprecipitation with anti-IRS-1 antibody and then immunoblotted with indicated antibodies. Experiments were performed in triplicate, and a representative picture is exhibited. Immunoblotting with antiphosphotyrosine (PY) antibody (lane a) did not augment phosphorylation of tyrosine in IRS-1 after stimulation with insulin in the core gene transgenic mice (Tg), in contrast to tyrosine phosphorylation markedly enhanced in control mice (nTg). Insulin-stimulated tyrosine phosphorylation was restored 40 min after treatment with anti-TNF-α antibody. Note differences in the intensity of bands 40 min after the administration of insulin (arrowheads). Immunoblotting with anti-IRS-1 antibody (lane b) served as control for the IRS-1 load.

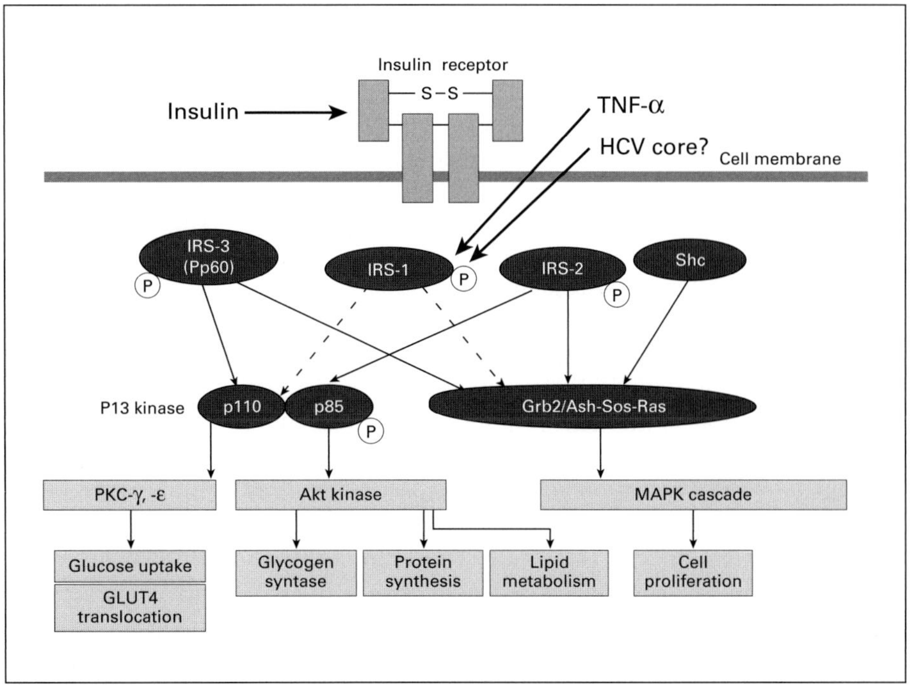

Fig. 6. A proposed mechanism for insulin resistance in HCV infection. HCV itself or elevated levels of cytokines such as TNF-α may inhibit tyrosine phosphorylation of IRS-1 in the liver, suppress intracellular transduction of insulin signal and lead to insulin resistance. PKC = Protein kinase C; MAPK = mitogen-activated protein kinase.

TNF-α in insulin resistance in transgenic mice, serum insulin was determined and an insulin tolerance test performed after they had received anti-TNF-α intraperitoneally. Pretreatment with anti-TNF-α partially improved insulin resistance in mice transgenic for the HCV core gene. Albeit a direct anti-insulin activity of core protein and direct or indirect factors for insulin resistance are not to be excluded, high levels of TNF-α in the liver would be one of the factors for expression of insulin resistance in this mouse model.

Insulin Resistance in Patients with Chronic Hepatitis C

Concurrently with our report in experimental systems, Aytug et al. [23] investigated insulin signaling in biopsied liver specimens from patients with chronic hepatitis C. Specifically, they evaluated changes in IRS-1, IRS-2 and phosphatidyl inositol (PI)3 kinase levels in the liver of patients. With insulin stimulation of biopsied liver samples, insulin receptor proteins and IRS-1 increased, while phosphorylation of tyrosines in IRS-1 decreased to one half of the baseline value, along with a diminished activity for PI3 kinase associated with IRS-1, in patients with chronic hepatitis C. The authors went on to propose a possibility for disturbed transduction of the insulin signaling pathway in the liver to induce insulin resistance in patients with chronic hepatitis C [23]. Their report is quite intriguing in that it opens up the way for evaluating an association between HCV infection and insulin resistance in clinical samples at the molecular level.

The results of Aytug et al. [23] inadvertently coincide with ours in analyzing the mechanism of insulin resistance with the experimental system in mice (vide supra). They unanimously incriminate impaired tyrosine phosphorylation in IRS-1 in the induction of insulin resistance by HCV infection. It struck us as a surprise that the mechanism of insulin resistance induced by HCV infection has been in agreement between clinical samples and experimental animals, in spite of hepatic IRS-2 that was preferred to IRS-1 for its role in development of insulin resistance in former studies [24]. HCV infection is peculiar in that IRS-1 weighs heavier than IRS-2 in the induction of hepatic insulin resistance.

Although our data strongly indicate a hepatic character of insulin resistance in HCV infection, they by no means exclude roles of other factors in the induction of this resistance. There is little expression of the HCV core gene in muscles of our animal model; it is not known if HCV infects muscular cells in patients with chronic hepatitis C. Factors not intrinsic to the liver would have to be evaluated to sort this out, including dysfunction of mitochondria for induction of insulin resistance [25].

Insulin Resistance for Advanced Hepatic Fibrosis

Insulin resistance in HCV infection may have an additional significant clinical implication. In 260 patients with chronic hepatitis C, Hui et al. [26] have tried to establish the relationship between liver histology and indicators of glucose metabolism, as well as insulin resistance represented by the homeostasis model assessment of insulin resistance. They have found that insulin resistance already exists in hepatitis C patients with stage 0 or 1 fibrosis in the liver. This indicates that insulin resistance in HCV infection is not attributable to advanced liver disease. In their study, independent predictors of insulin resistance in HCV infection were body mass index, nonresponse to antiviral treatment, intensity of portal inflammation and infection with HCV genotype 3 [26]. Furthermore, the homeostasis model assessment of insulin resistance was a significant and independent predictor of the stage and velocity of hepatic fibrosis. The results of the study are of much importance, because they implicate a role of insulin resistance and hyperinsulinemia by inference, in promoting the progression of hepatic fibrosis. Insulin has been proven as an aggravating factor not only in atherosclerosis, but also in systemic inflammation and fibrosis. The liver is no exception to this.

Conclusions: Hepatitis C Viewed as a Metabolic Disease and Outlook for Therapeutic Strategies in the Future

We have demonstrated that HCV per se induces insulin resistance in the animal model. Superimposed high-fat diet and obesity may lead to overt diabetes. Since insulin resistance accelerates the progression of chronic hepatitis C, it would naturally influence the development of HCC. Although the association has not been established between nonalcoholic steatohepatitis and HCC, it needs to be energetically pursued in view of the histological homology of nonalcoholic steatohepatitis to chronic hepatitis C. Drugs for improving glucose metabolism and insulin resistance need to be kept in store in the treatment of hepatitis C patients who have failed to respond to antivirals, because they may well prevent progression of fibrosis and development of HCC in such patients. Traditional 'high-protein and high-calorie' diet, especially advocated in Japan after World War II, is obviously detrimental, except in some patients with advanced cirrhosis. Consultation on the dietary habit with hepatitis C patients should include iron restriction [27] as well as weight control, because high-calorie intakes are likely to accelerate hepatic fibrosis by aggravating insulin resistance.

References

1 Saito I, Miyamura T, Ohbayashi A, Harada H, Katayama T, Kikuchi S, Watanabe Y, Koi S, Onji M, Ohta Y: Hepatitis C virus infection is associated with the development of hepatocellular carcinoma. Proc Natl Acad Sci USA 1990;87:6547–6549.

2 Simonetti RG, Camma C, Fiorello F, Cottone M, Rapicetta M, Marino L, Fiorentino G, Craxi A, Ciccaglione A, Giuseppetti R: Hepatitis C virus infection as a risk factor for hepatocellular carcinoma in patients with cirrhosis. A case-control study. Ann Intern Med 1992; 116:97–102.

3 Agnello V, Chung RT, Kaplan LM: A role for hepatitis C virus infection in type II cryoglobulinemia. N Engl J Med 1992;327:1490–1495.

4 Johnson RJ, Gretch DR, Yamabe H, Hart J, Bacchi CE, Hartwell P, Couser WG, Corey L, Wener MH, Alpers CE: Membranoproliferative glomerulonephritis associated with hepatitis C virus infection. N Engl J Med 1993;328: 465–470.

5 Haddad J, Deny P, Munz-Gotheil C, Ambrosini JC, Trinchet JC, Pateron D, Mal F, Callard P, Beaugrand M: Lymphocytic sialadenitis of Sjogren's syndrome associated with chronic hepatitis C virus liver disease. Lancet 1992; 339:321–323.

6 Pawlotsky JM, Benchiki H, Pellet C, Duval J, Dhumeaux D, Revuz J, Bagot M: Lichen planus and hepatitis C virus (HCV)-related chronic hepatitis: Evaluation of HCV genotypes. Br J Dermatol 1995;133:666–667.

7 Koike K, Moriya K, Ishibashi K, Yotsuyanagi H, Shintani Y, Fujie H, Kurokawa K, Matsuura Y, Miyamura T: Sialadenitis histologically resembling Sjogren syndrome in mice transgenic for hepatitis C virus envelope genes. Proc Natl Acad Sci USA 1997;94:233–236.

8 Gisbert JP, Garcia-Buey L, Pajares JM, Moreno-Otero R: Prevalence of hepatitis C virus infection in B-cell non-Hodgkin's lymphoma: Systematic review and meta-analysis. Gastroenterology 2003;125:1723–1732.

9 Choo QL, Kuo G, Weiner AJ, Overby LR, Bradley DW, Houghton M: Isolation of a cDNA clone derived from a blood-borne non-A, non-B viral hepatitis genome. Science 1989; 244:359–362.

10 Bach N, Thung SN, Schaffner F: The histological features of chronic hepatitis C and autoimmune chronic hepatitis: A comparative analysis. Hepatology 1992;15:572–577.

11 Lefkowitch JH, Schiff ER, Davis GL, Perrillo RP, Lindsay K, Bodenheimer HC Jr, Balart LA, Ortego TJ, Payne J, Dienstag JL, Gibas A, Jacobson IM, Tamburro CH, Carey W, O'Brien C, Sampliner R, van Thiel DH, Feit D, Albrecht J, Meschievitz C, Sanghvi V, Vaughan RD: Pathological diagnosis of chronic hepatitis C: A multicenter comparative study with chronic hepatitis B. Gastroenterology 1993; 104:595–603.

12 Moriya K, Yotsuyanagi H, Shintani Y, Fujie H, Ishibashi K, Matsuura Y, Miyamura T, Koike K: Hepatitis C virus core protein induces hepatic steatosis in transgenic mice. J Gen Virol 1997;78:1527–1531.

13 Moriya K, Fujie H, Shintani Y, Yotsuyanagi H, Tsutsumi T, Ishibashi K, Matsuura Y, Kimura S, Miyamura T, Koike K: The core protein of hepatitis C virus induces hepatocellular carcinoma in transgenic mice. Nat Med 1998;4:1065–1067.

14 Lerat H, Honda M, Beard MR, Loesch K, Sun J, Yang Y, Okuda M, Gosert R, Xiao SY, Weinman SA, Lemon SM: Steatosis and liver cancer in transgenic mice expressing the structural and nonstructural proteins of hepatitis C virus. Gastroenterology 2002;122:352–365.
15 Moriya K, Sintani Y, Fujie H, Miyoshi H, Tsutsumi T, Yotsuyanagi H, Yasuda K, Iino S, Kimura S, Koike K: Serum lipid profile of patients with genotype 1b hepatits C viral infection in Japan. Hepatol Res 2003;25:369–374.
16 Naeem M, Bacon BR, Mistry B, Britton RS, Di Bisceglie AM: Changes in serum lipoprotein profile during interferon therapy in chronic hepatitis C. Am J Gastroenterol 2001;96:2468–2472.
17 Lonardo A, Adinolfi LE, Loria P, Carulli N, Ruggiero G, Day CP: Steatosis and hepatitis C virus: Mechanisms and significance for hepatic and extrahepatic disease. Gastroenterology 2004;126:586–597.
18 Allison ME, Wreghitt T, Palmer CR, Alexander GJ: Evidence for a link between hepatitis C virus infection and diabetes mellitus in a cirrhotic population. J Hepatol 1994;21:1135–1139.
19 Mehta SH, Brancati FL, Sulkowski MS, Strathdee SA, Szklo M, Thomas DL: Prevalence of type 2 diabetes mellitus among persons with hepatitis C virus infection in the United States. Ann Intern Med 2000;133:592–599.
20 Shintani Y, Fujie H, Miyoshi H, Tsutsumi T, Tsukamoto K, Kimura S, Moriya K, Koike K: Hepatitis C virus infection and diabetes: Direct involvement of the virus in the development of insulin resistance. Gastroenterology 2004;126:840–848.
21 Kahn BB: Type 2 diabetes: When insulin secretion fails to compensate for insulin resistance. Cell 1998;92:593–596.
22 Tsutsumi T, Suzuki T, Moriya K, Yotsuyanagi H, Shintani Y, Fujie H, Matsuura Y, Kimura S, Koike K, Miyamura T: Alteration of intrahepatic cytokine expression and AP-1 activation in transgenic mice expressing hepatitis C virus core protein. Virology 2002;304:415–424.
23 Aytug S, Reich D, Sapiro LE, Bernstein D, Begum N: Impaired IRS-1/PI3-kinase signaling in patients with HCV: A mechanism for increased prevalence of type 2 diabetes. Hepatology 2003;38:1384–1392.
24 Suzuki R, Tobe K, Aoyama M, Inoue A, Sakamoto K, Yamauchi T, Kamon J, Kubota N, Terauchi Y, Yoshimatsu H, Matsuhisa M, Nagasaka S, Ogata H, Tokuyama K, Nagai R, Kadowaki T: Both insulin signaling defects in the liver and obesity contribute to insulin resistance and cause diabetes in Irs2(–/–) mice. J Biol Chem 2004;279:25039–25049.
25 Petersen KF, Befroy D, Dufour S, Dziura J, Ariyan C, Rothman DL, DiPietro L, Cline GW, Shulman GI: Mitochondrial dysfunction in the elderly: Possible role in insulin resistance. Science 2003;300:1140–1142.
26 Hui JM, Sud A, Farrell GC, Bandara P, Byth K, Kench JG, McCaughan GW, George J: Insulin resistance is associated with chronic hepatitis C virus infection and fibrosis progression. Gastroenterology 2003;125:1695–1704.
27 Kato J, Kobune M, Nakamura T, Kuroiwa G, Takada K, Takimoto R, Sato Y, Fujikawa K, Takahashi M, Takayama T, Ikeda T, Niitsu Y: Normalization of elevated hepatic 8-hydroxy-2′-deoxyguanosine levels in chronic hepatitis C patients by phlebotomy and low iron diet. Cancer Res 2001;61:8697–8702.

Pathophysiology

Intervirology

Intervirology 2006;49:58–63
DOI: 10.1159/000087264

Impaired Function of Dendritic Cells Circulating in Patients Infected with Hepatitis C Virus Who Have Persistently Normal Alanine Aminotransferase Levels

Tatsuya Kanto[a, b] Michiyo Inoue[a] Masanori Miyazaki[a] Ichiyo Itose[a] Hideki Miyatake[a] Mitsuru Sakakibara[a] Takayuki Yakushijin[a] Aki Kaimori[a] Chika Oki[a] Naoki Hiramatsu[a] Akinori Kasahara[c] Norio Hayashi[a]

Departments of [a]Molecular Therapeutics, [b]Dendritic Cell Biology and Clinical Applications, and [c]General Medicine, Osaka University Graduate School of Medicine, Osaka, Japan

Key Words
Cytokines · Dendritic cells · Hepatitis C virus · Progenitors · Th1/Th2

Abstract
Hepatitis C virus (HCV) induces chronic liver disease in hosts which can eventually progresses to liver cirrhosis and hepatocellular carcinoma. However, progression of liver disease is slower in patients with persistently normal levels of alanine aminotransferase (ALT) than in those with active hepatitis. Although distinct immune responses against HCV have been proposed in asymptomatic infection, the role of circulating dendritic cells (DC) in the pathogenesis of these patients remains obscure. To address this issue, we compared the number and function of myeloid DC (MDC) and plasmacytoid DC (PDC) between uninfected individuals and HCV-infected patients with or without elevated ALT levels. Numbers of DC and DC progenitors were significantly lower in patients with chronic active hepatitis than in control subjects. However, no differences were found in the number of DC between normal controls and HCV-infected patients with persistently normal ALT levels. MDC from patients with active hepatitis were less able to polarize naive CD4 T cells into the Th1 phenotype, while their MDC and PDC primed more CD4 T cells producing IL-10 than those from normal controls. Such dysfunction of DC was also observed in patients with persistently normal ALT levels. In conclusion, circulating DC decrease in number predominantly in HCV-infected patients with active hepatitis, and the function of DC is impaired even in those with normal ALT levels.

Introduction

Hepatitis C virus (HCV) is a double-stranded RNA virus and can cause a wide spectrum of chronic liver disease in humans, ranging from mild or active chronic hepatitis through cirrhosis to hepatocellular carcinoma (HCC) [1]. Therefore, HCV should be eradicated to prevent the progression of liver injuries and the subsequent development of HCC in some patients infected with HCV. To improve the prognosis of chronically infected patients, it needs to be elucidated why HCV can persistently infect human beings and resist the clearance even after repeated treatments with antiviral agents such as interferon (IFN) and ribavirin. It has been suggested that HCV has its own strategies to escape the immune surveillance of hosts, for example, by disabling the function of

KARGER
Fax +41 61 306 12 34
E-Mail karger@karger.ch
www.karger.com

0300–5526/06/0492–0058$23.50/0

Accessible online at:
www.karger.com/int

Norio Hayashi, MD
Department of Molecular Therapeutics
Osaka University Graduate School of Medicine
Suita, Osaka 565-0871 (Japan)
Tel. +81 6 6879 3442, Fax +81 6 6879 3449, E-Mail hayashin@moltx.med.osaka-u.ac.jp

antigen-presenting cells (APC) [2] or inhibiting responses of CD4 and CD8 T cells [3, 4].

Dendritic cells (DC) are professional APC that stimulate innate and adaptive immune reactions by priming other types of blood cells [5]. To date, ontogenetically distinct subsets of DC have been reported, and they are grouped into at least two types, i.e. myeloid DC (MDC) and lymphoid or plasmacytoid DC (PDC) [5]. In general, human MDC predominantly produce IL-12 or TNF-α following proinflammatory stimuli and preferentially drive the Th1 response, while human PDC release a considerable amount of type I IFN upon virus infection and preferentially induce Th2 polarization [5]. Several reports have focused on the dysfunction of DC and its involvement in the pathogenesis of a variety of disorders [6, 7]. In chronic HCV infection, we as well as others have shown that DC are impaired in the capacity to stimulate T cells [2, 8, 9], thereby suggesting that DC themselves would be a reciprocal target of HCV for inducing immune dysfunction.

It is well known that some HCV-infected patients have persistently normal levels of serum alanine aminotransferase (ALT); they are classified into asymptomatic carriers (ASC) of HCV. Progression from hepatitis to cirrhosis is much slower in ASC than in patients with active hepatitis [10]. Albeit distinct anti-HCV responses have been implicated in the maintenance of the asymptomatic carrier state, the exact mechanism is largely unknown. To clarify the role of DC subsets in the pathogenesis of ASC, we compared the number and function of circulating DC between uninfected individuals and HCV-infected patients who had or did not have elevated ALT levels. Our finding of note is that DC and DC progenitors in the circulation of ASC are comparable in number with those of uninfected individuals, while they are functionally impaired to the extent of patients with active hepatitis. Thus, HCV infection per se impairs the function of circulating DC, regardless of liver injuries, which may contribute to the persistence of HCV infection.

Materials and Methods

Patients

Sixty-seven patients infected with HCV were enrolled in this study. Of those, 49 had chronic hepatitis with persistently elevated or fluctuating ALT levels (male:female ratio 30:19; serum ALT 98 ± 70 IU/l). The remaining 18 patients were ASC and they continued to have normal ALT levels for more than 2 years (male:female ratio 9:9; ALT 21 ± 5 IU/l). In some of these patients, liver biopsy was carried out to diagnose their histological activity and grade of fibrosis. In ASC, only minimal mononuclear cell infiltration was found in portal areas, without apparent lobular inflammation or necrosis. These observations were in sharp contrast to patients with chronic hepatitis, who showed a higher degree of inflammation spanning the portal to venous areas with spotty lobular necrosis. Serving as normal controls were 26 age-matched healthy volunteers who were negative for serum markers of HCV, hepatitis B virus or human immunodeficiency virus type 1 infection (male:female ratio 20:6).

MDC and PDC in the Peripheral Blood

DC subsets and their progenitors in the blood were determined as reported previously [9]. In brief, DC were defined as lineage marker (Lin; CD3, CD14, CD16, CD20 and CD56)-negative and HLA-DR+ cells, and they were classified into MDC and PDC by the pattern of CD11c and CD123 expressions. MDC are Lin–/HLA-DR+/CD11c+/CD123^{low} and PDC are Lin–/HLA-DR+/CD11c–/CD123^{high} cells. Early and late progenitors of DC were defined by Lin–/CD34+/CD123+/CD45RA– and Lin–/CD34+/CD123+/CD45RA+ phenotypes, respectively. Based on the percentages of these cells determined by analyses in fluorescence-activated cell sorter, the absolute numbers of DC and their subsets in the blood were calculated by multiplying them by the number of peripheral blood mononuclear cells (PBMC).

Culture of DC

For functional analyses, MDC and PDC were isolated from PBMC by BDCA-1 and BDCA-4 separation kits (Miltenyi Biotec, Bergisch Gladbach, Germany) with some modifications [11]. Sorted MDC and PDC were cultured as reported previously [9]. To analyze cytokine production, MDC at day 3 of culture or fresh PDC were stimulated with human L cells transfected with CD40 ligand or 5 μM CpG oligodeoxynucleotide 2216, respectively. The culture supernatants were collected 24 h after the stimulation and were used for ELISA.

Polarization of Helper T Cell by Subsets of DC

The ability of DC to polarize naive CD4 T cells into Th1 or Th2 was analyzed as reported previously [9]. In brief, DC at day 3 were cultured with allogeneic naive CD4 T cells for an additional 7 days. On day 7, the cells were stimulated with phorbol 12-myristate 13-acetate and ionomycin, and then incubated for 24 h. Thereafter, supernatants of stimulated cells were tested for cytokines by ELISA.

Enzyme-Linked Immunosorbent Assay

Concentrations of cytokines were determined by ELISA with respective pairs of antibodies against human IFN-γ, IL-10 and IL-12 p70 (Endogen, Mass., USA) according to the manufacturer's instructions. IFN-α was determined by ELISA with a commercial kit (BioSource, Camarillo, Calif., USA).

Results

Circulating DC Decreased in Patients with Chronic Hepatitis C

MDC, PDC and their progenitors in the peripheral blood were clearly identified by flow cytometry (data not shown). Numbers of MDC and PDC were lower in patients with chronic hepatitis than in normal controls

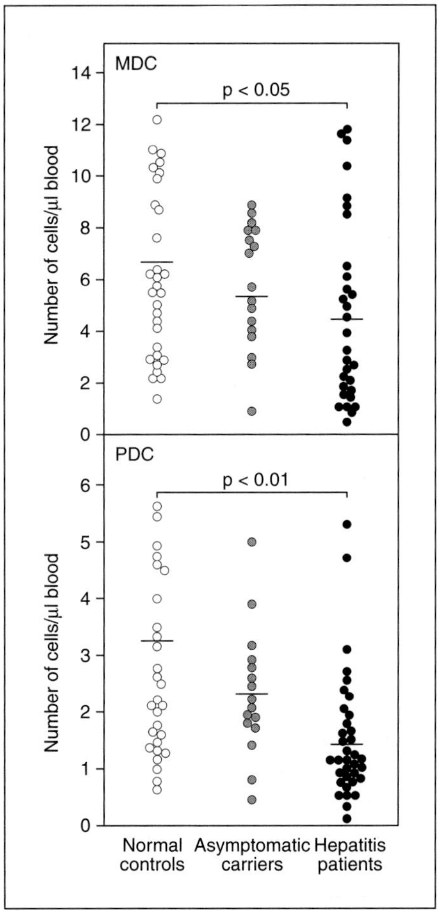

Fig. 1. DC in the circulation. MDC are characterized by Lin–/HLA-DR+/CD11c+/CD123^{low} and PDC by Lin–/HLA-DR+/CD11c–/CD123^{high}. They were determined based on their frequencies in peripheral blood mononuclear cells. Horizontal bars indicate the median. Statistical differences were evaluated by the Mann-Whitney U test.

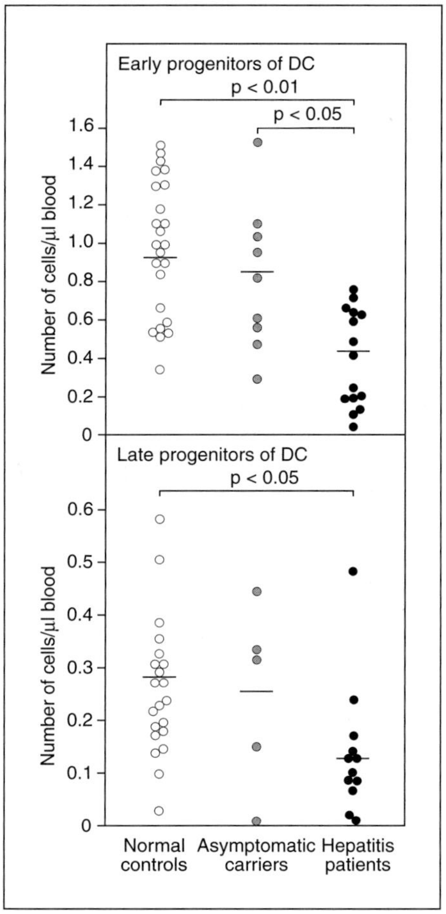

Fig. 2. Progenitors of DC in the circulation. Early and late progenitors of DC are characterized by Lin–/CD34+/CD123+/CD45RA– and Lin–/CD34+/CD123+/CD45RA+, respectively. They were determined based on their frequencies in peripheral blood mononuclear cells. Horizontal bars indicate the median. Statistical differences were evaluated by the Mann-Whitney U test.

(fig. 1). The number of DC tended to be lower in ASC than in normal controls, but the difference fell short of being significant. Numbers of early and late progenitors of DC were significantly lower in patients with chronic hepatitis than in normal controls, whereas they were no different between ASC and normal controls (fig. 2).

Functional Impairment in Subsets of Circulating DC from Patients Infected with HCV

After MDC and PDC had been sorted, we determined IL-12 p70 secreted by MDC and IFN-α by PDC. Upon stimulation, MDC and PDC from patients released these cytokines in less amounts than those from normal controls (fig. 3a). No differences were observed in levels of IL-12 and IFN-α between patients with chronic hepatitis and ASC.

DC prime naive CD4 T cells to differentiate them into two kinds of helper T cells, Th1 and Th2 cells; they produce IFN-γ and IL-10, respectively. MDC from patients infected with HCV were less able to drive the Th1 response than those from normal controls (fig. 3b). Both MDC and PDC from patients with chronic hepatitis primed more IL-10 producers than those from normal controls (fig. 3c). Such dysfunction of DC was also observed in ASC with persistently normal ALT levels. Thus, chronic HCV infection impairs the function of circulating DC toward the polarization of CD4 cells into type I helper T cells.

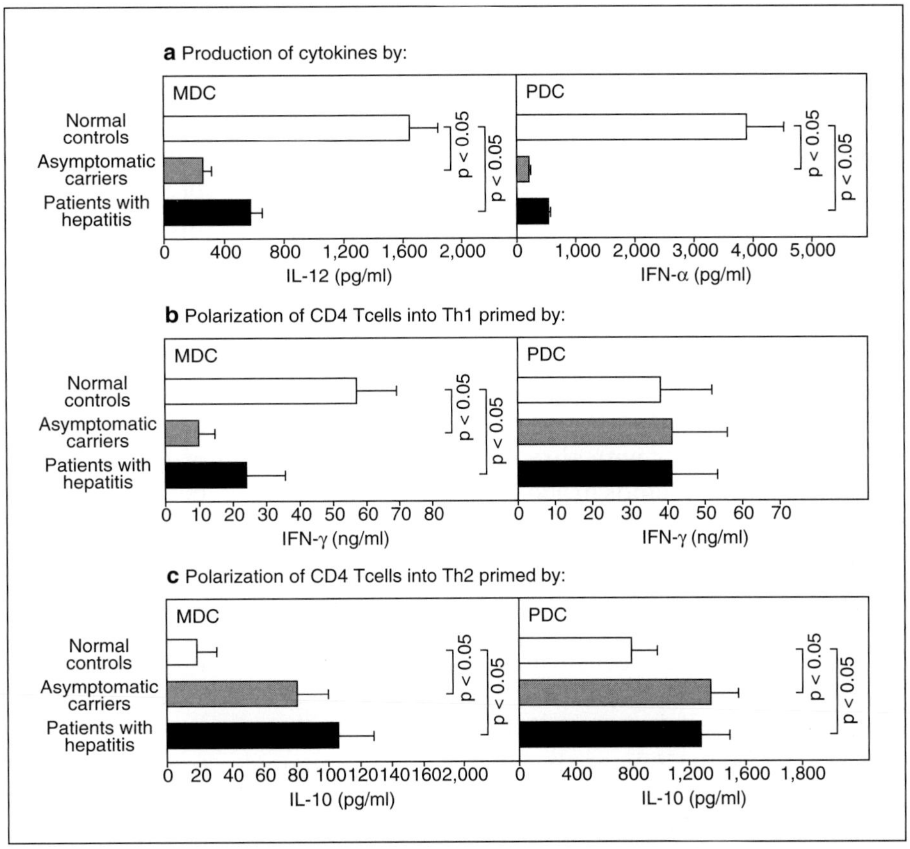

Fig. 3. Functions of MDC and PDC in the circulation. MDC harvested at day 3 of culture were stimulated with L cells expressing CD40 ligand for 24 h. PDC were harvested at day 1 and cultured for 24 h in the presence of 5 μ*M* CpG oligodeoxynucleotide 2216. Supernatants of both cultures were examined for IL-12 p70 and IFN-α by ELISA (**a**). Polarization of CD4 T cells into Th1 (**b**) and Th2 (**c**) primed by DC. MDC or PDC harvested at day 3 were cultured with allogeneic naive CD4 T cells for an additional 7 days. CD4 T cells were stimulated with phorbol 12-myristate 13-acetate and ionomycin for 24 h, and cytokines in supernatants were determined by ELISA. Columns indicate the mean, with a bar representing the SD.

Discussion

DC are well-known central regulators in innate as well as adaptive immune responses [5]. Several studies including our own have demonstrated the dysfunction of DC recovered from PBMC of patients infected with HCV and implicated it in the persistence of HCV infection [2, 8]. Very recently, we reported decreased numbers and impaired function of blood DC in patients with chronic hepatitis C in comparison with normal individuals [9]. In this study, we have extended these results to additional patients with chronic hepatitis. Furthermore, we have demonstrated the reduction in number and the dysfunction of circulating DC subsets in patients infected with HCV, even in those who do not have inflammation in the liver.

The impact of DC numbers on the pathogenesis of virus-related disorders has been well documented in infection with HIV. PDC decrease in parallel with an increase in HIV load as well as the severity of disease [12], suggesting that they would be able to control HIV replication as well as HIV-related disorders. In contrast, no correlation was observed between DC counts and titers of HCV RNA in patients with hepatitis C (data not shown), implying that the number of DC would not be a primary factor influencing the replication of HCV. Patients who had cleared HCV after IFN-α therapy possessed DC in numbers comparable with those of healthy blood donors (unpublished data). Hence, the infection with HCV by itself appears to lessen DC. However, numbers of DC which are lower in patients with active hepatitis than in ASC suggest that inflammation in the liver would decrease DC.

Several explanations are feasible for the mechanism of decreased DC in HCV infection. A hypothesis has been proposed for HCV to infect DC and enhance their susceptibility to apoptosis. In fact, HCV RNA detectable by polymerase chain reaction is reported in MDC or PDC recovered from some chronically infected patients [8, 13]. We have demonstrated that recombinant vesicular stomatitis virus coated with E1 and E2 proteins of HCV (pseudotype HCV) enter MDC but not PDC, suggesting that MDC would be susceptible to HCV infection [14]. Thus, the decreased number and dysfunction of MDC may be induced by HCV infection; however, reasons why PDC function is impaired are still unknown. The next possibility for low numbers of circulating DC is their enhanced mobilization to tissues, which is reported in patients with systemic lupus erythematosus or tuberculosis [15, 16]. Likewise, in HCV infection, DC may migrate from the periphery to inflamed liver or lymphoid tissues, which is supported by our observations that circulating DC decrease in patients with active hepatitis but not in those with normal ALT levels (fig. 1). Finally, the reduction in number of DC progenitors and/or precursors may eventually decrease the DC pool in the blood [9]. Our study has shown that early and late progenitor cells are decreased in patients with chronic hepatitis, but not in ASC (fig. 2), which stands in good agreement with the results of numerical analyses on DC.

Several lines of evidence have clearly demonstrated that a Th1 response is required for the eradication of HCV, either spontaneously or induced by IFN-α therapy [17, 18]. One of the mechanisms for defective Th1 responses to MDC from patients with chronic hepatitis would be a decreased amount of IL-12. Indeed, direct infection of DC with HCV may be involved in the impaired production of IL-12. This view is supported by the finding that the expression of HCV proteins in monocyte-derived DC suppresses the release of IL-12 [19]. Another feature in HCV infection is a strong ability of MDC and PDC to prime T cells producing IL-10, which in turn inhibits the antigen-specific T cell response by suppressing APC function or directly suppresses the ability of MDC for Th1 polarization. Further examination is required to study the mechanism for priming more IL-10-producing cells by PDC from patients than from healthy controls.

Long-term follow-ups of ASC have shown that the progression from hepatitis to cirrhosis is much slower than in patients with active hepatitis C [10]. These observations imply that, even in the presence of HCV, maintenance of a minimal activity of hepatitis would be beneficial for the prevention of HCC. In this respect, it is therapeutically rational to induce the ASC state in patients with chronic hepatitis. In the present study, the striking differences are demonstrated in the DC system, between ASC and patients with active hepatitis, in terms of higher counts of circulating DC and their progenitors. Although it is yet to be determined whether the decrease in circulating DC is the cause or effect of inflammation in the liver, recruitment of DC and/or DC progenitors from bone marrow to the periphery may be beneficial for alleviating liver disease.

Recently, doubts have been cast on the dysfunction of DC in the setting of chronic HCV infection [20]. However, the failure in demonstrating any defects of DC may have been attributable to different populations studied. Further, although functional impairment of DC was observed in some cases, cohort studies on chimpanzees with experimental HCV infection showed that it was not a prerequisite to persistent infection [21]. Evidently, further studies need to be planned and conducted to establish that DC, as a whole or in their subsets, are indeed disabled to promote persistence of HCV after primary infection in the setting of human chronic hepatitis C.

In summary, we have demonstrated that circulating DC from patients with chronic hepatitis C are functionally impaired, not only in those with elevated, but also in those with persistently normal ALT levels. Induction of disabled DC in the circulation may be one of the principle mechanisms for HCV to escape the immune surveillance of hosts, thus leading to the persistence of HCV.

References

1 Houghton M, Weiner A, Han J, Kuo G, Choo QL: Molecular biology of the hepatitis C viruses: Implications for diagnosis, development and control of viral disease. Hepatology 1991; 14:381–388.

2 Kanto T, Hayashi N, Takehara T, Tatsumi T, Kuzushita N, Ito A, Sasaki Y, Kasahara A, Hori M: Impaired allostimulatory capacity of peripheral blood dendritic cells recovered from hepatitis C virus-infected individuals. J Immunol 1999;162:5584–5591.

3 Wedemeyer H, He XS, Nascimbeni M, Davis AR, Greenberg HB, Hoofnagle JH, Liang TJ, Alter H, Rehermann B: Impaired effector function of hepatitis C virus-specific CD8+ T cells in chronic hepatitis C virus infection. J Immunol 2002;169:3447–3458.

4 Chang KM, Thimme R, Melpolder JJ, Oldach D, Pemberton J, Moorhead-Loudis J, McHutchison JG, Alter HJ, Chisari FV: Differential CD4(+) and CD8(+) T-cell responsiveness in hepatitis C virus infection. Hepatology 2001;33:267–276.

5 Liu YJ: Dendritic cell subsets and lineages, and their functions in innate and adaptive immunity. Cell 2001;106:259–262.

6 Fugier-Vivier I, Servet-Delprat C, Rivailler P, Rissoan MC, Liu YJ, Rabourdin-Combe C: Measles virus suppresses cell-mediated immunity by interfering with the survival and functions of dendritic and T cells. J Exp Med 1997; 186:813–823.

7 Chehimi J, Campbell DE, Azzoni L, Bacheller D, Papasavvas E, Jerandi G, Mounzer K, Kostman J, Trinchieri G, Montaner LJ: Persistent decreases in blood plasmacytoid dendritic cell number and function despite effective highly active antiretroviral therapy and increased blood myeloid dendritic cells in HIV-infected individuals. J Immunol 2002;168:4796–4801.

8 Bain C, Fatmi A, Zoulim F, Zarski JP, Trepo C, Inchauspe G: Impaired allostimulatory function of dendritic cells in chronic hepatitis C infection. Gastroenterology 2001;120:512–524.
9 Kanto T, Inoue M, Miyatake H, Sato A, Sakakibara M, Yakushijin T, Oki C, Itose I, Hiramatsu N, Takehara T, Kasahara A, Hayashi N: Reduced numbers and impaired ability of myeloid and plasmacytoid dendritic cells to polarize T helper cells in chronic hepatitis C virus infection. J Infect Dis 2004;190:1919–1926.
10 Persico M, Persico E, Suozzo R, Conte S, De Seta M, Coppola L, Palmentieri B, Sasso FC, Torella R: Natural history of hepatitis C virus carriers with persistently normal aminotransferase levels. Gastroenterology 2000;118:760–764.
11 Dzionek A, Fuchs A, Schmidt P, Cremer S, Zysk M, Miltenyi S, Buck DW, Schmitz J: BDCA-2, BDCA-3, and BDCA-4: Three markers for distinct subsets of dendritic cells in human peripheral blood. J Immunol 2000;165:6037–6046.
12 Donaghy H, Pozniak A, Gazzard B, Qazi N, Gilmour J, Gotch F, Patterson S: Loss of blood CD11c(+) myeloid and CD11c(–) plasmacytoid dendritic cells in patients with HIV-1 infection correlates with HIV-1 RNA virus load. Blood 2001;98:2574–2576.
13 Navas MC, Fuchs A, Schvoerer E, Bohbot A, Aubertin AM, Stoll-Keller F: Dendritic cell susceptibility to hepatitis C virus genotype 1 infection. J Med Virol 2002;67:152–161.
14 Kaimori A, Kanto T, Kwang Limn C, Komoda Y, Oki C, Inoue M, Miyatake H, Itose I, Sakakibara M, Yakushijin T, Takehara T, Matsuura Y, Hayashi N: Pseudotype hepatitis C virus enters immature myeloid dendritic cells through the interaction with lectin. Virology 2004;324:74–83.
15 Farkas L, Beiske K, Lund-Johansen F, Brandtzaeg P, Jahnsen FL: Plasmacytoid dendritic cells (natural interferon-alpha/beta-producing cells) accumulate in cutaneous lupus erythematosus lesions. Am J Pathol 2001;159:237–243.
16 Uehira K, Amakawa R, Ito T, Tajima K, Naitoh S, Ozaki Y, Shimizu T, Yamaguchi K, Uemura Y, Kitajima H, Yonezu S, Fukuhara S: Dendritic cells are decreased in blood and accumulated in granuloma in tuberculosis. Clin Immunol 2002;105:296–303.
17 Kamal SM, Fehr J, Roesler B, Peters T, Rasenack JW: Peginterferon alone or with ribavirin enhances HCV-specific CD4 T-helper 1 responses in patients with chronic hepatitis C. Gastroenterology 2002;123:1070–1083.
18 Gerlach JT, Diepolder HM, Jung MC, Gruener NH, Schraut WW, Zachoval R, Hoffmann R, Schirren CA, Santantonio T, Pape GR: Recurrence of hepatitis C virus after loss of virus-specific CD4(+) T-cell response in acute hepatitis C. Gastroenterology 1999;117:933–941.
19 Sarobe P, Lasarte JJ, Casares N, Lopez-Diaz de Cerio A, Baixeras E, Labarga P, Garcia N, Borras-Cuesta F, Prieto J: Abnormal priming of CD4(+) T cells by dendritic cells expressing hepatitis C virus core and E1 proteins. J Virol 2002;76:5062–5070.
20 Longman RS, Talal AH, Jacobson IM, Albert ML, Rice CM: Presence of functional dendritic cells in patients chronically infected with hepatitis C virus. Blood 2004;103:1026–1029.
21 Rollier C, Drexhage JA, Verstrepen BE, Verschoor EJ, Bontrop RE, Koopman G, Heeney JL: Chronic hepatitis C virus infection established and maintained in chimpanzees independent of dendritic cell impairment. Hepatology 2003;38:851–858.

Hepatocellular Carcinoma

Intervirology

Intervirology 2006;49:64–69
DOI: 10.1159/000087265

Early Detection and Characterization of Hepatocellular Carcinoma: Value of Imaging Multistep Human Hepatocarcinogenesis

Masatoshi Kudo

Department of Gastroenterology and Hepatology, Kinki University School of Medicine, Osaka, Japan

Key Words
Angiography · Computed tomography · Carbon dioxide · Dysplastic nodule hepatitis C virus · Hepatocellular carcinoma · Microbubbles · Ultrasonography

Abstract
The method for early detection of hepatocellular carcinoma (HCC) has been well established in Japan, by means of regularly screening patients at risk for developing HCC by imaging and serological markers of tumor. The principal screening protocol includes performing ultrasonography (US) every 3 months and testing for tumor markers every month in patients at high risk for HCC. There has been another important issue of accurate characterization of nodular lesions found in cirrhotic liver. This problem has been solved by the development of imaging modalities such as US angiography with intra-arterial injection of CO_2, computed tomography during hepatic arteriography and computed tomography during arterial portography. It is most important to differentiate the typical hemodynamic patterns of a low-grade dysplastic nodule having arterial hypovascularity with portal perfusion preserved from those of HCC characterized by arterial hypervascularity with decreased portal perfusion. At present, these findings are easily obtained by contrast-enhanced phase invasion harmonic imaging, which is a noninvasive US technology.

Introduction

Early detection of hepatocellular carcinoma (HCC) is important in improving prognosis of patients. Additionally, differentiation of nodular lesions found in cirrhotic liver is another important issue. In order to correctly characterize such nodular lesions, evaluation of intranodular hemodynamics is of utmost value, since pathological findings and malignancy grades of HCC are closely related to intranodular hemodynamics.

In this article, the methods for early detection of HCC and its differentiation from premalignant and/or borderline lesions are described.

Early Detection of HCC

In Japan, the screening protocol for early detection of HCC has been established during the past 2 decades. The patients with chronic viral hepatitis/liver cirrhosis induced by hepatitis B virus or hepatitis C virus infection are regarded with high risk for developing HCC. Regular follow-ups by ultrasonography (US) every 3 months and measurements of tumor markers including α-fetoprotein, as well as its activity to bind with *Lens culinaris* agglutinin A, and protein induced by vitamin K absence or antagonist-II every month have made it possible to detect HCC in an early stage, especially since 1989 (fig. 1). However, it has brought about another problematic issue: the

KARGER
Fax +41 61 306 12 34
E-Mail karger@karger.ch
www.karger.com

0300–5526/06/0492–0064$23.50/0

Accessible online at:
www.karger.com/int

Masatoshi Kudo, MD
Department of Gastroenterology and Hepatology, Kinki University School of Medicine
377-2, Ohno-Higashi
Osaka-Sayama, Osaka 589-8511 (Japan)
Tel. +81 723 66 0221, ext. 3149, Fax +81 723 67 2880, E-Mail m-kudo@med.kindai.ac.jp

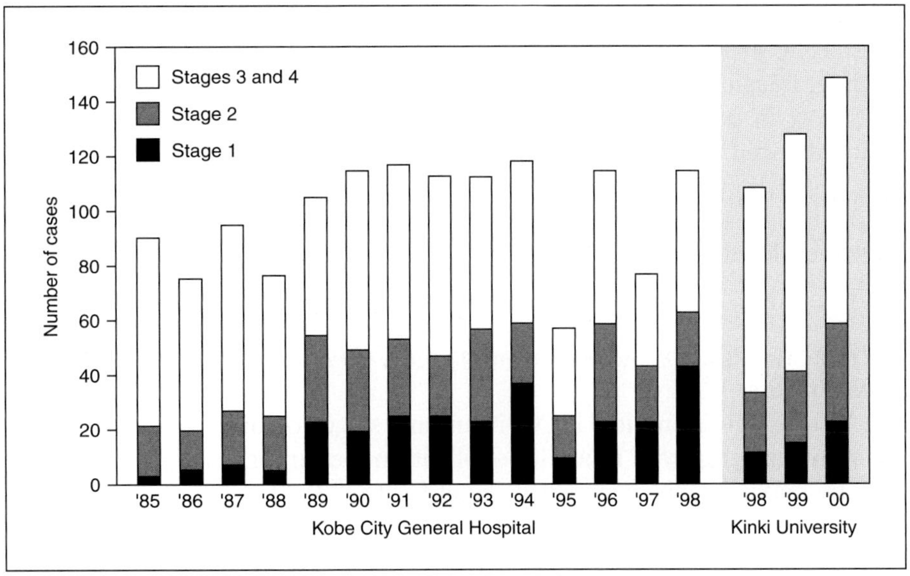

Fig. 1. Yearly trend of HCC in Japan stratified by the stage. Approximately 30–50% of HCCs detected in Japan are in stage I or stage II, presenting with a solitary tumor, and they are in a very early phase of disease.

more frequently US is performed, the more small nodular lesions are detected in the liver. Hence, lesions hardly diagnosed as overt HCC keep increasing with time. This is a very important clinicopathological problem that should be addressed and solved.

Intranodular Hemodynamics and Pathological Differentiation of HCC

As is well known, the biological characteristics of HCC are different from those of other malignant tumors, probably because the liver has dual blood supplies unlike any other organs. The liver parenchyma is supplied by both hepatic artery and portal vein, in contrast to the other organs which are fed only by the artery. The decrease of portal venous flow in the liver may partly affect human hepatocarcinogenesis, since a premalignant lesion has portal flow alone within the nodule, unlike an overt HCC that is perfused only by the hepatic artery [1, 2]. Therefore, intranodular hemodynamics are considered closely related to hepatocarcinogenesis during the multistep development.

Patterns of intranodular hemodynamics evaluated by intranodular hemodynamic imagings, such as US angiography with arterial infusion of CO_2 microbubbles [3, 4] and computed tomography during hepatic arteriography (CTHA), correlate well with the grade of histopathological differentiation (Edmondson-Steiner's grade). As the arterial vascularity increases, it has been shown that the grade of histological differentiation decreases. Therefore, US angiography and CTHA are useful tools in assessing the grade of differentiation of HCC, even when a histological specimen is not available [5, 6]. Portal perfusion within nodular lesions evaluated by CT during arterial portography (CTAP) also correlate well with the pathological differentiation of HCC.

Intranodular Hemodynamics of Overt HCC and Low-Grade Dsyplastic Nodule

Intranodular Hemodynamics of Overt HCC

Since afferent blood vessels of an overt HCC stem from the hepatic artery, intranodular hemodynamics in HCC are characterized by arterial neovascularization and absence of portal venous flow [7]. By contrast, the hemodynamic pattern of a premalignant lesion – low-grade dysplastic nodule (LGDN) – or a borderline lesion manifests itself with a poor arterial vascularity and the presence of portal supply or an increase thereof [1]. The imaging diagnosis of HCC and premalignant lesions is based on such characteristics of intranodular hemodynamics.

Angiography is not always efficient in demonstrating arterial hypovascularity or portal venous flow in small nodules less than 1.5 cm in diameter, as previously reported [8–11]. Rather, US angiography and CTHA are more informative in detecting intranodular arterial vascularity. CTAP is a sensitive tool in detecting portal perfusion within a nodule [12], enabling discrimination of overt HCC from premalignant lesions. Likewise, color Doppler imaging is useful in detecting afferent portal venous flow in premalignant lesions [13]. Recently, contrast-enhanced US with intravenous injection of a contrast agent, Levovist (Schering, Germany), is reported useful in evaluating portal perfusion within the nodule to improve the distinction of LGDN from overt HCC [14].

Hemodynamics of Well-Differentiated HCC in an Early Stage

Most well-differentiated HCCs in an early stage do not stain on angiography or retain lipiodol within the tumor, thereby making their diagnosis difficult [6, 15–23]. It is widely known that some well-differentiated HCCs in an early stage are fed by the portal vein and not by the hepatic artery, unlike typical HCCs (fig. 2) [2, 6, 8, 11, 24–26]. Therefore, some hypovascular HCCs (early-stage HCCs) show no perfusion defects on CTAP and may look like benign nodules with 'benign-appearing' patterns of the vasculature [27]. Color Doppler imaging picks up afferent portal flow signals as well [13, 28]. With the exception of the nodules which have a 'benign-appearing' hemodynamic pattern, the diagnosis of HCC is possible even in its early stage by a combined use of tomographic vascular imagings, including US angiography, CTHA and CTAP [2, 6, 8, 11, 15, 29, 30].

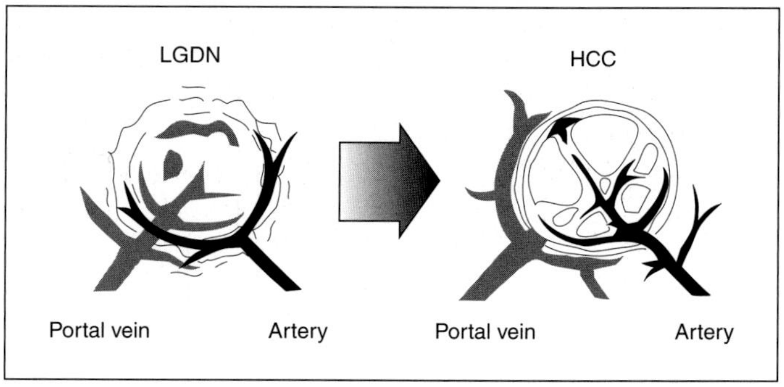

Fig. 2. Schematic presentation of blood supplies shifting from LGDN to HCC.

Intranodular Hemodynamic Transition during Multistep Human Hepatocarcinogenesis: Hypothesis Based on Comparison between Intranodular Hemodynamic Findings and Histopathological Studies

Hepatocarcinogenesis is a multistep process evolving from a hyperplastic nodule (LGDN) through early HCC and eventually leading to advanced overt hypervascular HCC [15, 20, 31–33]. During this process, changes in intranodular hemodynamics occur; they are hypothesized by associating radiologic findings with histopathologic pictures as described earlier [6]. At the initial phase of carcinogenesis, the hemodynamic pattern shows arterial *hypovascularity* with portal perfusion still present (type I). In the next step, both arterial and portal blood supplies decrease (type II). Subsequently, intranodular arterial vascularity increases to *isovascular* pattern (type III) and finally to *hypervascular* pattern (type IV). Another hemodynamic transition occurs from type I to type V (nodule-in-nodule type having partial spots of arterial vascularity in a hypovascular background of portal perfusion) [5, 6, 34, 35].

Fatty metamorphosis is frequently observed in the nodules hemodynamically classified into types II and III. This is attributed to a relative decrease in the blood supply due to diminished portal supply and immature arterial neovascularization [15]. Decreased arterial and portal supplies are supported by pathological evidence for decreased densities of arterial and portal vessels in well-differentiated HCCs in an early stage [36].

Natural Course of Nodular Lesions in Cirrhotic Liver

It has been demonstrated by close observation of the natural course of nodular lesions that an intranodular hemodynamic transition occurs from type I to type II, from type I to type IV and then from type II to type III, before proceeding from type III to type IV during the multistep human hepatocarcinogenesis. In some cases, the transition from type I to type V and that from type V to type IV were observed as well. This sequence has been confirmed by a 5-year clinical follow-up. It has supported the hypothesis that intranodular hemodynamic transition correlates well with pathological dedifferentiation in the clinical setting. It also suggests a possibility for determining the stage of a nodule, in the process of malignant transformation, based on blood supplies visualized by a combination of tomographic vascular imaging techniques. An accurate detection of intranodular hemodynamics by these means would enable us to reliably determine whether it is benign or malignant [5, 27].

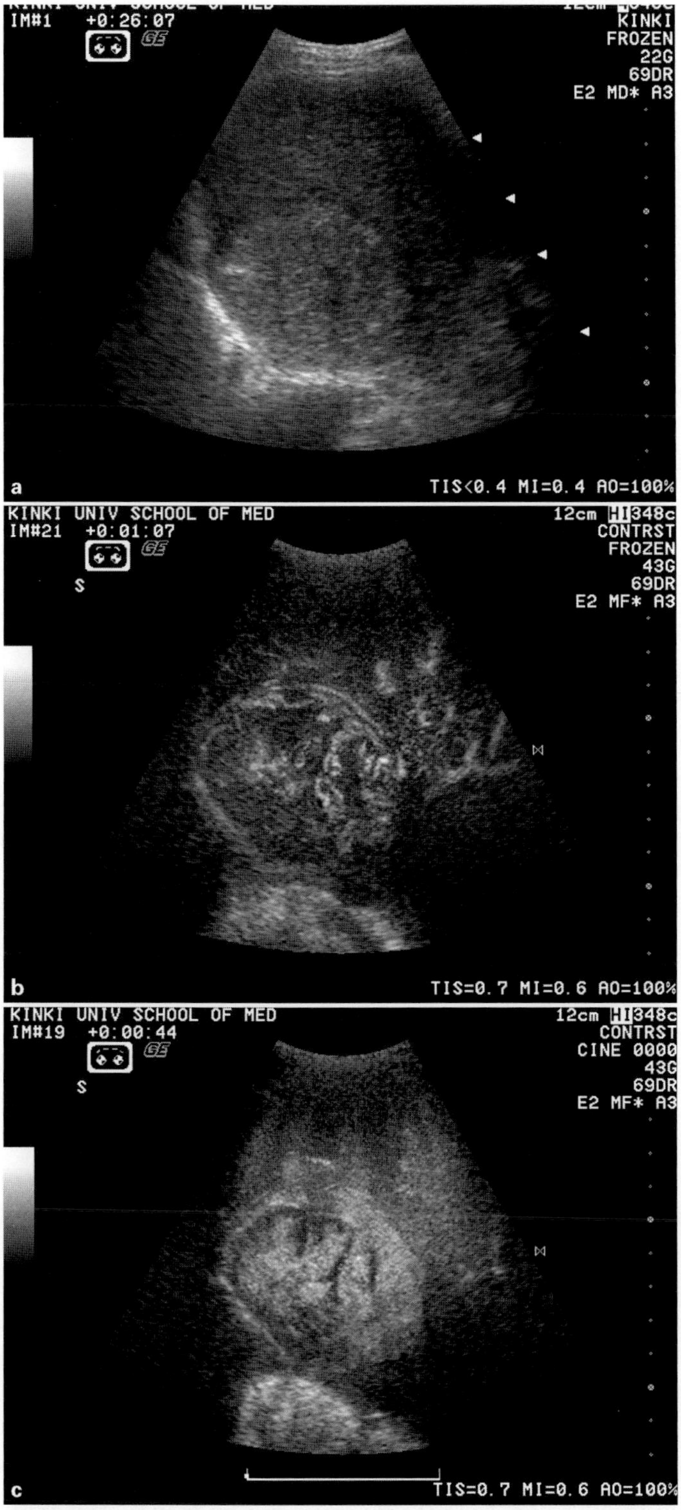

Fig. 3. Harmonic US of a typical HCC. Imagings of plain US (**a**), arterial phase of harmonic US clearly showing tumor vessels within the nodule (**b**) and tumor stain depicted by interval delay scan of harmonic US (**c**) are shown.

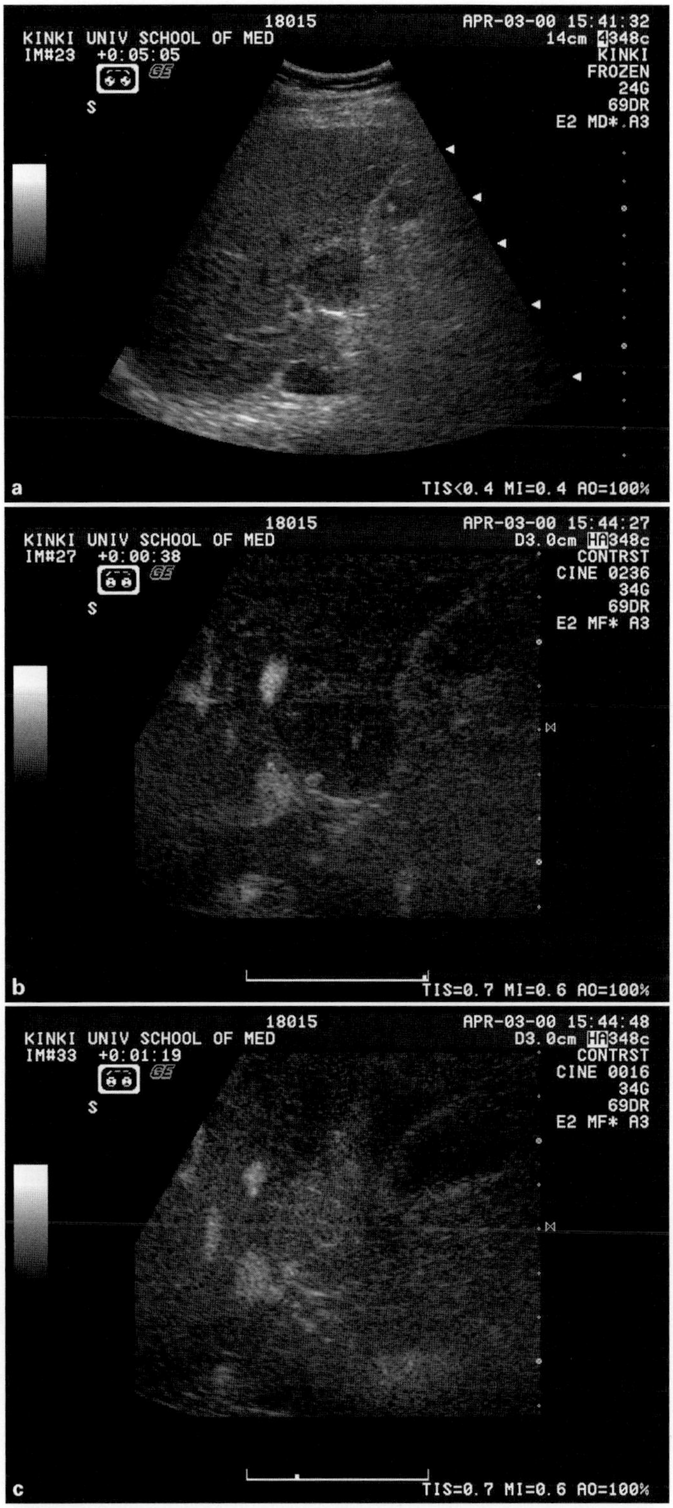

Fig. 4. Harmonic US of typical LGDN. Patterns of plain US (**a**), portal phase of harmonic US clearly showing portal flow within the nodule (**b**) and portal perfusion visualized within the nodule by intermittent scan of harmonic US (**c**) are shown.

Role of Harmonic Imaging in the Characterization of HCC and LGDN

Detection of Arterial and Portal Flows in HCC

Contrast-enhanced harmonic imaging [14, 37–40] detects intratumoral vascularity in more than 95% of HCCs; no blood signals are observed in the remaining 5%. Likewise, 98% of HCC nodules show hyper- and/or isovascularity on dynamic CT. Therefore, the detection rate of intratumoral vascularity is no different between contrast harmonic US and CT [14, 38].

In hypervascular HCCs, contrast-enhanced harmonic US images tumor vessels originating in the periphery, infiltrating into the center of tumors and having irregular branches (fig. 3). Most HCCs show heterogeneous or homogeneous staining of tumor parenchyma, which is hyperechoic on a gray background in comparison with surrounding liver parenchyma. Perfusion defects in the postvascular phase, due to rapid washout from the nodule, are other characteristics of these HCCs [38].

Contrast-enhanced harmonic US pictures most HCCs with the characteristic hemodynamic pattern of HCC. The sensitivity and specificity of this HCC pattern are 92.8 and 92.3%, with positive and negative predictive values of 97.9 and 76.6%, respectively [14, 38].

Low-Grade Dysplastic Nodule

Contrast-enhanced harmonic US in the early arterial phase depicts no blood vessels in any LGDN (fig. 4). In the late vascular phase and postvascular phase, it can detect isovascular staining in 75% and hypervascular staining in 12.5%, pointing to a portal venous supply. However, the remaining LGDN can present with a hypovascular pattern, with portal venous flow demonstrated by CTAP. The sensitivity and specificity of the LGDN pattern are 75 and 100%, with respective positive and negative predictive values of 100 and 99% [38]. In contrast, dynamic CT images low attenuation only in the arterial phase in all the dysplastic nodules; it is accompanied by isoattenuation in the portal and delayed phases in 75% of LGDN. Therefore, the rate of detecting intranodular vascularity in LGDN is comparable between contrast-enhanced harmonic US and dynamic CT [14, 38].

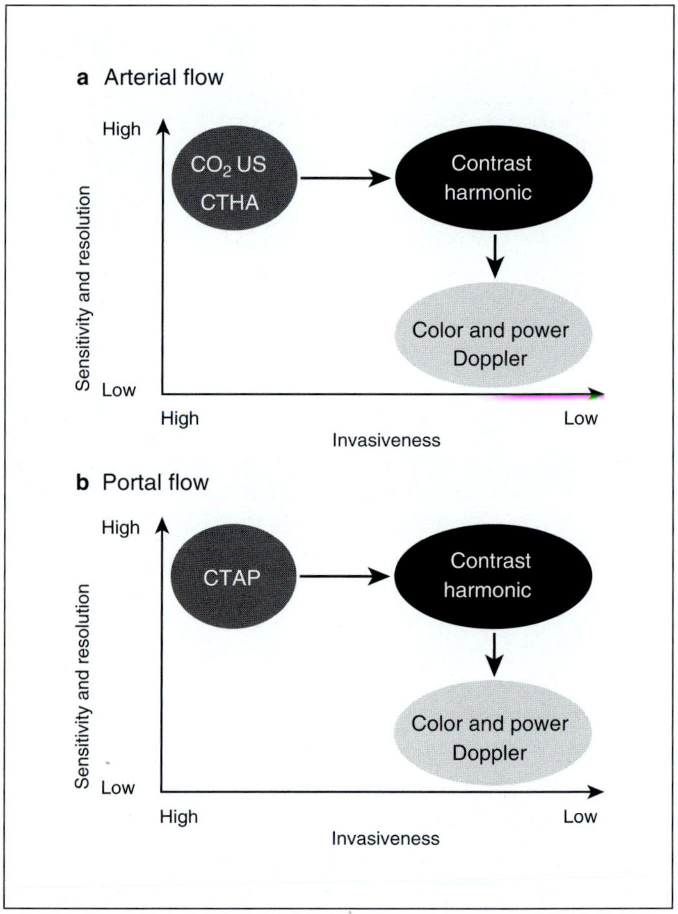

Fig. 5. a Invasiveness in comparison with sensitivity and resolution of imaging modalities for evaluating intranodular hemodynamics of arterial flow. Contrast harmonic imaging is as sensitive as CO_2 US or CTHA and still keeps less invasiveness. **b** Invasiveness in comparison with sensitivity and resolution of imaging modalities for evaluating intranodular hemodynamics of portal flow. Contrast harmonic imaging is as sensitive as CTAP and retains less invasiveness.

Conclusion

Early detection of HCC and accurate characterization of nodular lesions in cirrhotic liver are equally important. In this respect, it is of utmost importance to clearly detect intranodular hemodynamic alterations during multistep human hepatocarcinogenesis by precisely imaging intranodular hemodynamics with the use of invasive techniques including CO_2 US, CTHA and CTAP (fig. 5). Recent remarkable progresses in contrast-enhanced harmonic imaging have made it possible to determine the malignant grade in a high sensitivity, without resort to these invasive methods, which is very auspicious to cirrhotic patients and doctors in the clinical hepatology, especially in coping with frequent HCC development.

References

1 Sasaki K: Adenomatous hyperplasia in liver cirrhosis: An approach from a microangiographical point of view. Gann Monogr Cancer Res 1980;25:127–140.

2 Matsui O, Kadoya M, Kameyama T, Yoshikawa J, Takashima T, Nakanuma Y, Unoura M, Kobayashi K, Izumi R, Ida M, et al: Benign and malignant nodules in cirrhotic livers: Distinction based on blood supply. Radiology 1991;178:493–497.

3 Kudo M, Tomita S, Tochio H, Mimura J, Okabe Y, Kashida H, Hirasa M, Ibuki Y, Todo A: Small hepatocellular carcinoma: Diagnosis with US angiography with intraarterial CO_2 microbubbles. Radiology 1992;182:155–160.

4 Kudo M, Tomita S, Tochio H, Mimura J, Okabe Y, Kashida H, Hirasa M, Ibuki Y, Todo A: Sonography with intraarterial infusion of carbon dioxide microbubbles (sonographic angiography): Value in differential diagnosis of hepatic tumors. AJR Am J Roentgenol 1992; 158:65–74.

5 Kudo M: Imaging diagnosis of hepatocellular carcinoma and premalignant/borderline lesions. Semin Liver Dis 1999;19:297–309.

6 Kudo M, Tomita S, Kashida H, Mimura J, Okabe Y, Hirasa M, Ibuki Y, Komori H, Orino A, Todo A: Tumor hemodynamics in hepatic nodules associated with liver cirrhosis. Relationship between cancer progression and tumor hemodynamic change (in Japanese). Jpn J Gastroenterol 1991;88:1554–1565.

7 Nakashima T, Kojiro M: Angioarchitecture of hepatocellular carcinoma; in Nakashima T, Kojiro M (eds): Hepatocellular Carcinoma: An Atlas of Its Pathology, ed 1. Tokyo, Springer, 1997, pp 107–109.

8 Takayasu K, Muramatsu Y, Mizuguchi Y, Moriyama N, Ojima H: Imaging of early hepatocellular carcinoma and adenomatous hyperplasia (dysplastic nodules) with dynamic CT and a combination of CT and angiography: Experience with resected liver specimens. Intervirology 2004;47:199–208.

9 Sumida M, Ohto M, Ebara M, Kimura K, Okuda K, Hirooka N: Accuracy of angiography in the diagnosis of small hepatocellular carcinoma. AJR Am J Roentgenol 1986;147:531–536.

10 Yoshimatsu S, Inoue Y, Ibukuro K, Suzuki S: Hypovascular hepatocellular carcinoma undetected at angiography and CT with iodized oil. Radiology 1989;171:343–347.

11 Matsui O: Imaging of multistep human hepatocarcinogenesis by CT during intra-arterial contrast injection. Intervirology 2004;47:271–276.

12 Matsui O, Kadoya M, Suzuki M, Inoue K, Itoh H, Ida M, Takashima T: Work in progress: Dynamic sequential computed tomography during arterial portography in the detection of hepatic neoplasms. Radiology 1983;146:721–727.

13 Tochio H, Kudo M: Afferent and efferent vessels of premalignant and overt hepatocellular carcinoma: Observation by color Doppler imaging. Intervirology 2004;47:144–153.

14 Kudo M: Contrast Harmonic Imaging in the Diagnosis and Treatment of Hepatic Tumors. Springer, Tokyo, 2003.

15 Kudo M, Tomita S, Tochio H, Hamada M, Mimura J, Okabe Y, Kashida H, Hirasa M, Ibuki Y, Komori H, Orino A, Tani T, Kajiwara T, Hayashi M, Ishikawa T, Shirane H, Uchida H, Todo A: Hemodynamic characteristics of early stage hepatocellular carcinoma. In vivo evaluation with vascular imagings (in Japanese). Acta Hepatol Jpn 1992;33:283–291.

16 Kojiro M, Sugihara S, Nakashima O: Pathomorphologic characteristics of early hepatocellular carcinoma. Gann Monogr Cancer Res 1991;38:S29–S37.

17 Okuda K: Early recognition of hepatocellular carcinoma. Hepatology 1986;6:729–738.

18 Okuda K: Hepatocellular carcinoma: Recent progress. Hepatology 1992;15:948–963.

19 Choi B, Takayasu K, Han MC: Small hepatocellular carcinomas and associated nodular lesions of the liver. Pathology, pathogenesis, and imaging findings. Am J Roentgenol 1993;160: 1177–1187.

20 Muramatsu Y, Nawano S, Takayasu K, Moriyama N, Yamada T, Yamasaki S, Hirohashi S: Early hepatocellular carcinoma: MR imaging. Radiology 1991;181:209–213.

21 Sakamoto M, Hirohashi S, Shimosato Y: Early stages of multistep hepatocarcinogenesis: Adenomatous hyperplasia and early hepatocellular carcinoma. Hum Pathol 1991;22:172–178.

22 Krinsky G: Imaging of dysplastic nodules and small hepatocellular carcinomas: Experience with explanted livers. Intervirology 2004;47: 191–198.

23 Murakami T, Hori M, Kim T, Kawata S, Abe H, Nakamura H: Multidetector row CT and MR imaging in diagnosing hepatocellular carcinoma. Intervirology 2004;47:209–226.

24 Yoshimitsu K, Irie H, Aibe H, Tajima T, Nishie A, Asayama Y, Matake K, Nakayamka T, Kakihara D, Honda H: Pitfalls in the imaging diagnosis of hepatocellular nodules in the cirrhotic and noncirrhotic liver. Intervirology 2004;47:238–251.

25 Takayasu K, Wakao F, Moriyama N, Muramatsu Y, Sakamoto M, Hirohashi S, Makuuchi M, Kosuge T, Takayama T, Yamazaki S: Response of early-stage hepatocellular carcinoma and borderline lesions to therapeutic arterial embolization. AJR Am J Roentgenol 1993; 160:301–306.

26 Kudo M: Morphological diagnosis of hepatocellular carcinoma: Special emphasis on intranodular hemodynamic imaging. Hepatogastroenterology 1998;45(suppl 3):1226–1231.

27 Kudo M: Atypical large well-differentiated hepatocellular carcinoma with benign nature: A new clinical entity. Intervirology 2004;47: 227–237.

28 Kudo M, Tochio H, Zhou P: Differentiation of hepatic tumors by color Doppler imaging: Role of the maximum velocity and the pulsatility index of the intratumoral blood flow signal. Intervirology 2004;47:154–161.

29 Yamashita Y, Morishita S, Awai K, Kawanaka K: Imaging of the liver by helical CT and MR imaging. Intervirology 2004;47:125–133.

30 Ito K, Mitchell DG: Imaging diagnosis of cirrhosis and chronic hepatitis. Intervirology 2004;47:134–143.

31 Takayama T, Makuuchi M, Hirohashi S, Sakamoto M, Okazaki N, Takayasu K, Kosuge T, Motoo Y, Yamazaki S, Hasegawa H: Malignant transformation of adenomatous hyperplasia to hepatocellular carcinoma. Lancet 1990;336:1150–1153.

32 Kim SR, Hayashi Y, Kudo M, Imoto S, Song KB, Ando K, Shintani S, Koterazawa T, Kim KI, Taniguchi M: TTV positivity and transfusion history in non-B, non-C hepatocellular carcinoma compared with HBV- and HCV-positive cases. Intervirology 2000;43:13–15.

33 Kim SR, Hayashi Y, Kudo M, Matsuoka T, Imoto S, Song KB, Maekawa Y: Hepatocellular carcinoma transforming from dysplastic nodule with background of non-B non-C chronic persistent hepatitis. J Hepatol 2000;33:857–858.

34 Kojiro M: 'Nodule-in-nodule' appearance in hepatocellular carcinoma: Its significance as a morphologic marker of dedifferentiation. Intervirology 2004;47:179–183.

35 Zheng RQ, Zhou P, Kudo M: Hepatocellular carcinoma with nodule-in-nodule appearance: Demonstration by contrast-enhanced coded phase inversion harmonic imaging. Intervirology 2004;47:184–190.

36 Kutami R, Nakashima Y, Nakashima O, Shiota K, Kojiro M: Pathomorphologic study on the mechanism of fatty change in small hepatocellular carcinoma of humans. J Hepatol 2000;33:282–289.

37 Wen YL, Zhou P, Kudo M: Detection of intratumoral vascularity in small hepatocellular carcinoma by coded phase inversion harmonics. Intervirology 2004;47:169–178.

38 Wen YL, Kudo M, Zheng RQ, Ding H, Zhou P, Minami Y, Chung H, Kitano M, Kawasaki T, Maekawa K: Characterization of hepatic tumors: Value of contrast-enhanced coded phase-inversion harmonic angio. AJR Am J Roentgenol 2004;182:1019–1026.

39 Minami Y, Kudo M, Kawasaki T, Kitano M, Chung H, Maekawa K, Shiozaki H: Transcatheter arterial chemoembolization of hepatocellular carcinoma: Usefulness of coded phase-inversion harmonic sonography. AJR Am J Roentgenol 2003;180:703–708.

40 Choi BI, Lee JY, Han JK, Lee JM, Kim SH: Contrast-enhanced sonography for hepatocellular carcinoma. Intervirology 2004;47:162–168.

Hepatocellular Carcinoma

Intervirology

Intervirology 2006;49:70–75
DOI: 10.1159/000087266

Current Status of Hepatitis C Virus Infection in Korea

Dong Jin Suh[a] Sook-Hyang Jeong[b]

[a]Division of Gastroenterology, Department of Internal Medicine, Asan Medical Center, University of Ulsan College of Medicine, Seoul, and [b]Division of Gastroenterology, Department of Internal Medicine, Seoul National University, Bundang Hospital, Gyeonggido, Korea

Key Words
Genotypes · Hepatitis B virus · Hepatitis C virus · Hepatocellular carcinoma · Korea

Abstract
Chronic liver disease, including liver cirrhosis and hepatocellular carcinoma (HCC), has been a major cause of mortality in Korea. The prevalence rates of hepatitis C virus (HCV) and hepatitis B virus (HBV) infections in the general population of Korea are approximately 1 and 5%, respectively. The most common genotypes of HCV in Korea are 1b and 2a. The sustained virological response rates after antiviral therapies, including combined interferon-α and ribavirin, have been reported to be 38–59%. The annual incidence of HCC among HCV-related liver cirrhosis has been estimated at 5%, and approximately 12% of HCC is attributable to HCV and 68% to HBV in Korea. The mean age of patients with HCV-related HCC at the time of diagnosis was consistently 10 years older than that of patients with HBV-related HCC. Moreover, HCV-related HCC was accompanied by more advanced liver cirrhosis than HBV-related HCC. Coinfection with HBV seemed to increase the risk of developing HCC in chronic HCV infection. After the successful program of hepatitis B vaccination, HCV infection is now emerging as an important etiology of chronic liver disease in Korea, which warrants more detailed and large-scale studies.

Introduction

Hepatitis C virus (HCV) is a major public health problem, with about 170 million people infected with it, corresponding to approximately 3% of the world population. HCV causes a high rate of chronic infection, resulting in severe complications of chronic liver disease [1]. In Korea, chronic liver disease, including chronic hepatitis, liver cirrhosis and hepatocellular carcinoma (HCC), accounted for approximately 10% of total deaths in 2002, with a mortality rate of 45.1/100,000 people. It is the leading cause of death for men in their forties, and mortality due to HCC mounts to 17.7% of total cancer deaths in Korea [2].

The major etiologic agents of chronic liver disease in Korea have been hepatitis B virus (HBV) and HCV. However, early development of hepatitis B vaccine and the successful immunization program during the past 20 years have significantly reduced the prevalence of hepatitis B surface antigen (HBsAg) among the general population from 10 to 5%. Decrease in the HBsAg carrier rate among children has been so remarkable that it is now rather difficult to detect carriers in pediatric clinics. Moreover, a reduction of the incidence of HCC among adult vaccinees has been reported, confirming that hepatitis B vaccine is effective for prevention of HCC [3]. Since 1991, the Korean Red Cross has adopted an anti-HCV test for screening blood donors. Although the prevalence of anti-HCV seems to have been stable for the past 5 years, the relative importance of HCV as an etiology of chronic liver disease is expected to increase in Korea.

KARGER

Fax +41 61 306 12 34
E-Mail karger@karger.ch
www.karger.com

0300–5526/06/0492–0070$23.50/0

Accessible online at:
www.karger.com/int

Sook-Hyang Jeong, MD
Department of Internal Medicine, Seoul National University, Bundang Hospital
300 Gumi-dong, Seongnam-si
Gyeonggi-do 463-707 (Korea)
Tel. +82 31 787 7034, Fax +82 31 787 4052, E-Mail jsh@snubh.org

Here, we give an overview of HCV infection in Korea, with respect to its prevalence, etiologic role in liver cirrhosis and HCC, viral, immunological and clinical characteristics as well as the response to antiviral therapy in patients with chronic HCV infection.

Prevalence of HCV Infection in Korea

Prevalence of Anti-HCV in Blood Donors, Pregnant Women and Children

The estimated positive rate of anti-HCV tested by the third-generation enzyme immunoassay (EIA) among 2,040,151 Korean blood donors has been reported at 0.34% in 1997 (table 1). About half of the donors with anti-HCV were positive, measured by the confirmatory immunoblot test. There were some geographic differences ranging from 0.08 to 0.74%, with the highest prevalence in the southern harbor area and western harbor cities [4]. The prevalence of anti-HCV among 10,644 pregnant women was 0.89% by the second-generation EIA in the Pusan area where anti-HCV was most frequently detected in Korea. About one third of pregnant women with anti-HCV were positive for HCV RNA [5]. The prevalence of anti-HCV among 2,080 children (elementary school students) was 0.82% by the third-generation EIA in 1996. Only 6% of children with anti-HCV were positive for HCV RNA. In contrast to the anti-HCV prevalence, the prevalence of HBsAg among these children was zero [6].

Prevalence of Anti-HCV in Health Check Examinees

Park et al. [7] reported that among 21,291 adult health check examinees, the prevalence of anti-HCV changed slightly from 1.1 to 0.8% during 1997–2001, and the prevalence of HBsAg decreased from 7 to 5.2%. In their study, the prevalence of anti-HCV was not significantly different between men and women, while the prevalence of HBsAg was significantly higher in men than in women. The peak prevalence of anti-HCV was observed at the age of 60 or older, in contrast to the peak prevalence of HBsAg occurring in their forties. Among examinees positive for anti-HCV, 47% revealed abnormal liver function tests. Generally, the prevalence of anti-HCV in health check examinees was higher than that in blood donors, because a large proportion of blood donors were young military men, and history taking before blood donation might be able to screen out donors at high risk for HCV infection.

Table 1. Prevalence of anti-HCV in Korea

Subject	n	Year	Anti-HCV, %	Generation of EIA
Blood donors	2,040,151	1997	0.34	3rd
Health check examinees	6,790	2001	2.1	3rd
	21,291	2003	0.9	3rd
Pregnant women	10,644	1995	0.89	2nd
Children	2,080	1996	0.82	3rd
Hemophiliacs	104	2002	42.3	3rd
Patients on hemodialysis	224	1997	14.7	2nd
Leprotics	96	1997	67.7	2nd
Injection drug user	185	1997	80.0	2nd

Data retrieved from references [4–11].

Prevalence of Anti-HCV in High-Risk Groups

Hemophiliacs have a very high risk of HCV infection. The prevalence of anti-HCV determined by the third-generation EIA in 104 hemophiliacs was 42.3%, while the prevalence of HBsAg was 5.2%. The risk of HCV infection was significantly related to age of the patients and the severity of hemophilia [8].

The frequency of anti-HCV in 96 leprous patients examined by the second-generation EIA was 67.7%, in contrast to only 5.5% prevalence of HBsAg. Among anti-HCV-positive leprous patients, 82% were confirmed by the immunoblot assay, and this remarkably high prevalence might be related to the high frequency of skin lesions and incompetent immune response [9].

Bang et al. [10] reported that the prevalence of anti-HCV among patients with end-stage renal disease on hemodialysis in Korea was 13.7%, while that of HBsAg was 12.6%. Follow-up of 902 end-stage renal disease patients who received renal transplantation during 15 years showed that the 5-year survival rate among the HBsAg-positive group (72%) was significantly lower than that of the anti-HCV-positive group (92%) or the HBsAg-negative and anti-HCV-negative (non-B, non-C) group (94%). Reasons for such differences would include that the mortality related to liver disease is significantly higher in HBsAg-positive than in anti-HCV-positive or in non-B, non-C patients.

Recently, injection drug use has become the most common risk factor of HCV infection. Although injection drug use has not been common in Korea so far, Kim and Choo [11] reported anti-HCV prevalence in 80% of 185 drug abusers, in contrast to prevalence of HBsAg and anti-HIV in 4 and 0%, respectively.

Table 2. Clinical characteristics of Korean patients with hepatocellular carcinoma (HCC) who received surgical resection of HCC

Features	HBsAg positive	Anti-HCV positive	Both positive	Both negative	p value
Number of patients	275 (67%)	62 (15%)	13 (3%)	61 (15%)	
Mean age ± SD	50 ± 9*	62 ± 6*	53 ± 12	54 ± 11	0.001*
Serum albumin, g/dl	3.7 ± 0.4*	3.5 ± 0.3*	3.8 ± 0.4	3.8 ± 0.4	0.006*
Prothrombin time, %	91 ± 14*	83 ± 16*	90 ± 10	95 ± 13	0.001
ICG R_{15}[a], %	9 ± 8*	19 ± 9*	10 ± 10	7 ± 5	0.001
Mean tumor size, cm	4.6 ± 3.0*	3.5 ± 2.6*	4.8 ± 2.5	5.6 ± 3.6	0.005
Major hepatectomy[b], %	18*	5*	8	26	0.01
Survival at 5 years, %	54*	58	32*	60	0.029

Data retrieved from Kim et al. [16]. * Significance between groups.
[a] Indocyanine green retention rate at 15 min. [b] Lobectomy or more than lobectomy.

Risk Factors of HCV Infection

A case-control study on the risk factors of HCV infection among Koreans showed that transfusion was the main route of transmission, while operation, acupuncture, endoscopy, tooth extraction, tattooing and ear piercing were not associated with an increased risk [12]. The family history of hepatitis was not found to be significantly associated with HCV infection in this study, although other studies revealed a significantly high prevalence of anti-HCV (12.2–16.1%) among spouses of the index patients increasing with the duration of marriage.

Etiologic Role of HCV in Chronic Liver Disease

HCV in Liver Cirrhosis

Of the patients with liver cirrhosis, 56% were HBsAg-positive (HBV-related), 10% were anti-HCV-positive (HCV-related), 3% were both HBsAg- and anti-HCV-positive (coinfection with HBV and HCV) and 31% were non-B, non-C. About 90% of non-B, non-C cirrhotics were heavy alcohol drinkers. At the time of diagnosis, the mean age of patients with HBV-related cirrhosis was consistently 10 years younger than that of patients with HCV-related cirrhosis. This difference may be explained by the time of HBV infection during the perinatal period in the majority of Korean patients, in contrast to the time of HCV infection during adulthood. About one third of HCV-related cirrhotics were heavy alcohol drinkers, and diabetes mellitus was significantly associated with HCV-related liver cirrhosis [13].

HCV in HCC

The annual incidence of HCC was about 5% among HCV-related cirrhosis, 4% among HBV-related cirrhosis and 1% among non-B, non-C-related cirrhosis [13]. In Korea, approximately 64–70% of HCC were HBV related, 12–17% HCV related, 1.5–8% coinfected with HBV and HCV, and 16–18% were of a non-B, non-C etiology (fig. 2) [14]. We could detect occult viremia with HBV in 20% and with HCV in 16% of patients with non-B, non-C HCC [15].

In surgically resected HCC, HCV-related cases were found to accompany more advanced cirrhosis with a less functional reservoir of the liver than HBV-related cases, which prevented the majority of patients with HCV-related HCC from major liver resection, despite the mean tumor size smaller than that in HBV-related HCC (table 2). Tumor stage, presence of portal vein invasion and overall postoperative survival were not significantly different between HCV-related and HBV-related HCC [16]. The pattern of proteome expression closely reflected etiologic factors of HCC, suggesting the molecular mechanism of hepatocarcinogenesis different between HBV- and HCV-related HCC [17].

Virological Characteristics of HCV in Korea

HCV Genotypes

The most common HCV genotypes among the Korean patients with HCV-related chronic liver disease were genotype 1b (40–59%) and 2a (33–52%) (fig. 1) [18–20].

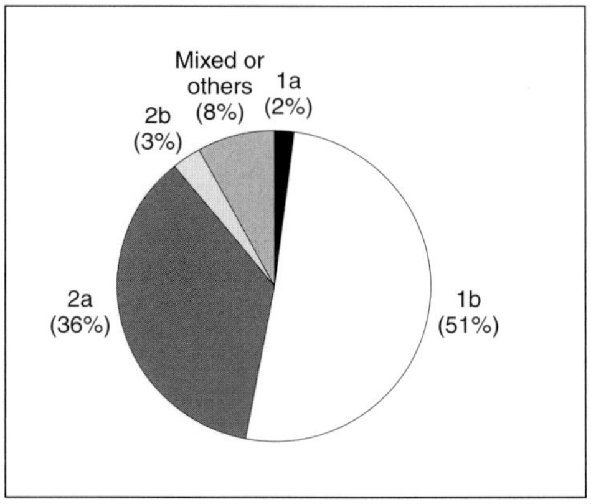

Fig. 1. Distribution of HCV genotypes in Korea. Data were adopted from references [18, 19].

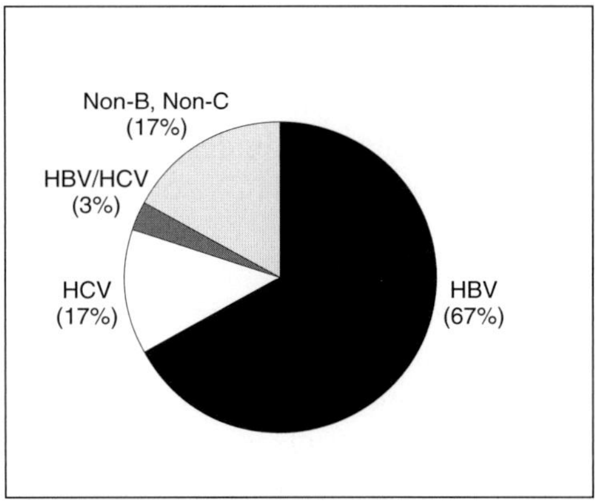

Fig. 2. The etiology of HCC in Korea. Data were adopted from references [13, 14].

There was no association between HCV genotype and disease severity. The patients' age, gender and the route of transmission were not significantly different among patients infected with HCV of distinct genotypes. However, serum levels of HCV RNA were significantly higher in the patients with genotype 1 than with genotype 2a infection [19].

Coinfection of HBV, Hepatitis G Virus or TT Virus with HCV Infection

Among anti-HCV-positive patients, coinfection with HBV diagnosed as HBsAg positive and anti-HCV positive was predominantly observed in HCC patients compared with non-HCC patients, including those with chronic hepatitis and liver cirrhosis as well as healthy carriers. When the risk factors associated with HCC were evaluated by multivariate analysis in comparison with non-HCC among the anti-HCV-positive patients, age (more than 50 years), male gender, HCV RNA and HBV DNA were found to be significant risk factors. The presence of serum HBV DNA showed the strongest association with HCC with an odds ratio of 83.5, suggesting that coinfection with HBV was a significant risk factor for the development of HCC in chronic HCV infection. About two thirds of coinfected patients had HBV viremia, about half had HCV viremia and one third had viremia with both HBV and HCV, reflecting a complicated replication status of each virus by viral interference and interaction [21].

Hepatitis G virus RNA and TT virus DNA were detected in 10.5 and 21.1% of patients with chronic hepatitis C. However, coinfection of either hepatitis G virus or TT virus with chronic HCV infection did not affect the severity of liver disease [22].

Immunological Characteristics of HCV Infection in Korea

Proliferation of Peripheral Lymphocytes and Pattern of Cytokine Production

Since HCV is not considered directly cytopathic in immune-competent hosts, the immune response would play a major role in the pathogenesis of chronic liver disease. When the proliferation of peripheral blood mononuclear cells (PBMCs) from 32 patients with HCV-related chronic liver disease was examined after in vitro stimulation with HCV core protein and NS3 protein, about 60% showed positive proliferation response (stimulation index >3) to NS3 protein and 15% to HCV core protein, while none of the healthy controls and patients infected with HBV showed positive response [23]. After stimulation with HCV NS3 and core proteins, PBMCs from about 60 and 30% of the patients were found to produce interferon (IFN)-γ, while the production of IL-4 was hardly detected, suggesting that NS3 protein was more immunogenic than core protein and that a Th1-biased cytokine profile was dominant in HCV-related chronic liver disease. Interestingly, when PBMCs were stimulated with a combination of HCV core and NS3 proteins, the proliferation response was significantly decreased compared with that after the stimulation with NS3 alone. The inhibition of a proliferative response by core protein was also observed when PBMCs were stimulated with phytohemagglutinin and core protein. The addition of core protein resulted in a marked dose-dependent reduction of the phytohemagglutinin stimulation index. This result was consistent with those of other studies, which have shown that HCV core protein interacts with the complement receptor (gC1qR) and suppresses T cell proliferation [24]. Lee et al. [25] also reported that the HCV core protein inhibits the production of IL-12 in activated macrophages, which could be a mechanism underlying the inhibition of T cell proliferation by the HCV core protein.

Autoantibodies in HCV Infection

HCV infection is associated with a wide range of extrahepatic manifestations, such as cryoglobulinemia, glomerulonephritis and sicca syndrome. Lee et al. [26] reported that 29 of the 49 (59%) patients with chronic hepatitis C had cryoglobulinemia, all of type III. Rheumatoid factors and antinuclear antibodies were detected in sera from 18–25% and 3.4–25% of patients with chronic hepatitis C. However, there were no differences in demographic features, liver function tests, HCV genotypes, antiviral response or rheumatological symptoms between autoantibody-positive and -negative patients. Therefore, the presence of autoantibodies does not seem to have any definite clinical significance, albeit HCV infection may cause unexplained rheumatological symptoms.

Results of Antiviral Therapy for HCV

The rate of sustained virological response (SVR) in Korean patients with chronic hepatitis C after treatment with IFN-α alone was less than 20%. The response rate significantly increased to 38–59% with a combination therapy of IFN-α and ribavirin. The predictive factors for SVR were viral genotype and pretreatment level of HCV RNA in serum. About 15% of treated patients had to discontinue the therapy, and about one third needed a reduction of the drug dose because of side effects [27–29]. Pegylated IFN with or without ribavirin is ongoing in a clinical trial and seems promising, gaining an early virological response at 12 weeks after the start of treatment.

Liver transplantation from living donors is actively performed in Korea. In a large transplantation center, only 16 of the 587 (2.7%) patients with liver transplants were found with HCV-related liver disease. After liver transplantation, reappearance of HCV RNA was detected in 91% of the recipients accompanied by histological recurrence of hepatitis in 50%. One recipient among the 16 patients with HCV infection died of fibrosing cholestatic hepatitis at 14 weeks after transplantation [30].

Conclusion

In this article, we presented an overview of HCV infection in Korea. The prevalence of HCV infection in the general population of Korea was about 1%, with common viral genotypes 1b and 2a. Approximately 15% of HCC were attributable to HCV infection, and the annual incidence of HCC in HCV-related liver cirrhosis was 5%. The patients with HCV-related HCC were 10 years older than those with HBV-related HCC at the time of diagnosis. HCV-related HCC seems to accompany more advanced cirrhosis and less reservoir of liver function than HBV-related HCC. Proteome expression profiles were also different between HCV-related and HBV-related HCC. Peripheral blood lymphocytes from two thirds of patients with HCV-related chronic liver disease exhibited proliferation response to NS3 protein along with Th1-biased cytokine production. SVR after combined IFN-α and ribavirin therapy reached about 45%, and factors predictive of the response were viral genotype and HCV RNA level in serum.

All in all, clinical features and the response to antiviral therapies of chronic HCV infection in Korea do not seem significantly different from those in other countries, although large-scale studies in more details need to be conducted. After the successful immunization program for HBV, HCV infection is emerging as an important etiology of chronic liver disease in Korea. In order to work out the standard approach to diagnostic, therapeutic and preventive care, the Korean Association for the Study of the Liver is now preparing the practice guideline for treatment of chronic hepatitis C.

References

1 Memon MI, Memon MA: Hepatitis C: An epidemiological review. J Viral Hepat 2002;9:84–100.
2 Korean National Statistical Office: Annual report on the causes of death statistics (in Korean). Seoul, Korean National Statistical Office, 2004.
3 Lee MS, Kim DH, Kim H, Lee HS, Kim CY, Park TS, Yoo KY, Park BJ, Ahn YO: Hepatitis B vaccination and reduced risk of primary liver cancer among male adults: A cohort study in Korea. Int J Epidemiol 1998;27:316–319.
4 Oh HB, Hwang YS, Cho YJ, Kim DS, Kim SI: Experience of anti-HCV antibody immunoblot test in Korean blood donors (in Korean). Korean J Blood Transfus 1997;8:1–8.
5 Park SJ, Lee EJ, Chun CH, Jeon SS, Kim H: The prevalence of anti-HCV in pregnant women and results on HCV-PCR (in Korean). Korean J Clin Pathol 1995;15:487–494.

6 Lee JM, Yoo HS, Jang UK, Kim DJ, Kim YB, Kim HY, Park CK, Yoo JY: The prevalence of anti-HCV positivity in healthy Korean children (in Korean). Korean J Hepatol 1996;2:160–165.

7 Park KS, Lee YS, Lee SG, Hwang JU, Chung WJ, Cho KB, Hwang HS, Ahn SH, Park SK: A study on markers of viral hepatitis in adults living in Daegu and Gyungbuk area (in Korean). Korean J Gastroenterol 2003;41:473–479.

8 Kim SY, Kook JH, Choi IS, Kim SJ, Kook H, Hwang TJ: Viral hepatitis and change of lymphocyte subpopulation in hemophiliacs in Chonnam Kwangju area (in Korean). Korean J Blood Transfus 2002;13:43–51.

9 Choi SH: The prevalence of hepatitis C virus infection in leprous patients (in Korean). Korean J Gastroenterol 1997;30:486–494.

10 Bang BK, Choi BS, Kim HW, Kim SK, Yang CW, Kim YS, Kim SY, Choi EJ, Chang YS: Retrospective study on the impact of hepatitis B and hepatitis C virus infection on renal transplantation recipients over 15 years (in Korean). Korean J Nephrol 2002;21:423–434.

11 Kim HS, Choo DH: Prevalence of hepatitis C, B, and human immunodeficiency virus among drug users and chronic alcoholic patients in Korea (in Korean). Korean J Intern Med 1997;52:754–762.

12 Kim YS, Ahn YO, Kim DW: A case-control study on the risk factors of hepatitis C virus infection among Koreans. J Korean Med Sci 1996;11:38–43.

13 Kim YS, Um SH, Ryu HS, Lee JB, Lee JW, Park DK, Jin YT, Chun HJ, Lee HS, Lee SW, Choi JH, Kim CD, Hyun JH: The prognosis of liver cirrhosis in recent years in Korea. J Korean Med Sci 2003;18:833–841.

14 Lee HS, Han CJ, Kim CY: Predominant etiologic association of hepatitis C virus with hepatocellular carcinoma compared with hepatitis B virus in elderly patients in a hepatitis B-endemic area. Cancer 1993;72:2564–2567.

15 Cho HH, Kim YH, Jun JM, Cho KW, Cho SH, Choi DH, Jeong SH, Lee JH, Han CJ, Kim YC, Lee JO, Kim CM: Clinical characteristics of Non-B, non-C hepatocellular carcinoma and detection of HBV, HCV and TTV viremia (in Korean). Korean J Hepatol 2001;7:439–448.

16 Kim SB, Sub KS, Lee MK, Lee KW, Lee KU: Comparison of the clinicopathologic features and surgical outcomes of hepatocellular carcinoma related with hepatitis B and C (in Korean). Korean J HBP Surg 2000;4:62–66.

17 Kim W, Oe Lim S, Kim JS, Ryu YH, Byeon JY, Kim HJ, Kim YI, Heo JS, Park YM, Jung G: Comparison of proteome between hepatitis B virus- and hepatitis C virus-associated hepatocellular carcinoma. Clin Cancer Res 2003;9:5493–5500.

18 Han CJ, Lee HS, Kim HS, Choe JH, Kim CY: Hepatitis C virus genotypes in Korea and their relationship to clinical outcome in type C chronic liver diseases. Korean J Intern Med 1997;12:21–27.

19 Lee GC, Kim HG, Park NH, Won SY, Chung YH, Lee YS, Suh DJ: Distribution of hepatitis C virus genotypes determined by line probe assay in Korean patients with chronic HCV infection (in Korean). Korean J Hepatol 1998;4:244–253.

20 Lee DS, Sung YC, Whang YS: Distribution of HCV genotypes among blood donors, patients with chronic liver disease, hepatocellular carcinoma, and patients on maintenance hemodialysis in Korea. J Med Virol 1996;49:55–60.

21 Hong HJ, Kwag JY, Lee YW, Lee SW, Lee EJ, Cho JA, Jeong SH, Han CJ, Kim YD, Kim CM, Lee JO: The role of hepatitis B infection in the development of hepatitis C virus-related hepatocellular carcinoma (in Korean). Korean J Gastroenterol 2000;35:82–92.

22 Jeon MJ, Shin JH, Suh SP, Lim YC, Ryang DW: TT virus and hepatitis G virus infections in Korean blood donors and patients with chronic liver disease. World J Gastroenterol 2003;9:741–744.

23 Jeong SH, Yang MJ, Lee KH, Yun YS, Choi YH: Immune response of peripheral blood mononuclear cells to core and NS3 protein in chronic hepatitis C infection (in Korean). Korean J Hepatol 2001;7:292–298.

24 Kittlesen DJ, Chianese-Bullock KA, Yao ZQ, Braciale TJ, Hahn YS: Interaction between complement receptor gC1qR and hepatitis C virus core protein inhibits T-lymphocyte proliferation. J Clin Invest 2000;106:1239–1249.

25 Lee CH, Choi YH, Yang SH, Lee CW, Ha SJ, Sung YC: Hepatitis C virus core protein inhibits interleukin 12 and nitric oxide production from activated macrophages. Virology 2001;279:271–279.

26 Lee YH, Ji JD, Yeon JE, Byun KS, Lee CH, Song GG: Cryoglobulinaemia and rheumatic manifestations in patients with hepatitis C virus infection. Ann Rheum Dis 1998;57:728–731.

27 Choi WH, Paik SW, Choi MS, Lee JH, Ko KC, Yoo BC: Treatment of hepatitis C naïve patients according to EASL recommendations in Korea (abstract in Korean). Korean J Hepatol 2003;99:S53.

28 Yun BC, Kim HJ, Kim KS, Yoo HD, Lee SU, Han BS: Therapeutic efficacy of combination therapy with alpha interferon and ribavirin in chronic hepatitis C (in Korean). Korean J Gastroenterol 2001;37:203–209.

29 Suh DJ, Park NH, Chung YH, Lee YS: Efficacy of combination of interferon alpha2a, ribavirin and UDCA in the treatment of chronic hepatitis C (in Korean). Korean J Hepatol 1998;4:109–119.

30 Oh KB, Lee SG, Lee YJ, Park KM, Hwang S, Kim KU, Ahn CS, Moon DB, Chu CW, Yang HS, Ha TY, Cho SH: Recurrence and management of hepatitis C after liver transplantation (in Korean). Korean J Hepatol 2003;9:180–187.

Hepatocellular Carcinoma

Intervirology

Intervirology 2006;49:76–81
DOI: 10.1159/000087267

Viral Etiology of Hepatocellular Carcinoma and HCV Genotypes in Taiwan

Chuan-Mo Lee[a] Chao-Hung Hung[a] Sheng-Nan Lu[a] Jing-Houng Wang[a] Hung-Da Tung[a] Wu-Shiung Huang[a] Chao-Long Chen[b] Wei-Jen Chen[c] Chi-Sin Changchien[a]

[a]Division of Hepatogastroenterology, Department of Internal Medicine, and Departments of [b]Surgery and [c]Pathology, Kaohsiung Chang Gung Memorial Hospital, Kaohsiung, Taiwan, ROC

Key Words
Genotypes · Hepatitis C virus · Hepatocellular carcinoma · Interferon

Abstract
Etiologic variations of hepatocellular carcinoma (HCC) exist in different geographic areas of the world. Hepatitis B virus infection is associated with HCC. However, hepatitis C virus (HCV) infection plays an increasingly more important role in the development of HCC and is associated with more than 30% of HCC in Taiwan. The prevalence of HCV infection and HCV genotypes vary in different geographic areas. The prevalence of HCV genotype 1b (HCV-1b) was around 50–70% in Taiwan and even varied in different townships. In addition to host factors, HCV genotypes may be associated with the development of HCC. In our study, the prevalence of HCV-1b in patients with HCC was significantly higher than in those with liver cirrhosis and chronic hepatitis; multivariate analysis revealed that the disease severity was significantly correlated with age and HCV-1b. Furthermore, HCV-1b was associated with a lower response rate to interferon (IFN) therapy than HCV-2. Our study has demonstrated that mutations in the IFN sensitivity-determining region, spanning nucleotides 2,209–2,248 in the NS5A region, correlate with the sustained virological response to combination therapy with IFN and ribavirin in patients with chronic HCV-1b infection in Taiwan. A third-generation enzyme immunoassay for antibody to HCV can be used to predict viremia and monitor the virological response.

Introduction

Worldwide, hepatocellular carcinoma (HCC) is one of the most common malignancies and a major cause of cancer death [1]. Chronic hepatitis B virus (HBV) infection has been well documented for its major role in the development of HCC [1]. Chronic infection with hepatitis C virus (HCV) has been causally associated with HCC as well [2–4]. The prevalence of anti-HCV in HCC patients varies considerably in distinct regions of the world from 6.2 to 75% [5, 6]. Localized areas endemic for HCV have also been reported in Japan, Egypt and Cameroon [7–9].

Prevalence of Chronic HCV Infection and HCV-Related HCC in Taiwan

In the general adult population of Taiwan, the rate of HBV carriers is 15–20% [10] and the prevalence of anti-HCV around 1–5% [11, 12]. In some villages, more than

KARGER
Fax +41 61 306 12 34
E-Mail karger@karger.ch
www.karger.com

0300–5526/06/0492–0076$23.50/0

Accessible online at:
www.karger.com/int

Chuan-Mo Lee, MD
Division of Hepatogastroenterology, Department of Internal Medicine
Kaohsiung Chang Gung Memorial Hospital
123 Ta Pei Road, Kaohsiung, Taiwan (ROC)
Tel. +886 7 7317123, Fax +886 7 7322402, E-Mail chmolee@ms15.hinet.net

50% of the population is positive for anti-HCV [13, 14]. In Taiwan, 80% of HCC was reported to be related to HBV infection [10], and 10–30% of HCC was documented to be anti-HCV positive [4, 15, 16].

In our previous study in southern Taiwan, we collected data of HCC patients from Paisha and Tzukuan townships where both HBV and HCV are endemic and found that HCV was the main cause of HCC in the Tzukuan township [17]. Furthermore, we analyzed data of HCC patients from the Kaohsiung Chang Gung Memorial Hospital in southern Taiwan and the Linko Chang Gung Memorial Hospital in northern Taiwan and found that the prevalence of anti-HCV in male patients in Chiayi county was much higher than that of Taiwan as a whole (52 vs. 27%) [4]. Recently, Lu et al. [17] studied HCC patients from seven medical centers scattered from southern to northern Taiwan and found the highest prevalence of HCV-related HCC around the Chiayi areas (Chiayi county, Chiayi city, Yunlin county and Tainan county) at 40–50%. The lowest was found in Taitung county and Taoyuan county, which was below 20% (unpublished data).

So far, chronic HBV infection has played a major role in the development of HCC in Taiwan [4, 10, 11, 13–16]. It is quite possible that HCV will replace HBV in the induction of HCC within the next one or two decades, because we have been carrying on with both a national vaccination program for preventing HBV infection [18] and blood donor screening for HBV, HCV and HIV. Lu et al. [17] found that the mortality due to liver cancer increased in the last two decades in Taiwan, while the rate of HBV-related HCC decreased (unpublished data). In total, the number of estimated cases of HBsAg-positive HCC is almost the same as before, but that of HBsAg-negative HCC has increased. The majority of HBsAg-negative HCC is related to HCV, which means that HCV-related HCC has increased in the last two decades.

Unfortunately, illegal medical services (such as the use of nondisposable needles as well as sharing syringes and fluid for injection) are still offered in Taiwan, which may spread HCV infection [14, 19, 20]. Chronic HCV infection can result in cirrhosis and HCC 20 and 30 years after the transmission through transfusion [21]. The mechanism of hepatocarcinogenesis induced by chronic HCV infection is still unclear. Unlike HBV that integrates into the host's DNA, HCV may not have direct carcinogenic effects and cause HCC as a consequence of cirrhosis or chronic necroinflammation [22].

Prevalence of HCV Genotypes and Their Influence on the Progression of Liver Disease

Major cofactors of disease progression in chronic hepatitis C are: age at infection, male gender, HBV/HIV coinfection, alcohol intake, iron overload, steatosis, obesity, smoking and genetic as well as viral factors [3]. The viral factor includes quasispecies and genotypes of HCV.

There are 6 major HCV genotypes separated by a sequence divergence in the entire genome exceeding 30%. Different HCV genotypes are prevalent in different geographical areas [23–25]. Thus, genotypes 1, 2 and 3 are widely distributed throughout the United States, Europe and the Far East (Japan, China, Taiwan and Thailand). Other genotypes are geographically more restricted, with type 4 found predominantly in Central Africa, the Middle East and Egypt, type 5 mainly in South Africa and type 6 principally in Hong Kong and Southeast Asia [24].

In previous studies utilizing reverse transcription polymerase chain reaction (RT-PCR) with type-specific primers [26–28], 58–73% of HCV isolates from northern Taiwan were found to be genotype 1b and 7.4–16.5% genotype 2a [27–29], while around 48–64.3% were genotype 1b and 35–41% genotype 2a in southern Taiwan [27, 30].

Some studies demonstrated HCV genotypes in association with the development of HCC [29, 31], while other reports have argued against this [32, 33]. We investigated the prevalence and clinical implication of HCV genotypes in 491 patients positive for both anti-HCV and HCV RNA and 263 patients with chronic hepatitis proven histologically or cytologically, including 98 with cirrhosis and 130 with HCC from southern Taiwan (unpublished data). Using an HCV line probe assay for genotyping (INNO-LiPA HCV, Innogenetics, Ghent, Belgium), HCV genotypes were mainly genotype 1b (46.4%), followed by 2a (31.0%) and 2b (7.3%). There were trends for genotype 1b to increase with age and disease severity. The frequency of genotype 1b in patients with HCC (66.9%) was significantly higher than that in patients with cirrhosis (48.7%) or chronic hepatitis (43.3%). Using the multiple logistic regression analysis, disease severity was significantly associated with age and genotype 1b. The predominance of genotype 1b in the elderly and specific properties of HCV genotypes may be responsible for disease progression related to HCV genotypes. Large-scale studies and long-term follow-up are needed to clarify this hypothesis.

HCV Genotypes and Treatment Response

Interferon (IFN) is widely used for the treatment of chronic HCV infection and reported to have a preventive effect on the development of HCC, especially in patients with sustained virological and biochemical responses [34–37]. IFN-α or pegylated (peg)-IFN-α in combination with ribavirin is the currently available and approved therapy for chronic hepatitis C [38–41]. IFN-α monotherapy has accomplished sustained virological response (SVR) in only about 15–25% of treated patients, whereas combination therapy with IFN and ribavirin has doubled it. Two recent randomized controlled trials in large scales have demonstrated that combined peg-IFN-α and ribavirin is superior to the standard IFN-α and ribavirin, achieving SVR in 56–63% of treated patients [40, 41].

Not only is the cost of combination therapy with IFN and ribavirin high, but it has several adverse effects as well. Therefore, it is important to identify a reliable predictor of the response to combination therapy. Several factors predictive of the response to IFN therapy have been evaluated, such as age, duration of disease, histological changes, pretreatment virus load, HCV RNA at week 12 and genotypes [42–44]. In general, patients infected with HCV-2 and HCV-3 respond better to IFN-α than those with HCV-1 [44, 45]. Genotype 1b has also been associated with increased severity and progression of chronic liver disease [31, 45]. Thus, it is important to identify predictors of IFN response in patients infected with HCV-1b.

Effects of IFN-α are mediated through diverse inducible cellular proteins, typified by double-stranded RNA-activated protein kinase (PKR) [46]. In turn, the activated PKR phosphorylates the α-subunit of the eukaryotic translation initiation factor (eIF-2α) which inhibits protein synthesis, thereby blocking viral replication in a way nonspecific for the virus [46]. So far, at least two distinct HCV proteins, NS5A and the second envelope protein (E2), are found with a potential to block the IFN-induced PKR, and therefore, they might interfere with the response to IFN therapy [46, 47]. Previous data obtained from Japanese patients suggested that the response to IFN in individuals infected with HCV-1b would be correlated with the amino acid sequence stretching nucleotides (nt) 2,209–2,248 in the NS5A region, which was named 'interferon sensitivity-determining region' (ISDR) [48]. However, results from the United States and Europe did not support such a correlation [49–51].

Combination therapy with IFN or peg-IFN and ribavirin has been considered the most effective in treatment of chronic HCV infection. Addition of ribavirin is very useful to achieve virus eradication in patients who initially respond to IFN, but it has gained limited effects in nonresponders. Thus, the responsiveness to IFN is the major determinant of outcome, even for combined IFN and ribavirin [52]. In our previous study, the mean number of amino acid substitutions in the PKR-binding domain of NS5A (nt 2,209–2,274), ISDR and the PKR-eIF-2α phosphorylation homology domain (nt 659–670) in patients with and without SVR was 4.53 ± 3.31 versus 2.83 ± 1.78 ($p = 0.094$), 2.45 ± 2.74 versus 1.03 ± 1.32 ($p = 0.042$) and 0.25 ± 0.70 versus 0.03 ± 0.17 ($p = 0.109$), respectively [53]. Patients with a mutant-type NS5A-ISDR having ≥ 4 amino acid substitutions gained SVR (67%, 6/9) more frequently ($p = 0.038$) than those with the wild type (23%, 5/22). Stepwise multiple logistic regression analysis of possible influencing factors (age, gender, viral load, cirrhosis rate, IFN dosage and amino acid substitutions) has revealed that the mutation in NS5A-ISDR (substitutions ≥ 4 vs. <4) was the only independent variable in treatment outcomes. Our data have shown that NS5A-ISDR mutations correlate with SVR to combined IFN and ribavirin in patients with chronic HCV-1b infection in Taiwan. These data stand in agreement with the study by Sarrazin et al. [54] who reported a correlation between a mutant type of ISDR and SVR in European patients receiving combined therapy with IFN and ribavirin. However, controversy still exists regarding the association between ISDR and response to IFN plus ribavirin [55–57].

Anti-HCV for Predicting Viremia and Monitoring Treatment Efficacy

Anti-HCV detected by enzyme immunoassays (EIAs) decreases or disappears after HCV RNA has been cleared from serum in treated or spontaneously resolved infection. In our data, subjects (10.7%) with sample/cut-off (S/CO) values less than or equal to 10 tended to have resolved a past infection or had nonspecific reaction, whereas most subjects with S/CO above 40 possessed a concurrent or persistent infection [58]. To date, the gold standard for accurate evaluation of the response to antiviral therapies in patients with chronic hepatitis C is still lacking. Negative HCV RNA by RT-PCR at 6 months after the completion of IFN is frequently used as a surrogate marker of virological response, since the overall likelihood of late (>18 months) biochemical relapse in sustained virological responders is only 8.7% [59]. Many variations in PCR assays for HCV RNA have been described, while the standardization of these assays has been difficult [60]. Intensive training of qualified clinical technicians, appropriate quality control measures and proficient testing are necessary to ensure the accuracy of PCR. On the other hand, EIAs are easy to use with less costs. They can be partly or fully automated and are easily adapted to testing in a large scale. In our previous studies, in which we used the ratio of 9-month to 6-month anti-HCV titers as an index and a receiver operator characteristic curve analysis with the cut-off point at 90%, we could differentiate sustained virological responders from nonresponders with a sensitivity and specificity of 91.7 and 90.9% 3 months after the end of treatment [61]. The titer by this third-generation anti-HCV EIA decreased progressively in sustained virological responders, and therefore, this assay may be used for monitoring and predicting the response to antiviral treatments.

Conclusion

There are variations in the etiology of HCC in different areas in Taiwan. HCV infection has recently taken an increasingly more important role in the development of HCC in Taiwan. Genotypes in 60–70% of HCV isolates from northern Taiwan are reported to be genotype 1b, while around 50% from southern Taiwan were genotype 1b and 30–41% genotype 2a. HCV-1b was associated with HCC in Taiwan. The anti-HCV S/CO ratio determined by a newly developed third-generation EIA can be used to predict viremia and is related to SVR. Patients with HCV-1b infection had a response rate lower than that in patients with HCV-2a infection. NS5A mutations are associated with the response to combination therapy with IFN and ribavirin.

Acknowledgments

This study was supported by research grants CMRP 1131 from the Chang Gung Memorial Hospital and PMRP 2057 from the Department of Health of Executive Yuan of Taiwan to C.-M.L.

References

1 Beasley RP: Hepatitis B virus as the etiologic agent in hepatocellular carcinoma: Epidemiological consideration. Hepatology 1982;2:S21–S26.

2 Hasan F, Jeffers LJ, De Medina M, Reddy KR, Parker T, Schiff ER, Houghton M, Choo QL, Kuo G: Hepatitis C-associated hepatocellular carcinoma. Hepatology 1990;12:589–591.

3 Hassan MM, Hwang LY, Hatten CJ, Swaim M, Li D, Abbruzzese JL, Beasley P, Patt YZ: Risk factors for hepatocellular carcinoma: Synergism of alcohol with viral hepatitis and diabetes mellitus. Hepatology 2002;36:1206–1213.

4 Lee CM, Lu SN, Changchien CS, Yeh CT, Hsu TT, Tang JH, Wang JH, Lin DY, Chen CL, Chen WJ: Age, gender, and local geographic variations of viral etiology of hepatocellular carcinoma in a hyperendemic area for hepatitis B virus infection. Cancer 1999;86:1143–1150.

5 Dazza MC, Meneses LV, Girard PM, Astagneau P, Villaroel C, Delaporte E, Larouze B: Absence of a relationship between antibodies to hepatitis C virus and hepatocellular carcinoma in Mozambique. Am J Trop Med Hyg 1993;48:237–242.

6 Bruix J, Barrera JM, Calvet X, Ercilla G, Costa J, Sanchez-Tapias JM, Ventura M, Vall M, Bruguera M, Bru C, Castillo R, Rodes J: Prevalence of antibodies to hepatitis C virus in Spanish patients with hepatocellular carcinoma and hepatic cirrhosis. Lancet 1989;ii:1004–1006.

7 Kiyosawa K, Tanaka E, Sodeyama T, Yoshizawa K, Yabu K, Furuta K, Imai H, Nakano Y, Usuda S, Uemura K, Furuta S, Watanabe Y, Watanabe J, Fukuda Y, Takayama T: Transmission of hepatitis C in an isolated area in Japan: Community-acquired infection. Gastroenterology 1994;106:1596–1602.

8 Abdel-Wahab MF, Zakaria S, Kamel M, Abdel-Khaliq MK, Mabrouk MA, Salama H, Esmat G, Thomas DL, Strickland GT: High seroprevalence of hepatitis C infection among risk groups in Egypt. Am J Trop Med Hyg 1994;51:563–567.

9 Louis FJ, Maubert B, Le Hesran JY, Kemmegne J, Delaporte E, Louis JP: High prevalence of anti-hepatitis C virus antibodies in a Cameroon rural forest area. Trans R Soc Trop Med Hyg 1994;88:53–54.

10 Tong MJ, Sun SC, Schaeffer BT, Chang NK, Lo KJ, Peters RL: Hepatitis-associated antigen and hepatocellular carcinoma in Taiwan. Ann Intern Med 1971;75:687–691.

11 Chen DS, Kuo GC, Sung JL, Lai MY, Sheu JC, Chen PJ, Yang PM, Hsu HM, Chang MH, Chen CJ, Hahn, LC, Choo QL, Wang TH, Houghton M: Hepatitis C virus infection in an area hyperendemic for hepatitis B and chronic liver disease: The Taiwan experience. J Infect Dis 1990;162:817–822.

12 Sheu JC, Wang JT, Wang TH, Wang CY, Yang PM, Huang GT, Shih LN, Lee HS, Chen DS: Prevalence of hepatitis C viral infection in a community in Taiwan. Detection by synthetic peptide-based assay and polymerase chain reaction. J Hepatol 1993;17:192–198.

13 Lu SN, Chue PY, Chen HC, Wu MH, Chen IL, Huang JF, Wang JH, Peng CF, Shih CH, You SL, Lu CF, Chen CJ, Chang WY: Different viral aetiology of hepatocellular carcinoma between two hepatitis B and C endemic townships in Taiwan. J Gastroenterol Hepatol 1997;12:547–550.

14 Wang JH, Lu SN, Wu JC, Huang JF, Yu ML, Chen SC, Chuang WL: A hyperendemic community of hepatitis B virus and hepatitis C virus infection in Taiwan. Trans R Soc Trop Med Hyg 1999;93:253–254.

15 Lee SD, Lee FY, Wu JC, Hwang SJ, Wang SS, Lo KJ: The prevalence of anti-hepatitis C virus among Chinese patients with hepatocellular carcinoma. Cancer 1992;69:342–345.

16 Liaw YF, Chien RN, Sheen IS, Lin DY, Lin HH, Chu CM: Hepatitis C virus infection in patients with chronic liver diseases in an endemic area for hepatitis B virus infection. Gastroenterol Jpn 1991;26:S167–S169.
17 Lu SN, Lee CM, Changchien CS, Chen CJ: Excess mortality from hepatocellular carcinoma in an HCV-endemic township of an HBV-endemic country (Taiwan). Trans R Soc Trop Med Hyg 1999;93:600–602.
18 Chang MH, Chen CJ, Lai MS, Hsu HM, Wu TC, Kong MS, Liang DC, Shau WY, Chen DS: Universal hepatitis B vaccination in Taiwan and the incidence of hepatocellular carcinoma in children. N Engl J Med 1997;336:1855–1859.
19 Chang SJ, Chen HC, Ying J, Lu CF, Ko YC: Risk factors of hepatitis C virus infection in a Taiwanese aboriginal community. Kaohsiung J Med Sci 1996;12:241–247.
20 Lu SN, Chue PY, Chen IL, Wang JH, Huang JF, Peng CF, Shih CH, Chang WY: Incidence of hepatitis C infection in a hepatitis C endemic township in southern Taiwan. Kaohsiung J Med Sci 1997;13:605–608.
21 Tong MJ, el-Farra NS, Reikes AR, Co RL: Clinical outcomes after transfusion-associated hepatitis C. N Engl J Med 1995;332:1463–1466.
22 Zignego AL, De Carli M, Monti M, Careccia G, La Villa G, Giannini C, D'Elios MM, Del Prete G, Gentilini P: Hepatitis C virus infection of mononuclear cells from peripheral blood and liver infiltrates in chronically infected patients. J Med Virol 1995;47:58–64.
23 Simmonds P: Clinical relevance of hepatitis C virus genotypes. Gut 1997;40:291–293.
24 Agha S, Tanaka Y, Saudy N, Kurbanov F, Abo-Zeid M, El-Malky M, Khalaf M, Ohta N, Yoshizawa H, Mizokami M: Reliability of hepatitis C virus core antigen assay for detection of viremia in HCV genotypes 1, 2, 3, and 4 infected blood donors: A collaborative study between Japan, Egypt, and Uzbekistan. J Med Virol 2004;73:216–222.
25 McOmish F, Yap PL, Dow BC, Follett EA, Seed C, Keller AJ, Cobain TJ, Krusius T, Kolho E, Naukkarinen R, Lin C, Lai C, Leong S, Medgyesi GA, Hejjas M, Kiyokawa H, Fukada K, Cuypers T, Saeed AA, Al-Rasheed AM, Lin M, Simmonds P: Geographical distribution of hepatitis C virus genotypes in blood donors: An international collaborative survey. J Clin Microbiol 1994;32:884–892.
26 Okamoto H, Tokita H, Sakamoto M, Horikita M, Kojima M, Iizuka H, Mishiro S: Characterization of the genomic sequence of type V (or 3a) hepatitis C virus isolates and PCR primers for specific detection. J Gen Virol 1993;74:2385–2390.
27 Wu JS, Lee HF, Hsiau HL, Lu HY, Chou WH, Lu CF, Chen HY, Lee FN, Chen PY, Tam KM: Genotype distribution of hepatitis C virus infection in Taiwan. J Med Virol 1994;44:74–79.
28 Chan CY, Lee SD, Hwang SJ, Lu RH, Lu CL, Lo KJ: Quantitative branched DNA assay and genotyping for hepatitis C virus RNA in Chinese patients with acute and chronic hepatitis C. J Infect Dis 1995;171:443–446.
29 Chen CH, Sheu JC, Wang JT, Huang GT, Yang PM, Lee HS, Lee CZ, Chen DS: Genotypes of hepatitis C virus in chronic liver disease in Taiwan. J Med Virol 1994;44:234–236.
30 Yu ML, Chuang WL, Chen SC, Dai CY, Hou C, Wang JH, Lu SN, Huang JF, Lin ZY, Hsieh MY, Tsai JF, Wang LY, Chang WY: Changing prevalence of hepatitis C virus genotypes: Molecular epidemiology and clinical implications in the hepatitis C virus hyperendemic areas and a tertiary referral center in Taiwan. J Med Virol 2001;65:58–65.
31 Ikeda K, Kobayashi M, Someya T, Saitoh S, Tsubota A, Akuta N, Suzuki F, Suzuki Y, Arase Y, Kumada H: Influence of hepatitis C virus subtype on hepatocellular carcinogenesis: A multivariate analysis of a retrospective cohort of 593 patients with cirrhosis. Intervirology 2002;45:71–78.
32 Reid AE, Koziel MJ, Aiza I, Jeffers L, Reddy R, Schiff E, Lau JY, Dienstag JL, Liang TJ: Hepatitis C virus genotypes and viremia and hepatocellular carcinoma in the United States. Am J Gastroenterol 1999;94:1619–1626.
33 Yotsuyanagi H, Koike K, Yasuda K, Moriya K, Hino K, Kurokawa K, Iino S: Hepatitis C virus genotypes and development of hepatocellular carcinoma. Cancer 1995;76:1352–1355.
34 Nishiguchi S, Kuroki T, Nakatani S, Morimoto H, Takeda T, Nakajima S, Shiomi S, Seki S, Kobayashi K, Otani S: Randomised trial of effects of interferon-alpha on incidence of hepatocellular carcinoma in chronic active hepatitis C with cirrhosis. Lancet 1995;346:1051–1055.
35 Mazzella G, Accogli E, Sottili S, Festi D, Orsini M, Salzetta A, Novelli V, Cipolla A, Fabbri C, Pezzoli A, Roda E: Alpha interferon treatment may prevent hepatocellular carcinoma in HCV-related liver cirrhosis. J Hepatol 1996; 24:141–147.
36 Hino K, Kitase A, Satoh Y, Fujiwara D, Yamaguchi Y, Korenaga M, Shingai Y, Konishi T, Yamashita S, Uchida K, Mori K, Hanada H, Kodama T, Nukui K, Okita K: Interferon retreatment reduces or delays the incidence of hepatocellular carcinoma in patients with chronic hepatitis C. J Viral Hepat 2002;9:370–376.
37 Omata M, Yoshida H: Resolution of liver cirrhosis and prevention of hepatocellular carcinoma by interferon therapy against chronic hepatitis C. Scand J Gastroenterol 2003;237:S47–S51.
38 Poynard T, Marcellin P, Lee SS, Niederau C, Minuk GS, Ideo G, Bain V, Heathcote J, Zeuzem S, Trepo C, Albrecht J: Randomised trial of interferon alpha2b plus ribavirin for 48 weeks or for 24 weeks versus interferon alpha2b plus placebo for 48 weeks for treatment of chronic infection with hepatitis C virus. Lancet 1998;352:1426–1432.
39 McHutchison JG, Gordon SC, Schiff ER, Shiffman ML, Lee WM, Rustgi VK, Goodman ZD, Ling MH, Cort S, Albrecht JK: Interferon alfa-2b alone or in combination with ribavirin as initial treatment for chronic hepatitis C. N Engl J Med 1998;339:1485–1492.
40 Fried MW, Shiffman ML, Reddy KR, Smith C, Marinos G, Goncales FL Jr, Haussinger D, Diago M, Carosi G, Dhumeaux D, Craxi A, Lin A, Hoffman J, Yu J: Peginterferon alfa-2a plus ribavirin for chronic hepatitis C virus infection. N Engl J Med 2002;347:975–982.
41 Hadziyannis SJ, Sette H Jr, Morgan TR, Balan V, Diago M, Marcellin P, Ramadori G, Bodenheimer H Jr, Bernstein D, Rizzetto M, Zeuzem S, Pockros PJ, Lin A, Ackrill AM: Peginterferon-alpha2a and ribavirin combination therapy in chronic hepatitis C: A randomized study of treatment duration and ribavirin dose. Ann Intern Med 2004;140:346–355.
42 Lin R, Liddle C, Byth K, Farrell GC: Virus and host factors are both important determinants of response to interferon treatment among patients with chronic hepatitis C. J Viral Hepat 1996;3:85–96.
43 Hung CH, Lee CM, Lu SN, Wang JH, Tung HD, Chen TM, Chen CH, Changchien CS: Is delayed normalization of alanine aminotransferase a poor prognostic predictor in chronic hepatitis C patients treated with a combined interferon and ribavirin therapy? J Gastroenterol Hepatol 2002;17:1307–1311.
44 Shiratori Y, Kato N, Yokosuka O, Imazeki F, Hashimoto E, Hayashi N, Nakamura A, Asada M, Kuroda H, Tanaka N, Arakawa Y, Omata M: Predictors of the efficacy of interferon therapy in chronic hepatitis C virus infection. Gastroenterology 1997;113:558–566.
45 Zein NN, Rakela J, Krawitt EL, Reddy KR, Tominaga T, Persing DH: Hepatitis C virus genotypes in the United States: Epidemiology, pathogenicity, and response to interferon therapy. Ann Intern Med 1996;125:634–639.
46 Gale M Jr, Blakely CM, Kwieciszewski B, Tan SL, Dossett M, Tang NM, Korth MJ, Polyak SJ, Gretch DR, Katze MG: Control of PKR protein kinase by hepatitis C virus nonstructural 5A protein: Molecular mechanisms of kinase regulation. Mol Cell Biol 1998;18:5208–5218.
47 Taylor DR, Shi ST, Romano PR, Barber GN, Lai MM: Inhibition of the interferon-inducible protein kinase PKR by HCV E2 protein. Science 1999;285:107–110.
48 Enomoto N, Sakuma I, Asahina Y, Kurosaki M, Murakami T, Yamamoto C, Ogura Y, Izumi N, Marumo F, Sato C: Mutations in the nonstructural protein 5A gene and response to interferon in patients with chronic hepatitis C virus 1b infection. N Engl J Med 1996;334:77–81.
49 Khorsi H, Castelain S, Wyseur A, Izopet J, Canva V, Rombout A, Capron D, Capron JP, Lunel F, Stuyver L, Duverlie G: Mutations of hepatitis C virus 1b NS5A 2209–2248 amino acid sequence do not predict the response to recombinant interferon-alfa therapy in French patients. J Hepatol 1997;27:72–77.

50 Squadrito G, Orlando ME, Cacciola I, Rumi MG, Artini M, Picciotto A, Loiacono O, Siciliano R, Levrero M, Raimondo G: Long-term response to interferon alpha is unrelated to 'interferon sensitivity determining region' variability in patients with chronic hepatitis C virus-1b infection. J Hepatol 1999;30:1023–1027.
51 Chung RT, Monto A, Dienstag JL, Kaplan LM: Mutations in the NS5A region do not predict interferon-responsiveness in American patients infected with genotype 1b hepatitis C virus. J Med Virol 1999;58:353–358.
52 Cavalletto L, Chemello L, Donada C, Casarin P, Belussi F, Bernardinello E, Marino F, Pontisso P, Gatta A, Alberti A: The pattern of response to interferon alpha (alpha-IFN) predicts sustained response to a 6-month alpha-IFN and ribavirin retreatment for chronic hepatitis C. J Hepatol 2000;33:128–134.
53 Hung CH, Lee CM, Lu SN, Lee JF, Wang JH, Tung HD, Chen TM, Hu TH, Chen WJ, Changchien CS: Mutations in the NS5A and E2-PePHD region of hepatitis C virus type 1b and correlation with the response to combination therapy with interferon and ribavirin. J Viral Hepat 2003;10:87–94.
54 Sarrazin C, Berg T, Lee JH, Teuber G, Dietrich CF, Roth WK, Zeuzem S: Improved correlation between multiple mutations within the NS5A region and virological response in European patients chronically infected with hepatitis C virus type 1b undergoing combination therapy. J Hepatol 1999;30:1004–1013.
55 Macquillan GC, Niu X, Speers D, English S, Garas G, Harnett GB, Reed WD, Allan JE, Jeffrey GP: Does sequencing the PKRBD of hepatitis C virus NS5A predict therapeutic response to combination therapy in an Australian population? J Gastroenterol Hepatol 2004;19: 551–557.
56 Cappiello G, Abbate I, Lo Iacono O, Longo R, Solmone M, Ferraro D, Antonucci G, Di Marco V, Di Stefano R, Craxi A, Ippolito G, Capobianchi MR: ISDR pattern and evolution in patients with chronic hepatitis C treated with standard or PEG-IFN plus ribavirin. Antivir Ther 2003;8:105–110.
57 Yang SS, Lai MY, Chen DS, Chen GH, Kao JH: Mutations in the NS5A and E2-PePHD regions of hepatitis C virus genotype 1b and response to combination therapy of interferon plus ribavirin. Liver Int 2003;23:426–433.
58 Huang WS, Lu SN, Wang JH, Lee CM, Tung HD, Chen TM, Changchien CS: Prediction of viremia for cases of hepatitis C virus (HCV) infection using a third-generation anti-HCV enzyme immunoassay test. Hepatogastroenterology, in press.
59 Craxi A, Camma C, Giunta M: Definition of response to antiviral therapy in chronic hepatitis C. J Hepatol 1999;31:S160–S167.
60 Pawlotsky JM: Diagnostic tests for hepatitis C. J Hepatol 1999;31:S71–S79.
61 Tung HD, Lu SN, Lee CM, Wang JH, Chen TM, Hung CH, Huang WS, Changchien CS: Antiviral treatment responses in patients with chronic hepatitis C virus infection evaluated by a third generation anti-hepatitis C virus assay. J Viral Hepat 2002;9:304–308.

Hepatocellular Carcinoma

Intervirology

Intervirology 2006;49:82–90
DOI: 10.1159/000087268

Anticarcinogenic Impact of Interferon on Patients with Chronic Hepatitis C: A Large-Scale Long-Term Study in a Single Center

Kenji Ikeda Yasuji Arase Satoshi Saitoh Masahiro Kobayashi
Takashi Someya Tetsuya Hosaka Hitomi Sezaki Norio Akuta
Fumitaka Suzuki Yoshiyuki Suzuki Hiromitsu Kumada

Department of Gastroenterology, Toranomon Hospital, and Okinaka Memorial Institute for Medical Research, Tokyo, Japan

Key Words
Cirrhosis · Fibrosis · Hepatitis C virus · Hepatocellular carcinoma · Interferon

Abstract
Background: The anticarcinogenic capacity of interferon (IFN) was assessed in a cohort of Japanese patients with chronic hepatitis C en masse. ***Patients and Methods:*** The rate of hepatocarcinogenesis was analyzed in 2,166 patients with chronic hepatitis C, of whom 1,654 had received IFN therapy while 512 had not. ***Results:*** Crude rates of hepatocarcinogenesis in treated and untreated patients were 2.6 and 4.6% at the end of the 5th year, 5.8 and 12.7% at the 10th year and 13.9 and 23.9% at the 15th year (after completion of IFN therapy for those treated) ($p < 0.001$). IFN decreased the hazard ratio of carcinogenesis to 0.42 ($p < 0.001$) in multivariate analysis with adjustments for significant covariates including fibrotic stage, γ-glutamyl transpeptidase level, gender, platelet count and age. Among the 1,654 patients treated with IFN, 606 (36.6%) achieved persistent loss of hepatitis C virus (HCV) RNA and an additional 266 (16.1%) gained normal levels of alanine aminotransferase without loss of HCV RNA for 6 months or longer after the completion of IFN therpay. Cumulative rates of hepatocarcinogenesis in sustained virological responders and biochemical responders were 1.4 and 2.0% at the end of the 5th year, 1.9 and 3.6% at the 10th year and 1.9 and 7.5% at the 15th year, respectively. The hazard ratio of sustained virological response was 0.10 ($p < 0.001$), and that of biochemical response was 0.12 ($p < 0.001$). Normalization of aminotransferase levels after IFN therapy without loss of serum HCV RNA decreased hepatocarcinogenesis. ***Conclusion:*** IFN significantly decreased the rate of hepatocarcinogenesis in patients with chronic hepatitis C as a whole in Japan, even in those who fail to clear HCV RNA from serum.

Introduction

In most developed countries, hepatitis B virus (HBV) and hepatitis C virus (HCV) infections account for the great majority of hepatocellular carcinoma (HCC), with incidence rates dependent on the regional prevalence of these hepatitis viruses. HCV-associated HCC typically develops through a sequence of events that progress from chronic inflammation through fibrosis and cirrhosis accompanying dysplasia and ultimately to HCC. In our previous cohort study on Japanese patients with HCV-related cirrhosis [1], cumulative rates of developing HCC at 5, 10 and 15 years were 21.5, 53.2 and 75.2%, respectively. According to our observations of untreated patients with chronic hepatitis C [2], rates of hepatocarcino-

KARGER
Fax +41 61 306 12 34
E-Mail karger@karger.ch
www.karger.com

0300–5526/06/0492–0082$23.50/0

Accessible online at:
www.karger.com/int

Kenji Ikeda, MD
Department of Gastroenterology, Toranomon Hospital
Toranomon 2-2-2, Minato-ku
Tokyo 105-8470 (Japan)
Tel. +81 44 877 5111, Fax +81 44 860 1623, E-Mail ikedakenji@tora.email.ne.jp

genesis at 5, 10 and 15 years were estimated to be 4.8, 13.6 and 26.0%, respectively. The life expectancy of patients with HCV-related cirrhosis is largely influenced by the development of HCC in the clinical course. As the efficacy of radically curative therapies for HCC remains limited at best, and since a severe organ shortage does not provide with sufficient chances for liver transplantation, the prevention of HCC in patients with chronic liver disease is of great importance at the present.

Interferon (IFN) is effective in eliminating HCV and reducing serum levels of alanine aminotransferase (ALT) in some patients with chronic hepatitis C [3–6]. Reduced incidence of HCC in HCV-associated cirrhosis by IFN has been reported by many investigators including ourselves [7–14]; only a few studies have failed to find its benefit [15, 16]. However, many published studies had shortcomings in the study design, in terms of pooling patients who received IFN in diverse regimens, relatively short periods of follow-up despite a long incubation period of HCC, large numbers of dropouts and retrospective studies with historical controls. Moreover, almost all studies evaluated the activity of IFN to prevent HCC by comparing responders and nonresponders to the treatment. Due to difficulties in studying patients with chronic hepatitis C, a number of nonrandomized studies examined the effect of IFN on the incidence of hepatocarcinogenesis [17–20]. With invariable limitations in study design and interpretation of the results, these studies have disclosed useful information as regards the treatment of patients with chronic HCV infection.

In order to evaluate whether IFN can reduce the rate of carcinogenesis in patients with chronic hepatitis C, we compared 1,654 patients with IFN therapy with 512 patients without treatment in a single clinical center, who were adjusted for background features by the multivariate analysis. Therefore, the principal aims of our study were to show the role of IFN in preventing HCC in chronic hepatitis type C en masse and to establish the extent to which IFN decreases the rate of carcinogenesis as a sequel to chronic hepatitis C in a society.

Patients and Methods

Study Population

A total of 2,166 patients with chronic hepatitis were examined, whose initial sera tested negative for hepatitis B surface antigen by radioimmunoassay (Ausria, Dainabot, Tokyo, Japan) and positive for anti-HCV by the second-generation enzyme-linked immunosorbent assay (Dainabot); anti-HCV was tested in sera that had been stored frozen at –80°C. They included 1,421 men and 745 women aged 14–78 with a median of 50 years. They were all diagnosed with chronic hepatitis by liver biopsy with or without peritoneoscopy between 1970 and 2000 at the Department of Gastroenterology in Toranomon Hospital, Tokyo, Japan. Patients who had possibly developed HCC already at the time of diagnosis of hepatitis were strictly excluded from the study. In order to exclusively investigate hepatocarcinogenesis in HCV-related cirrhosis, patients coinfected with HBV were excluded.

Among the 2,166 patients with HCV-related hepatitis, 1,654 (76.4%) received IFN therapy, mostly since 1987 when IFN was available in Japan; new antivirals or anticarcinogenic treatments of viral cirrhosis, except for IFN, were not introduced in 1987 or thereafter in Japan. The remaining 512 patients did not receive IFN or any other antiviral therapies. This is a retrospective cohort study with historical controls composed of patients before 1987 and those who refused or could not receive IFN for various reasons since 1987.

Background and Laboratory Findings

Table 1 shows demographic profiles and laboratory data for the 1,654 patients treated with IFN and the 512 without receiving IFN since they were diagnosed with chronic hepatitis. There were more males, with a median age 3 years lower in treated than in nontreated patients. There were 299 treated patients (18.1%) with a history of alcohol intake ≥500 kg until the diagnosis of chronic hepatitis (corresponding to daily consumption of 3,000 ml of beer or 300 ml of whiskey for 20 years) and 113 (22.1%) untreated patients ($p < 0.001$). Because IFN was introduced to our hospital in 1987, the observation period was significantly shorter in the treated than in untreated patients (median 10.4 vs. 12.3 years; $p < 0.0001$).

Although all patients tested positive for HCV RNA during their clinical courses, tests for the concentration of HCV RNA in the initial serum was possible in 1,863 (86.5%) patients. HCV genotypes were analyzed by the serological typing method with a commercial kit (Kokusai Diagnostic Corporation, Kobe, Japan) in which the serological group 1 represented genotypes 1a and 1b, and group 2 stood for 2a and 2b genotypes. HCV in the serological group 2 was significantly more frequent in patients with IFN treatment than in those without. Concentration of HCV RNA was determined in the initial sera from 1,873 (86.5%) patients by the competitive polymerase chain reaction (PCR) method with the HCV probe assay (Chiron Corp., Emeryville, Calif., USA) or by PCR with Amplicor HCV Monitor kits (Roche Diagnostics Japan Co., Tokyo, Japan). High concentration of HCV ($\geq 10^6$ copies/ml by the competitive PCR or $\geq 10^6$ equivalents/ml by the HCV probe assay) was significantly more frequent in untreated than in treated patients ($p < 0.0001$). The stage of hepatic fibrosis was not different between the two groups.

Interferon Treatment and Judgment of the Effect

A total of 1,654 patients underwent IFN therapy in one or more treatment courses: 1,358 patients (82.1%) received IFN once, 240 patients (14.5%) twice, and the remaining 56 patients (3.4%) three times or more. Initial treatment was performed with natural or recombinant IFN-α (n = 1,238), natural IFN-β (n = 386) or both (n = 30). Regimens of IFN were variable: 926 (56.0%) patients received IFN 6–9 million units (MU) daily for 8 weeks, followed by 2 or 3 times per week for 16 weeks; 329 (20.0%) received IFN 6–9 MU daily for 2–4 weeks, followed by 3 times per week for 20–22 weeks; 185 (11.2%) underwent a short-course therapy with IFN

Table 1. Patient profiles and laboratory data at the diagnosis of chronic hepatitis

Factors	Interferon therapy		p value
	yes (n = 1,654)	no (n = 512)	
Male	1,110 (67.1%)	311 (60.7%)	0.024
Age, years	50 (16–72)	53 (21–78)	<0.001
History of transfusion	607 (36.7%)	229 (44.7%)	0.001
Family member with liver disease	426 (25.8%)	140 (27.3%)	0.47
Alcohol intake ≥500 kg	299 (18.1%)	113 (22.1%)	0.044
Observation period, year	10.4 (0.1–33.6)	12.3 (0.1–33.6)	<0.001
Laboratory data			
ALT, IU/l	63 (4–1,266)	67 (4–704)	0.098
AST, IU/l	106 (9–1,660)	96 (12–832)	0.0001
γ-GTP, IU/ml	62 (6–1,118)	70 (3–850)	0.39
Platelet counts, $\times 1{,}000/mm^3$	169 (27–433)	165 (35–560)	0.091
ICG R_{15}, %	14 (1–90)	16 (1–95)	0.003
AFP, ng/ml	4 (1–90)	5 (1–1,180)	0.42
HCV serological group			
Group 1, genotypes 1a/1b	1,021 (66.1%)	259 (81.4%)	<0.0001
Group 2, genotypes 2a/2b	488 (31.6%)	48 (15.1%)	
Undetermined	36 (2.3%)	11 (3.5%)	
HCV RNA concentration			
High[a]	937 (58.4%)	191 (71.3%)	<0.0001
Low[b]	668 (41.6%)	77 (28.7%)	
Histological stage of hepatitis			
F1, slight fibrosis	1,029 (62.2%)	298 (58.2%)	0.10
F2/F3, moderate/severe fibrosis	625 (37.8%)	214 (41.6%)	

AST = Aspartate aminotransferase; AFP = α-fetoprotein; ICG R_{15} = retention of indocyanine green at 15 min.

[a] HCV RNA concentration $\geq 10^6$ copies/ml by the competitive PCR or $\geq 10^6$ equivalents/ml by the HCV probe assay.

[b] HCV RNA concentrations less than high concentrations.

daily for 4–8 weeks; 128 (7.7%) were administered with intermittent IFN 3 times per week for 24 weeks; 72 (4.4%) had a prolonged course of IFN for 8–36 months; 8 (0.5%) received IFN-β 6 MU daily for 6–18 months, and the remaining 6 (0.4%) were given IFN-α combined with IFN-β for 4 months. The median dose of 624 MU was administered during the median period of 24 weeks. IFN for 24 weeks or longer was given to 83.2% of the patients. IFN therapy was usually initiated within a few months after the diagnosis of chronic hepatitis, and all patients were started on it within 12 months. The median interval between liver biopsy and initiation of IFN was 9 days.

Almost all the patients given IFN showed varied degrees of fever, chills, myalgia, headache and general malaise after the first injection. Most patients developed leukocytopenia and thrombocytopenia in various degrees. A significant thrombocytopenia $\leq 40{,}000/mm^3$ required a reduction of the IFN dose in 39 patients. IFN therapy was discontinued due to psychosis in 35 patients and ophthalmological symptoms in 12 patients. None of the patients developed decompensated liver disease with ascites, encephalopathy, jaundice or variceal bleeding. Although only 88 (5.3%) patients could not continue injection with IFN, studies for carcinogenesis were analyzed on the intention-to-treat basis.

The efficacy of IFN was judged by the clearance of HCV RNA from serum and ALT levels 12 months after the completion of treatment. Sustained virological response (SVR) was defined as persistent disappearance of HCV RNA after therapy, biochemical response (BR) as normal ALT levels without elimination of HCV RNA for at least 6 months after therapy, and no response (NR) as persistently elevated or transiently normalized ALT levels without loss of HCV RNA lasting for less than 6 months.

Follow-Up of Patients and Diagnosis of HCC

Patients were followed up monthly after diagnosis of chronic hepatitis in our outpatient clinic and monitored for hematological, biochemical and virological parameters. With their admission, during and after the treatment with IFN, weekly or biweekly follow-up was performed in almost all patients who received IFN. Imaging diagnosis was made once or twice per year in the majority of patients with ultrasonography or computed tomography. Angiography was performed only when HCC was highly suspected on imaging by ultrasonography or computed tomography.

When angiography pictured a characteristic hypervascular nodule specific for HCC in patients, histological confirmation was not required in the majority of them. Microscopic examinations of liv-

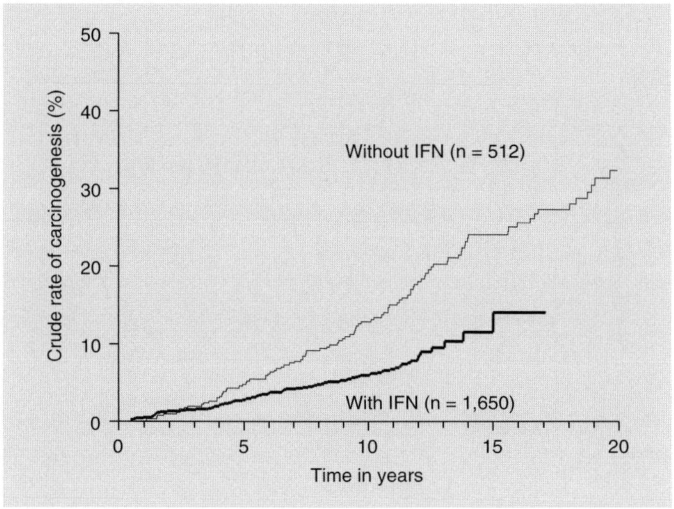

Fig. 1. Crude rates of hepatocarcinogenesis in patients treated with IFN and those untreated. The carcinogenesis rate was significantly lower in treated than in untreated patients (log-rank test, $p < 0.0001$).

er tissues obtained by a fine-needle biopsy were performed in 14 patients whose angiogram could not portray a typical image of HCC. There were 89 patients in whom HCC was confirmed histologically on liver specimens obtained at surgery or autopsy. Detection of serological tumor markers and increase with time were also taken into account in the diagnosis of HCC.

There were 223 (10.3%) patients lost to follow-up, including 164 (9.9%) treated and 59 (11.5%) untreated. Rates of annual dropouts in treated and untreated patients were 0.95 and 0.93%, respectively. In 9 patients, the response to IFN was judged by information on aminotransferase levels determined in other clinics and by persistent HCV RNA, as well as aminotransferase levels at 6 months after the completion of therapy in an additional 3 patients. Therefore, the response to IFN could be judged in all patients including the 12 who were lost to our follow-up early. Since the eventual outcome with respect to the development of HCC was not confirmed in these patients, their data were censored in statistical analyses [21]. Deaths unrelated to liver disease were censored and withdrawn from the analysis. The date of the last follow-up in this study was May 1, 2004, and the median observation period of studied patients was 10.7 years, with a range of 0.1–33.6 years.

Statistical Analysis

Nonparametric Mann-Whitney U test and χ^2 test were used for analysis of background characteristics of patients. The rate of HCC development was calculated by the Kaplan-Meier method [22]; it was based on the duration between diagnosis of chronic hepatitis by liver biopsy and detection of HCC. Differences in slopes of carcinogenesis curves were evaluated by the log-rank test. To gain a robust statistical power for the anticarcinogenic activity of IFN, observation of treated patients was initiated at the commencement of IFN therapy, in lieu of the diagnosis of chronic hepatitis. Independent factors associated with the development of HCC were studied using the stepwise Cox regression analysis [23]. The following 18 variables were analyzed for potential covariates in hepatocarcinogenesis at the time when hepatitis was diagnosed: age, sex, total alcohol intake, family history of liver disease, history of blood transfusion, stage of hepatic fibrosis, aspartic aminotransferase, ALT, albumin, bilirubin, globulin, γ-glutamyl transpeptidase (γ-GTP), platelet count, retention of indocyanine green at 15 min, serological grouping of HCV, HCV RNA level and IFN treatment.

Although continuous variables without conversion of data were evaluated in multivariate analyses, several variables were transformed into categorical data consisting of two or three ordinal numbers in calculating hazard ratios. All factors found to be marginally associated with hepatocarcinogenesis with p values <0.15 were tested by the multivariate Cox proportional hazard model. All analyses of data were performed with the computer program SPSS version 11 [24], and a p value <0.05 was considered significant.

Results

Response to IFN

Response to IFN was judged 12 months after the completion of therapy by both HCV RNA and serial ALT readings. Among the 1,654 patients with IFN treatment, SVR (elimination of HCV RNA) was achieved by 606 (36.6%), BR (ALT normalized for at least 6 months without clearance of HCV RNA from serum) in 266 (16.1%) and NR (elevated or transiently decreased ALT levels without loss of serum HCV RNA) in 782 (47.3%).

Crude Rates of Hepatocarcinogenesis

During the median observation period of 10.7 years, HCC developed in 199 of the 2,166 (9.2%) patients, including 96 of the 1,654 (5.8%) patients treated with IFN and 103 of the 512 (20.1%) patients without IFN (fig. 1). Among the 199 patients with HCC, 140 (70.4%) imaged a typical hypervascular stain on angiography and dynamic computed tomography, while 59 failed to exhibit tumor stains on angiography. HCC in these 59 patients was confirmed histologically on liver specimens obtained at surgery or by fine-needle biopsy.

Crude rates of hepatocarcinogenesis in patients treated with IFN and those untreated were 1.3 and 1.8% at the end of the 3rd year (after the completion of therapy), 2.6 and 4.6% at the end of the 5th year, 5.8 and 12.7% at the 10th year and 13.9 and 23.9% at the 15th year, respectively (fig. 1). The carcinogenesis rate was significantly lower in patients treated with IFN than in untreated patients (log-rank test, $p < 0.0001$).

Impact of IFN on Hepatocarcinogenesis

During the observation period, HCC developed in 96 of the 1,654 (5.8%) patients treated with IFN, including

11 patients (1.8%) with SVR, 10 (3.8%) with BR and 75 (9.6%) with NR to IFN. Rates of hepatocarcinogenesis in patients with SVR, BR and NR were 0.7, 0.8 and 2.0% at the end of the 3rd year, 1.4, 2.0 and 3.8% at the 5th year, 1.6, 2.9 and 6.5% at the 7th year, 1.9, 3.6 and 9.6% at the 10th year and 1.9, 7.5 and 27.6% at the end of 15th year (fig. 2). Hepatocarcinogenesis was significantly less frequent in patients with SVR or BR than in patients with NR and those untreated (log-rank test, $p < 0.0001$).

Factors Influencing Hepatocarcinogenesis

Univariate analysis identified 9 factors significantly associated with carcinogenesis. They were fibrotic stage ($p < 0.001$), age ($p < 0.001$), α-fetoprotein ($p < 0.001$), aspartic aminotransferase ($p = 0.001$), retention of indocyanine green at 15 min ($p = 0.002$), total alcohol intake ($p = 0.002$), γ-GTP ($p = 0.005$) and HCV serotype ($p = 0.045$). IFN therapy ($p = 0.064$), histological activity of hepatitis ($p = 0.069$) and ALT ($p = 0.70$) were marginally associated with carcinogenesis.

In order to prove the role of IFN on carcinogenesis in patients with chronic hepatitis type C en masse, multivariate analysis was performed by non-time-dependent proportional hazard analysis. Fibrotic stage, γ-GTP, gender, IFN therapy, platelet count and age independently influenced the development of HCC in the cohort (table 2). Advanced liver fibrosis in F2/F3 stages imposed a higher risk for carcinogenesis with a hazard ratio of 8.68, 95% confidence interval (CI) 5.08–14.81, compared with the F1 stage. Similarly, higher γ-GTP levels (hazard ratio 2.64), male sex (2.38), low platelet count (2.22) and older age (1.90) posed higher carcinogenesis risks. After adjusting background clinical biases between treated and untreated patients for the 5 significant covariates identified in the multivariate analysis, IFN therapy significantly decreased the hepatocarcinogenesis rate in the entire patients with chronic hepatitis C with a hazard ratio of 0.42 (95% CI 0.29–0.61) in comparison with untreated patients.

Based on the multivariate analysis, curves of carcinogenesis rates were theoretically illustrated in treated and untreated patients with the average histological stage, average γ-GTP value, average ratio of male to female, average platelet count and average age (fig. 3).

Hazard of Hepatocarcinogenesis Stratified by the Response to IFN

Since the carcinogenesis rate in patients with SVR or BR was significantly lower than that of patients with NR or untreated patients by the product limit method, a mul-

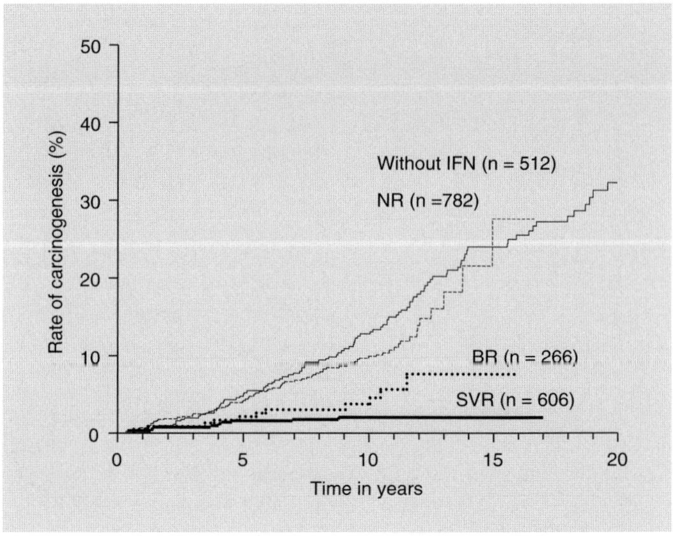

Fig. 2. Rates of hepatocarcinogenesis in patients with SVR, BR and NR to IFN. The rate in patients with NR (persistently elevated ALT or transiently normalized ALT for less than 6 months) was significantly higher than that in patients with SVR or BR.

Table 2. Factors associated with hepatocarcinogenesis in patients with chronic hepatitis C[a]

Factors	HR	95% CI	p value
Fibrosis stage			
F1	1		
F2–F3	8.68	(5.08–14.81)	<0.001
γ-GTP, IU/ml			
<50	1		
≥50	2.64	(1.58–4.42)	<0.001
Gender			
Women	1		
Men	2.38	(1.56–3.70)	<0.001
IFN therapy			
No	1		
Yes	0.42	(0.29–0.61)	<0.001
Platelet count, $\times 10^3/mm^3$			
≥100	1		
<100	2.22	(1.47–3.44)	<0.001
Age, years			
<50	1		
≥50	1.90	(1.27–2.85)	0.002

HR = Hazard ratio.
[a] Evaluated by the Cox proportional hazard analysis.

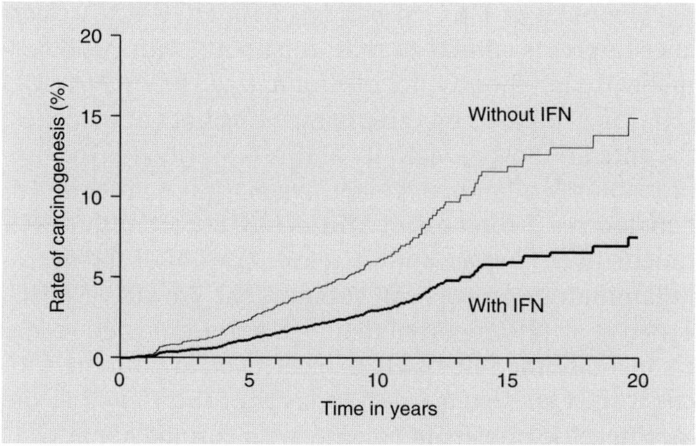

Fig. 3. Theoretical curves of hepatocarcinogenesis in patients treated with IFN and those untreated who have the average histological stage, average γ-GTP value, average ratio of male to female, average platelet count and average age. They are based on the analysis of 1,654 patients treated with IFN and 512 untreated patients.

Table 3. Factors associated with hepatocarcinogenesis in patients with chronic hepatitis C who had distinct responses to IFN therapy[a]

Factors	HR	95% CI	p value
Fibrosis stage			
F1	1		
F2–F3	9.90	(4.19–23.40)	<0.001
Gender			
Women	1		
Men	3.44	(1.89–6.25)	<0.001
γ-GTP, IU/ml			
<50	1		
≥50	2.68	(1.30–5.54)	0.008
Age, years			
<50	1		
≥50	2.56	(1.50–4.38)	0.001
AFP, ng/ml			
<20	1		
≥20	2.32	(1.34–4.02)	0.003
Platelet count, $\times 10^3/mm^3$			
≥100	1		
<100	2.09	(1.14–3.75)	0.013
Response to IFN			
Without IFN	1		<0.001
NR	0.57	(0.13–2.56)	0.46
BR	0.12	(0.04–0.35)	<0.001
SVR	0.10	(0.03–0.30)	<0.001

HR = Hazard ratio; AFP = α-fetoprotein.
[a] Evaluated by the Cox proportional hazard analysis.

tivariate analysis was performed taking into account the response to IFN. Hazard ratios of patients with SVR and BR to IFN therapy were 0.10 (95% CI 0.03–0.30, $p < 0.001$) and 0.12 (95% CI 0.04–0.35, $p < 0.001$), respectively, in comparison with that of untreated patients, when the other 5 factors served as significant covariates (table 3). The hazard ratio of NR at 0.57 (95% CI 0.13–2.56) was less than 1, but fell short of making a significant difference against untreated patients.

Mortality and Causes of Death

During the observation period, 116 of the 2,166 (5.4%) patients died, including 52 of the 1,654 (3.1%) subjects treated with IFN and 64 of the 512 (12.5%) subjects without IFN. Estimated survival rates in the treated and untreated patients were 99.3 and 98.3% at 5 years, 97.8 and 96.0% at 10 years and 93.8 and 86.9% at 15 years, respectively. The survival rate of treated patients was significantly higher than that of untreated patients (log-rank test, $p < 0.0001$).

Discussion

Based on our epidemiological data obtained by long-term observations of patients with chronic hepatitis [2] and patients with cirrhosis [1], the life expectancy of patients with HCV-related chronic liver disease heavily depends on the development of HCC. The possibility of eventually developing HCC in patients with HCV infection and cirrhosis is staggeringly high at 75% [1]. Theoretically, the treatment of chronic HCV infection with IFN can prevent the development of HCC. From the ethical point of view, a prospective randomized trial with control untreated patients is not to be allowed at present when IFN has become the standard radical therapy for chronic hepatitis C; everyone can receive IFN, as expenses are being covered for by the medical insurance in Japan. Another difficulty involves the informed consent in prospective randomized studies. It requires at least 5 years in order that IFN can decrease the incidence of carcinogenesis in chronic hepatitis C, with a statistical difference in the carcinogenesis rate between treated and 'untreated' patients. Since any randomized studies are considered extremely difficult in the future, we attempted to carry out this retrospective study by the multivariate analysis with statistical adjustments for possible covariates.

In the product limit analysis, IFN significantly decreased the crude rate of hepatocarcinogenesis in the entire cohort of 2,166 patients with chronic hepatitis C. Since there were some background differences between treated and untreated patients, we tried to correct for biases including stage of fibrosis, γ-GTP value, sex, platelet count and age, which significantly affect the carcinogenesis rate. Demographic, histological and biochemical factors having been adjusted, IFN is proven to bring about a significant decrease in the hazard of carcinogenesis in patients with chronic hepatitis C en masse (hazard ratio 0.42, $p < 0.001$ by the non-time-dependent model). Taking into consideration that a significant number of patients without IFN had received anti-inflammatory medicines, which might have contributed to suppression of hepatocarcinogenesis, the actual anticarcinogenic activity of IFN may be higher than the observed. Having published results of a similar study on a cohort of 1,643 patients with a median observation period of 5.4 years in 1999 [18], we could not establish the anticarcinogenic activity of IFN because of a low risk of carcinogenesis in untreated patients (1.2% per year). Nevertheless, we expected a significant statistical difference if we could extend the median observation period to longer than 7 or 10 years in our studied patients. This has been realized in the present study, in which 2,166 patients with and without IFN therapy were observed for a median of more than 10 years. As far as we are aware, it represents the first study that has demonstrated preventive effects of IFN on the carcinogenesis rate in a large cohort of patients in a single center, in correlation with distinct responses to it, such as SVR, BR and NR.

Treatment of patients with chronic HCV infection using IFN-α and ribavirin has led to sustained loss of serum HCV RNA in 40–50% of recipients with HCV genotype 1 and 75–80% with HCV genotype 2 or 3. However, to date, the combination therapy with IFN-α and ribavirin has not been evaluated for its impact on the risk of developing HCC. Monotherapy with IFN-α achieves sustained clearance of serum HCV RNA in only 20–30% of patients; the impact of IFN-α on the development of HCC has been evaluated only in patients who had received IFN-α without ribavirin [17–20, 25–27].

Multivariate analysis definitively demonstrated that IFN lessens the carcinogenesis risk in the patients whose ALT levels decreased after therapy. Furthermore, the anticarcinogenic capacity of IFN was demonstrated not only in the patients with persistent aminotransferase normalization, but also in those with transient normalization of ALT for at least 6 or 12 months. Many authors have already described that the activity of IFN to suppress the development of HCC in patients with HCV RNA clearance (SVR) is similar to that in patients with ALT normalization in the absence of eliminating HCV RNA (BR) [18, 25–27]. Based on these compelling lines of evidence, the anticarcinogenic activity of IFN is ascribed to the suppression of inflammatory and regenerative processes in hepatocytes. Moreno and Muriel [28] reported that IFN reverts liver fibrosis, and therefore, control of the necroinflammatory process can suppress the growth of HCC. Tarao et al. [29] reported that high aminotransferase levels increase the rate of HCC recurrence in patients with cirrhosis. Our results stand in favor of the view that the carcinogenic process in patients with chronic hepatitis C would be enhanced by fluctuating as well as persistently elevated levels of aminotransferases. It does seem that IFN exerts suppressive effects on HCC through reduction or complete remission of inflammatory activity. Recently, a few authors reported that even transient disappearance of HCV RNA during IFN therapy contributed to a low carcinogenesis rate in the clinical course of hepatitis [17, 27]. The significance of transient HCV in decreasing hepatocarcinogenesis should be further explored and confirmed by multicenter clinical studies with rigorous virological assessments.

HCC developed in a few patients with SVR 5 years after the HCV infection had been terminated by IFN, along with normalized ALT levels. These patients would have developed minute HCC in their livers already while receiving IFN which escaped the detection by imaging modalities or screening for serological tumor markers. This would indicate the limitation of IFN in preventing HCC. IFN will not be able to suppress HCC once it has developed, even when it succeeds in eliminating HCV and suppressing necroinflammatory processes in the liver.

With many difficulties in vaccine development, the recent progress in treatment of chronic HCV infection, from IFN monotherapy to combination therapy with ribavirin, is very auspicious. SVR and BR can be achieved in up to 56% of patients with combined IFN and ribavirin [30]. There is evidence that a sustained virological response can lead to decrease in fibrosis and even reversal of cirrhosis [31]. Because HCV-associated HCC occurs almost exclusively in patients with cirrhosis, successful treatment for SVR in patients without cirrhosis is likely to prevent future development of HCC [32]. However, once cirrhosis has been established, a preventive benefit of IFN monotherapy is restricted to the patients who can achieve SVR or BR. In their meta-analysis of 3 randomized and 11 nonrandomized controlled trials, Camma et al. [33] have reported a low but statistically significant preventive effect.

In conclusion, IFN significantly decreases the rate of hepatocarcinogenesis in patients with chronic hepatitis C, irrespective of the response to it.

Acknowledgement

This study was supported in part by a research grant from the Ministry of Health, Labour and Welfare in Japan.

References

1 Ikeda K, Saitoh S, Koida I, Arase Y, Tsubota A, Chayama K, Kumada H, Kawanishi M: A multivariate analysis of risk factors for hepatocellular carcinogenesis: A prospective observation of 795 patients with viral and alcoholic cirrhosis. Hepatology 1993;18:47–53.

2 Ikeda K, Saitoh S, Suzuki Y, Kobayashi M, Tsubota A, Koida I, Arase Y, Fukuda M, Chayama K, Murashima N, Kumada H: Disease progression and hepatocellular carcinogenesis in patients with chronic viral hepatitis: A prospective observation of 2,215 patients. J Hepatol 1998;28:930–938.

3 Davis GL, Balart LA, Schiff ER, Lindsay K, Bodenheimer HC Jr, Perrillo RP, Carey W, Jacobson IM, Payne J, Dienstag JL, van Thiel DH, Tamburro C, Lefkowitch J, Albrecht J, Meschievitz C, Ortego T: Treatment of chronic hepatitis C with recombinant interferon alfa. A multicenter randomized, controlled trial. N Engl J Med 1989;321:1501–1506.

4 Di Bisceglie AM, Martin P, Kassianides C, Lisker-Melman M, Murray L, Waggoner J, Goodman Z, Banks SM, Hoofnagle JH: Recombinant interferon alfa therapy for chronic hepatitis C. A randomized, double-blind, placebo-controlled trial. N Engl J Med 1989;321:1506–1510.

5 Causse X, Godinot H, Chevallier M, Chossegros P, Zoulim F, Ouzan D, Heyraud JP, Fontanges T, Albrecht J, Meschievitz C, Trepo C: Comparison of 1 or 3 MU of interferon alfa-2b and placebo in patients with chronic non-A, non-B hepatitis. Gastroenterology 1991;101:497–502.

6 Chayama K, Saitoh S, Arase Y, Ikeda K, Matsumoto T, Sakai Y, Kobayashi M, Unakami M, Morinaga T, Kumada H: Effect of interferon administration on serum hepatitis C virus RNA in patients with chronic hepatitis C. Hepatology 1991;13:1040–1043.

7 Nishiguchi S, Kuroki T, Nakatani S, Morimoto H, Takeda T, Nakajima S, Shiomi S, Seki S, Kobayashi K, Otani S: Randomised trial of effects of interferon-alpha on incidence of hepatocellular carcinoma in chronic active hepatitis C with cirrhosis. Lancet 1995;346:1051–1055.

8 Mazzella G, Accogli E, Sottili S, Festi D, Orsini M, Salzetta A, Novelli V, Cipolla A, Fabbri C, Pezzoli A, Roda E: Alpha interferon treatment may prevent hepatocellular carcinoma in HCV-related liver cirrhosis. J Hepatol 1996;24:141–147.

9 Schalm SW, Fattovich G, Brouwer JT: Therapy of hepatitis C: Patients with cirrhosis. Hepatology 1997;26:S128–S132.

10 Benvegnu L, Chemello L, Noventa F, Fattovich G, Pontisso P, Alberti A: Retrospective analysis of the effect of interferon therapy on the clinical outcome of patients with viral cirrhosis. Cancer 1998;83:901–909.

11 Niederau C, Lange S, Heintges T, Erhardt A, Buschkamp M, Hurter D, Nawrocki M, Kruska L, Hensel F, Petry W, Haussinger D: Prognosis of chronic hepatitis C: Results of a large, prospective cohort study. Hepatology 1998;28:1687–1695.

12 International Interferon-alpha Hepatocellular Carcinoma Study Group: Effect of interferon-alpha on progression of cirrhosis to hepatocellular carcinoma: A retrospective cohort study. Lancet 1998;351:1535–1539.

13 Hu KQ, Tong MJ: The long-term outcomes of patients with compensated hepatitis C virus-related cirrhosis and history of parenteral exposure in the United States. Hepatology 1999;29:1311–1316.

14 Ikeda K, Saitoh S, Kobayashi M, Suzuki Y, Suzuki F, Tsubota A, Arase Y, Murashima N, Chayama K, Kumada H: Long-term interferon therapy for 1 year or longer reduces the hepatocellular carcinogenesis rate in patients with liver cirrhosis caused by hepatitis C virus: A pilot study. J Gastroenterol Hepatol 2001;16:406–415.

15 Fattovich G, Giustina G, Degos F, Tremolada F, Diodati G, Almasio P, Nevens F, Solinas A, Mura D, Brouwer JT, Thomas H, Njapoum C, Casarin C, Bonetti P, Fuschi P, Basho J, Tocco A, Bhalla A, Galassini R, Noventa F, Schalm SW, Realdi G: Morbidity and mortality in compensated cirrhosis type C: A retrospective follow-up study of 384 patients. Gastroenterology 1997;112:463–472.

16 Valla DC, Chevallier M, Marcellin P, Payen JL, Trepo C, Fonck M, Bourliere M, Boucher E, Miguet JP, Parlier D, Lemonnier C, Opolon P: Treatment of hepatitis C virus-related cirrhosis: A randomized, controlled trial of interferon alfa-2b versus no treatment. Hepatology 1999;29:1870–1875.

17 Kasahara A, Hayashi N, Mochizuki K, Takayanagi M, Yoshioka K, Kakumu S, Iijima A, Urushihara A, Kiyosawa K, Okuda M, Hino K, Okita K: Risk factors for hepatocellular carcinoma and its incidence after interferon treatment in patients with chronic hepatitis C. Hepatology 1998;27:1394–1402.

18 Ikeda K, Saitoh S, Arase Y, Chayama K, Suzuki Y, Kobayashi M, Tsubota A, Nakamura I, Murashima N, Kumada H, Kawanishi M: Effect of interferon therapy on hepatocellular carcinogenesis in patients with chronic hepatitis type C: A long-term observation study of 1,643 patients using statistical bias correction with proportional hazard analysis. Hepatology 1999;29:1124–1130.

19 Shindo M, Ken A, Okuno T: Varying incidence of cirrhosis and hepatocellular carcinoma in patients with chronic hepatitis C responding differently to interferon therapy. Cancer 1999;85:1943–1950.

20 Yoshida H, Shiratori Y, Moriyama M, Arakawa Y, Ide T, Sata M, Inoue O, Yano M, Tanaka M, Fujiyama S, Nishiguchi S, Kuroki T, Imazeki F, Yokosuka O, Kinoyama S, Yamada G, Omata M: Interferon therapy reduces the risk for hepatocellular carcinoma: National surveillance program of cirrhotic and noncirrhotic patients with chronic hepatitis C in Japan. IHIT Study Group. Inhibition of Hepatocarcinogenesis by Interferon Therapy. Ann Intern Med 1999;131:174–181.

21 Harrington DP, Fleming TR: A class of rank test procedures for censored survival data. Biometrica 1982;69:553–566.

22 Kaplan EL, Meier P: Nonparametric estimation for incomplete observation. J Am Stat Assoc 1958;53:457–481.

23 Cox DR: Regression models and life tables. J R Stat Soc 1972;34:248–275.

24 SPSS Incorporation: SPSS for Windows Version 11.0 Manual. Chicago, SPSS Inc., 2001.

25 Kasahara A, Hayashi N, Mochizuki K, Hiramatsu N, Sasaki Y, Kakumu S, Kiyosawa K, Okita K: Clinical characteristics of patients with chronic hepatitis C showing biochemical remission, without hepatitis C virus eradication, as a result of interferon therapy. The Osaka Liver Disease Study Group. J Viral Hepat 2000;7:343–351.

26 Yabuuchi I, Imai Y, Kawata S, Tamura S, Noda S, Inada M, Maeda Y, Shirai Y, Fukuzaki T, Kaji I, Ishikawa H, Matsuda Y, Nishikawa M, Seki K, Matsuzawa Y: Long-term responders without eradication of hepatitis C virus after interferon therapy: Characterization of clinical profiles and incidence of hepatocellular carcinoma. Liver 2000;20:290–295.

27 Okanoue T, Itoh Y, Minami M, Sakamoto S, Yasui K, Sakamoto M, Nishioji K, Murakami Y, Kashima K: Interferon therapy lowers the rate of progression to hepatocellular carcinoma in chronic hepatitis C but not significantly in an advanced stage: A retrospective study in 1,148 patients. J Hepatol 1999;30:653–659.
28 Moreno MG, Muriel P: Remission of liver fibrosis by interferon-alpha 2b. Biochem Pharmacol 1995;50:515–520.
29 Tarao K, Takemiya S, Tamai S, Sugimasa Y, Ohkawa S, Akaike M, Tanabe H, Shimizu A, Yoshida M, Kakita A: Relationship between the recurrence of hepatocellular carcinoma (HCC) and serum alanine aminotransferase levels in hepatectomized patients with hepatitis C virus-associated cirrhosis and HCC. Cancer 1997;79:688–694.
30 Fried MW, Shiffman ML, Reddy KR, Smith C, Marinos G, Goncales FL Jr, Haussinger D, Diago M, Carosi G, Dhumeaux D, Craxi A, Lin A, Hoffman J, Yu J: Peginterferon alfa-2a plus ribavirin for chronic hepatitis C virus infection. N Engl J Med 2002;347:975–982.
31 Shiratori Y, Imazeki F, Moriyama M, Yano M, Arakawa Y, Yokosuka O, Kuroki T, Nishiguchi S, Sata M, Yamada G, Fujiyama S, Yoshida H, Omata M: Histologic improvement of fibrosis in patients with hepatitis C who have sustained response to interferon therapy. Ann Intern Med 2000;132:517–524.
32 Di Bisceglie AM, Carithers RL Jr, Gores GJ: Hepatocellular carcinoma. Hepatology 1998;28:1161–1165.
33 Camma C, Giunta M, Andreone P, Craxi A: Interferon and prevention of hepatocellular carcinoma in viral cirrhosis: An evidence-based approach. J Hepatol 2001;34:593–602.

Treatment

Intervirology

Intervirology 2006;49:91–95
DOI: 10.1159/000087269

Combined Interferon and Ribavirin Therapy for Chronic Hepatitis C in Taiwan

Ming-Yang Lai

Graduate Institute of Clinical Medicine, Department of Internal Medicine, Hepatitis Research Center, National Taiwan University College of Medicine and National Taiwan University Hospital, Taipei, Taiwan, ROC

Key Words
Chronic hepatitis · Hepatitis B virus · Hepatitis C virus · Hepatocellular carcinoma · Interferon · Ribavirin

Abstract
Chronic hepatitis C virus (HCV) infection, including its sequelae, is an important healthcare problem in Taiwan. The seroprevalence of HCV infection in first-time blood donors in Taiwan is 1.2% and an estimated 2–5% in the general population, with a great geographic variation. Genotype 1b is the most prevalent HCV genotype in Taiwan, with a prevalence rate of 50–70%. An increasing incidence of hepatocellular carcinoma (HCC) is mainly attributed to HCV infection, while the declining role of HBV is observed in Taiwan. The seroprevalence of hepatitis B surface antigen among patients with HCC was 90% three decades ago, while recently, chronic HCV infection accounts for more than 30% of HCC patients in the National Taiwan University Hospital. With the advent of a combined conventional interferon (IFN)-α and ribavirin therapy, to which Taiwan has contributed in the early study phase, the sustained virological response rate has been greatly improved compared with IFN monotherapy. The sustained virological response rate in Taiwanese patients treated with the combination therapy for 6 months has reached up to 50–60%, which is higher than that reported in patients from the Western countries receiving a 12-month regimen. It is necessary to searche for the underlying mechanisms for the better treatment outcome with IFN plus ribavirin combination therapy in Taiwanese patients. Whether long-term effects of IFN plus ribavirin therapy can reduce the incidence of HCC needs to be established.

Introduction

Chronic infection with hepatitis C virus (HCV) is a major healthcare problem and a leading cause of chronic liver disease worldwide. After acute infection with HCV, 50–85% of patients develop chronic infection that can lead to liver cirrhosis, hepatic decompensation and hepatocellular carcinoma (HCC) in 20–30 years [1–3]. The rate of sustained virological response (SVR) to therapy with interferon (IFN)-α is limited and has been reported to range from 10 to 20% [4], except in Japan where a higher dose of IFN induced SVR in up to 33% [5]. Combination of IFN with ribavirin improved SVR to 33–41%

KARGER

Fax +41 61 306 12 34
E-Mail karger@karger.ch
www.karger.com

0300–5526/06/0492–0091$23.50/0

Accessible online at:
www.karger.com/int

Ming-Yang Lai, MD
Graduate Institute of Clinical Medicine, National Taiwan University College of Medicine
7, Chung-Shan South Road, Taipei, 100 Taiwan (ROC)
Tel. +886 2 2312 3456, ext. 7073, Fax +886 2 2382 5962
E-Mail mylai@ha.mc.ntu.edu.tw

[6, 7]. The recently developed pegylated (peg)-IFN, when used in combination with ribavirin, resulted in an even higher SVR of 54–56% [8, 9].

In Taiwanese patients with chronic hepatitis C, clinical observations indicate that SVR obtained with IFN plus ribavirin is higher than that in studies conducted in Western countries. This paper comprehensively reviews the epidemiology of HCV infection and the results obtained with conventional IFN plus ribavirin therapy in patients with chronic hepatitis C as well as in those coinfected with HCV and hepatitis B virus (HBV). Additionally, it examines the long-term effects of combination therapy in reducing the incidence of HCC.

Table 1. Prevalence of anti-HCV among first-time blood donors in six regional blood centers in Taiwan (January–October 2004)[a]

Blood center	Donors	Anti-HCV positive	Percentage
Taipei	45,443	425	0.94
Hsinchu	26,457	302	1.14
Taichung	37,548	499	1.33
Tainan	33,705	456	1.35
Kaoshiung	29,100	393	1.35
Hualien	9,330	102	1.09
Total	181,583	2,177	1.20

[a] Courtesy of the Taiwan Blood Services Foundation.

HCV Infection in Taiwan

Taiwan is an area endemic for chronic HBV infection, with a prevalence of hepatitis B surface antigen (HBsAg) in 15–20% of the general population [10]. The first survey of anti-HCV in Taiwan, conducted in 420 volunteer adults, indicated a prevalence of 0.95% [11]. A recent study among first-time blood donors from six regional blood centers across Taiwan in 2004 detected anti-HCV at the average of 1.2% (range 0.94–1.35%) (table 1), which is higher than that in blood donors in Japan [12]. Several community surveys [13–17] identified hyperendemic villages with the prevalence of anti-HCV higher than 20% (table 2) [13, 15, 16]. A nationwide epidemiological study on HCV infection and transmission routes in the general population of the community has revealed a significant geographic variation in seroprevalence of anti-HCV (from 1.6 to 19.6%, with a mean of 4.3%) [18]. Age is significantly associated with increased prevalence of anti-HCV [18], and iatrogenic factors were common vehicles for HCV infection [19]. Genotype 1b is the most prevalent genotype and accounts for 50–70% in Taiwan [20, 21].

An increasing incidence of HCC has been reported in Japan and Western countries, which has been mainly attributed to HCV infection, while the role of HBV is steadily declining [22–25]. Three decades ago, the seroprevalence of HBsAg among patients with HCC in Taiwan was about 90% [26]. By contrast, a recent study of HBV and HCV status in 1,002 patients with HCC treated at the National Taiwan University Hospital during 1994–2000 found seropositive rates of HBsAg, anti-HCV

Table 2. Seroprevalence of anti-HCV in Taiwan

Year	Authors	Region	Population	Samples	Anti-HCV positive, %
1990	Chen et al. [11]	Taipei	Blood donors	420	0.95
1991	Wu et al. [13]	Eastern Taiwan	Aborigines	3,709	14.2–35.1
1993	Sheu et al. [14]	Northern Taiwan	Community	1,500	2.5
1997	Lu et al. [15]	Tzukuan	Community	244	37–38
1997	Lu et al. [15]	Paisha	Community	1,365	19–26
1997	Ho et al. [16]	Eastern Taiwan	Aborigines	80	41.3
1998	Hwu et al. [17]	Hsin-Chu	Health examinees	890	1.6–19.6
1999	Sun et al. [18]	Seven townships	Community	11,904	4.3 (mean)

Table 3. HCV and HBV status of 1,002 patients with HCC in the National Taiwan University Hospital (1994–2000)

Anti-HCV	HBsAg	Men	Women	Total
+	–	159 (20.5)	105 (46.7)	264 (26.3)
–	+	448 (62.8)	73 (32.5)	561 (56.0)
+	+	56 (7.2)	17 (7.5)	73 (7.3)
–	–	74 (9.5)	30 (13.3)	104 (10.3)
Total		777	225	1,002

Figures in parentheses are percentages.

and both HBsAg and anti-HCV at 56.0, 26.3 and 7.3%, respectively (table 3, based on data kindly provided by Dr. Chien-Hong Chen). Thus, chronic HCV infection is also playing an increasingly important role in the development of HCC in Taiwan as in other developed countries.

IFN and Ribavirin Therapy for Chronic Hepatitis C

The combination of IFN with ribavirin is more efficacious than IFN alone as the initial treatment for chronic hepatitis C. Using conventional IFN-α 3 million units three times per week along with daily ribavirin 1,200 mg for 6 months, three randomized, controlled trials from Taiwan, Italy and Sweden were the first to show SVR significantly higher (43, 47 and 40%, respectively) than that of IFN-α monotherapy (6, 13 and 20%, respectively) [27–29]. Later, large-scale multicenter studies from Europe [6] and the United States [7] compared IFN monotherapy with combination therapy for 24–48 weeks. Overall, SVR with combination therapy was 33% for the 24-week treatment and 41% for the 48-week treatment.

Recently, combination treatment with long-acting peg-IFN-α and oral ribavirin has improved SVR to 54–56% [8, 9]. A multicenter randomized trial in Taiwan has achieved a response to peg-IFN-α_{2b} plus ribavirin and conventional IFN-α_{2b} 3 million units three times per week plus ribavirin for 24 weeks in 67 and 64% of patients with chronic hepatitis C, by intent-to-treat analysis [21]. In patients with HCV genotype 1 infection, a significantly higher SVR was gained by peg-IFN plus ribavirin than by conventional IFN plus ribavirin (66 vs. 41%), but no significant difference was found in SVR among patients infected with HCV of non-1 genotypes [21]. The mechanism of ribavirin in enhancing the efficacy of IFN in treatment of chronic hepatitis C remains to be established, but one of our previous studies has indicated that ribavirin enhances IFN-γ levels in patients with chronic hepatitis C who had been treated with IFN-α [30].

Combined IFN and Ribavirin for Patients Coinfected with HCV and HBV

In areas endemic for both HCV and HBV, the percentage of patients with dual infection can be substantial. In Taiwan, anti-HCV was detected in 11% of patients with HBV-related chronic liver disease [11], and HBsAg prevailed in 12% of anti-HCV-positive patients [31]. A study for the efficacy of conventional IFN combined with ribavirin for 6 months in Taiwan accomplished SVR in 43% of patients coinfected with HCV and HBV, which compares with that of 60% in patients with HCV infection alone [32, 33].

Long-Term Efficacy of IFN plus Ribavirin Therapy and Incidence of HCC

Several studies have indicated that monotherapy with the conventional IFN-α can reduce the risk of HCC in patients with chronic hepatitis C, with or without cirrhosis, in comparison with untreated patients [5, 34–36]. However, other studies failed to demonstrate such a reduction [37–40]. Whether combination therapy with the conventional IFN-α plus ribavirin is superior to IFN monotherapy for reducing the risk of HCC in patients with chronic hepatitis C remains to be established. We have compared the incidence of HCC among some 300 patients with chronic hepatitis C receiving IFN plus ribavirin, IFN monotherapy or no treatment with a follow-up duration of nearly 8 years. We found the incidence of HCC significantly different among these groups as well as between groups of combination and IFN monotherapy (unpublished observations). None of the sustained viral responders treated with combination therapy developed HCC during follow-ups longer than 7 years.

Conclusion

The seroprevalence of HCV infection in first-time blood donors has been reported at 1.2% and in the general population of Taiwan with a wide geographic variation ranging from 2 to 5%. With the advent of combined conventional IFN-α and ribavirin, the outcome of chronic hepatitis C has been greatly improved. The fact that the SVR rate in Taiwanese patients treated with the combination therapy for 6 months has reached up to 50–60% [21, 28, 32], which is higher than that reported in patients from the Western countries receiving a 12-month regimen, is important and intriguing. Differences in the average body weight, viral loads, HCV genotypes, liver histology and racial or ethnic factors [41, 42] may play a role. A multicenter, randomized trial comparing 6- versus 12-month regimen of peg-IFN plus ribavirin needs to be conducted in Taiwan.

References

1 Di Bisceglie AM: Hepatitis C and hepatocellular carcinoma. Hepatology 1997;26:S34–S38.
2 Kiyosawa K, Sodeyama T, Tanaka E, Gibo Y, Yoshizawa K, Nakano Y, Furuta S, Akahane Y, Nishioka K, Purcell RH, Akahane Y, Nishioka K, Purcell RH, Alter HJ: Interrelationship of blood transfusion, non-A, non-B hepatitis and hepatocellular carcinoma: Analysis by detection of antibody to hepatitis C virus. Hepatology 1990;12:671–675.
3 Seeff LB: Natural history of chronic hepatitis C. Hepatology 2002;36:S35–S46.
4 Lindsay KL: Therapy of hepatitis C: Overview. Hepatology 1997;26:S71–S77.
5 Yoshida H, Shiratori Y, Moriyama M, Arakawa Y, Ide T, Sata M, Inoue O, Yano M, Tanaka M, Fujiyama S, Nishiguchi S, Kuroki T, Imazeki F, Yokosuka O, Kinoyama S, Yamada G, Omata M: Interferon therapy reduces the risk for hepatocellular carcinoma: National surveillance program of cirrhotic and noncirrhotic patients with chronic hepatitis C in Japan. Ann Intern Med 1999;131:174–181.
6 Poynard T, Marcellin P, Lee SS, Niederau C, Minuk GS, Ideo G, Bain V, Heathcote J, Zeuzem S, Trepo C, Albrecht J: Randomised trial of interferon alpha2b plus ribavirin for 48 weeks or for 24 weeks versus interferon alpha2b plus placebo for 48 weeks for treatment of chronic infection with hepatitis C virus. Lancet 1998;352:1426–1432.
7 McHutchison JG, Gordon SC, Schiff ER, Shiffman ML, Lee WM, Rustgi VK, Goodman ZD, Ling MH, Cort S, Albrecht JK: Interferon alfa-2b alone or in combination with ribavirin as initial treatment for chronic hepatitis C. Hepatitis Interventional Therapy Group. N Engl J Med 1998;339:1485–1492.
8 Manns MP, McHutchison JG, Gordon SC, Rustgi VK, Shiffman M, Reindollar R, Goodman ZD, Koury K, Ling M, Albrecht JK: Peginterferon alfa-2b plus ribavirin compared with interferon alfa-2b plus ribavirin for initial treatment of chronic hepatitis C: A randomised trial. Lancet 2001;358:958–965.
9 Fried MW, Shiffman ML, Reddy KR, Smith C, Marinos G, Goncales FL Jr, Haussinger D, Diago M, Carosi G, Dhumeaux D, Craxi A, Lin A, Hoffman J, Yu J: Peginterferon alfa-2a plus ribavirin for chronic hepatitis C virus infection. N Engl J Med 2002;347:975–982.
10 Chen DS: From hepatitis to hepatoma: Lessons from type B viral hepatitis. Science 1993;262: 369–370.
11 Chen DS, Kuo GC, Sung JL, Lai MY, Sheu JC, Chen PJ, Yang PM, Hsu HM, Chang MH, Chen CJ, et al: Hepatitis C virus infection in an area hyperendemic for hepatitis B and chronic liver disease: The Taiwan experience. J Infect Dis 1990;162:817–822.
12 Moriya T, Koyama T, Tanaka J, Mishiro S, Yoshizawa H: Epidemiology of hepatitis C virus in Japan. Intervirology 1999;42:153–158.
13 Wu JS, Lu CF, Liu WT, Lin SY: Prevalence of antibodies to hepatitis C virus (anti-HCV) in different populations in Taiwan. Chinese J Microbiol Immunol 1991;24:55–60.
14 Sheu JC, Wang JT, Wang TH, Wang CY, Yang PM, Huang GT, Shih LN, Lee HS, Chen DS: Prevalence of hepatitis C viral infection in a community in Taiwan. Detection by synthetic peptide-based assay and polymerase chain reaction. J Hepatol 1993;17:192–198.
15 Lu SN, Chue PY, Chen HC, Wu MH, Chen IL, Huang JF, Wang JH, Peng CF, Shih CH, You SL, Lu CF, Chen CJ, Chang WY: Different viral aetiology of hepatocellular carcinoma between two hepatitis B and C endemic townships in Taiwan. J Gastroenterol Hepatol 1997;12:547–550.
16 Ho MS, Hsu CP, Yuh Y, King CC, Tsai JF, Mau YC, Hsu LC, Chao WH: High rate of hepatitis C infection in an isolated community: Persistent hyperendemicity or period-related phenomena. J Med Virol 1997;52:370–376.
17 Hwu NY, Fan CK, Chung WC, Wang CY, Hsueh YM, Chen HH, Lin CF, Su TT, Jang YS: Seroepidemiological study of hepatitis C virus infection in the Hsin-Chu Area, Taiwan. Tsu Chi Med J 1998;10:305–310.
18 Sun CA, Chen HC, Lu CF, You SL, Mau YC, Ho MS, Lin SH, Chen CJ: Transmission of hepatitis C virus in Taiwan: Prevalence and risk factors based on a nationwide survey. J Med Virol 1999;59:290–296.
19 Sun CA, Chen HC, Lu SN, Chen CJ, Lu CF, You SL, Lin SH: Persistent hyperendemicity of hepatitis C virus infection in Taiwan: The important role of iatrogenic risk factors. J Med Virol 2001;65:30–34.
20 Kao JH, Chen PJ, Lai MY, Yang PM, Sheu JC, Wang TH, Chen DS: Genotypes of hepatitis C virus in Taiwan and the progression of liver disease. J Clin Gastroenterol 1995;21:233–237.
21 Lee SD, Yu ML, Cheng PN, Lai MY, Chao YC, Hwang SJ, Chang WY: Comparison of a six-month course of peginterferon-α_{2b} plus ribavirin and interferon-$2\alpha_{2b}$ plus ribavirin in treating Chinese patients with chronic hepatitis C in Taiwan. J Viral Hepat 2005;12:283–291.
22 Okuda K, Fujimoto I, Hanai A, Urano Y: Changing incidence of hepatocellular carcinoma in Japan. Cancer Res 1987;47:4967–4972.
23 El-Serag HB, Mason AC: Rising incidence of hepatocellular carcinoma in the United States. N Engl J Med 1999;340:745–750.
24 Taylor-Robinson SD, Foster GR, Arora S, Hargreaves S, Thomas HC: Increase in primary liver cancer in the UK, 1979–94. Lancet 1997;350:1142–1143.
25 El-Serag HB, Davila JA, Petersen NJ, McGlynn KA: The continuing increase in the incidence of hepatocellular carcinoma in the United States: An update. Ann Intern Med 2003;139:817–823.
26 Sung JL, Chen DS: Hepatitis B surface antigen and antibody in liver disease in Taiwan. Proc 5th Asian-Pacific Congr Gastroenterol, Singapore, 1976, pp 265–269.
27 Chemello L, Cavalletto L, Bernardine E, Guido M, Pontisso P, Alverti A: The effect of interferon alfa and ribavirin combination therapy in naïve patients with chronic hepatitis C. J Hepatol 1995;23:S8–S12.
28 Lai MY, Kao JH, Yang PM, Wang JT, Chen PJ, Chan KW, Chu JS, Chen DS: Long-term efficacy of ribavirin plus interferon alfa in the treatment of chronic hepatitis C. Gastroenterology 1996;111:1307–1312.
29 Reichard O, Norkrans G, Fryden A, Braconier JH, Sonnerborg A, Weiland O: Randomised, double-blind, placebo-controlled trial of interferon alpha-2b with and without ribavirin for chronic hepatitis C. Lancet 1998;351:83–87.
30 Fang SH, Lai MY, Hwang LH, Yang PM, Chen PJ, Chiang BL, Chen DS: Ribavirin enhances interferon-gamma levels in patients with chronic hepatitis C treated with interferon-alpha. J Biomed Sci 2001;8:484–491.

31 Liaw YF: Role of hepatitis C virus in dual and triple hepatitis virus infection. Hepatology 1995;22:1101–1108.
32 Liu CJ, Chen PJ, Lai MY, Kao JH, Jeng YM, Chen DS: Ribavirin and interferon is effective for hepatitis C virus clearance in hepatitis B and C dually infected patients. Hepatology 2003;37:568–576.
33 Liu CJ, Chen PJ, Chen DS: A forgotten population with chronic hepatitis C infection: Subjects coinfected with hepatitis B virus. Hepatology 2004;40:266.
34 Mazzella G, Accogli E, Sottili S, Festi D, Orsini M, Salzetta A, Novelli V, Cipolla A, Fabbri C, Pezzoli A, Roda E: Alpha interferon treatment may prevent hepatocellular carcinoma in HCV-related liver cirrhosis. J Hepatol 1996; 24:141–147.
35 Imai Y, Kawata S, Tamura S, Yabuuchi I, Noda S, Inada M, Maeda Y, Shirai Y, Fukuzaki T, Kaji I, Ishikawa H, Matsuda Y, Nishikawa M, Seki K, Matsuzawa Y: Relation of interferon therapy and hepatocellular carcinoma in patients with chronic hepatitis C. Osaka Hepatocellular Carcinoma Prevention Study Group. Ann Intern Med 1998;129:94–99.
36 Benvegnu L, Chemello L, Noventa F, Fattovich G, Pontisso P, Alberti A: Retrospective analysis of the effect of interferon therapy on the clinical outcome of patients with viral cirrhosis. Cancer 1998;83:901–909.
37 Niederau C, Lange S, Heintges T, Erhardt A, Buschkamp M, Hurter D, Nawrocki M, Kruska L, Hensel F, Petry W, Haussinger D: Prognosis of chronic hepatitis C: Results of a large, prospective cohort study. Hepatology 1998;28: 1687–1695.
38 Fattovich G, Giustina G, Degos F, Diodati G, Tremolada F, Nevens F, Almasio P, Solinas A, Brouwer JT, Thomas H, Realdi G, Corrocher R, Schalm SW: Effectiveness of interferon alfa on incidence of hepatocellular carcinoma and decompensation in cirrhosis type C. J Hepatol 1997;27:201–205.
39 Ikeda K, Saitoh S, Arase Y, Chayama K, Suzuki Y, Kobayashi M, Tsubota A, Nakamura I, Murashima N, Kumada H, Kawanishi M: Effect of interferon therapy on hepatocellular carcinogenesis in patients with chronic hepatitis type C: A long-term observation study of 1,643 patients using statistical bias correction with proportional hazard analysis. Hepatology 1999;29:1124–1130.
40 Aizawa Y, Shibamoto Y, Takagi I, Zeniya M, Toda G: Analysis of factors affecting the appearance of hepatocellular carcinoma in patients with chronic hepatitis C. A long term follow-up study after histologic diagnosis. Cancer 2000;89:53–59.
41 McHutchison JG, Poynard T, Pianko S, Gordon SC, Reid AE, Dienstag J, Morgan T, Yao R, Albrecht J: The impact of interferon plus ribavirin on response to therapy in black patients with chronic hepatitis C. Gastroenterology 2000;119:1317–1323.
42 Cheng PN, Marcellin P, Bacon B, Farrell G, Parsons I, Wee T, Chang TT: Racial differences in responses to interferon-beta-1a in chronic hepatitis C unresponsive to interferon-alpha: A better response in Chinese patients. J Viral Hepat 2004;11:418–426.

Intervirology

Intervirology 2006;49:96–98
DOI: 10.1159/000087270

Response to Combined Interferon and Ribavirin Is Better in Patients Infected with Hepatitis C Virus Genotype 6 than Genotype 1 in Hong Kong

Man-Fung Yuen Ching-Lung Lai

Department of Medicine, University of Hong Kong, Queen Mary Hospital, Hong Kong, SAR, China

Key Words
Hepatitis C virus · Hong Kong · Genotypes · Interferon · Ribavirin

Abstract
Data on the treatment efficacy of interferon (IFN)-α and ribavirin in patients with chronic hepatitis infected with hepatitis C virus (HCV) of genotype 6 are lacking. A study has been reported from Hong Kong which compared the treatment efficacy of IFN-α and ribavirin in the treatment of chronic HCV infection with genotypes 1 and 6. Twenty-four patients with HCV genotype 1 and 16 patients with HCV genotype 6 were studied. The baseline demographic data including median age, gender ratio, alanine aminotransferase levels, bilirubin levels, HCV RNA levels and histological scores were comparable between the two groups of patients. All patients received IFN-α 5 million units three times per week and ribavirin (1,000 mg for those weighing ≤75 kg and 1,200 mg for those weighing >75 kg) for 1 year. Patients infected with HCV genotype 6 achieved virological response significantly higher than those with HCV genotype 1 (67 vs. 33% at week 24, $p = 0.02$; 75 vs. 42% at the end of treatment, $p = 0.05$; 63 vs. 29% at 6 months after completion of treatment, $p = 0.04$). Histological improvement in inflammatory activity and fibrosis in the liver were observed in 25% and 25% of patients infected with HCV genotype 6 in contrast to only 13 and 8% in patients infected with HCV genotype 1; however, the differences were not statistically significant. In conclusion, patients with HCV genotype 6 gain a better response to combined treatment with IFN-α and ribavirin than those with HCV genotype 1 and achieve a significantly higher rate of sustained virological response.

Introduction

Genotypes of hepatitis C virus (HCV) have different geographic distributions in the world. In Asian countries, unique distribution patterns are also observed. For instance, HCV genotypes 1b, 2a and 2b are common in Japan and Taiwan [1]. Hong Kong differs from Japan and Taiwan in that HCV genotype 6 is found, in addition to genotypes 1a, 1b, 2b and 3 [2–5]. According to an international collaborative study on the distribution of HCV genotypes in blood donors [2], those from Japan and Taiwan were infected only with HCV genotypes 1 or 2, in remarkable contrast to those from Hong Kong who were infected with HCV genotypes 1, 2 or 6. In spite of the geographical proximity between Hong Kong and the Mainland China, HCV genotype 6 was not found in China where 1b and 2a were the only HCV genotypes identified [3]. Based on the results of these two studies, Hong Kong has a greater diversity of HCV genotypes. According to the study conducted by Prescott et al. [4], the prevalence of HCV genotypes in Hong Kong was as follows: 1a, 6.2%; 1b, 58.8%; 2a, 1.4%; 2b, 1.4%; 3a, 1.9%, and 6a, 27%. In addition, this study reports that serum levels of alanine aminotransferase (ALT) are lower in patients infected with HCV genotype 6 than in patients with ge-

KARGER

Fax +41 61 306 12 34
E-Mail karger@karger.ch
www.karger.com

0300–5526/06/0492–0096$23.50/0

Accessible online at:
www.karger.com/int

Man-Fung Yuen, MD
Department of Medicine, the University of Hong Kong, Queen Mary Hospital
Pokfulam Road
Hong Kong, SAR (China)
Tel. +852 28553984, Fax +852 28725828, E-Mail mfyuen@hkucc.hku.hk

Table 1. Response to IFN-α at 3 different time points in patients infected with HCV genotypes 1 and 6

Time points of treatment	Genotype 1 (n = 24)	Genotype 6 (n = 16)	p value	Odds ratio	95% confidence interval
24 weeks	8 (33)	11 (69)	0.02	4.4	1.1–17.1
52 weeks (end of treatment)	10 (42)	12 (75)	0.05	4.2	1.0–16.9
6 months after treatment	7 (29)	10 (63)	0.04	4.1	1.0–15.5

Figures in parentheses are percentages.

notype 1. From the combined results of various studies, genotypes 1 and 6 are the two predominant genotypes accounting for approximately 60–70 and 25% of patients with chronic HCV infection in Hong Kong. HCV genotype 6 occurs even more prevalently in, respectively, subgroups, including patients with thalassemia (50%), and intravenous drug users (60%) [4, 5]. Furthermore, HCV genotype 6 is also found in Macau, Vietnam and Thailand [6]. There are wide virological differences between HCV genotype 6 and the other genotypes. In comparison of a nucleotide sequence of 194 base pairs in the center of the HCV core gene, homologies between genotype 6a and genotypes 1a, 1b, 2a, 2b, 3a and 5 were 81.1, 82.1, 73.8, 77.3, 81.4 and 78.9%, respectively [3].

It has been shown that high level of viremia, genotype 1b, degree of genetic diversity (quasispecies) and infection through blood transfusion are associated with more progressive liver disease. As far as the treatment response to interferon (IFN)-α and ribavirin is concerned, both host factors (gender, age of the patients, duration of infection, pretreatment ALT level, degree of fibrosis, presence or absence of cirrhosis) and viral factors (viral genotype, level of viremia and degree of viral heterogeneity) are important and influential. Previous studies have consistently shown that HCV genotype 1b has a poorer treatment response than genotype 2 or 3. However, data on the efficacy of IFN-α and ribavirin in patients infected with HCV genotype 6 are largely deficient.

A Study of Hepatitis C Virus Infection in Hong Kong

A study comparing the effect of combination therapy with IFN-α and ribavirin between patients infected with HCV genotype 1 and genotype 6 was conducted in the Department of Medicine, University of Hong Kong, Queen Mary Hospital, Hong Kong [7]. To the best of our knowledge, it was the first study to compare these two HCV genotypes.

The inclusion criteria comprised antibody to HCV detected by the third-generation enzyme-linked immunosorbent assay (Ortho Diagnostic Systems), HCV RNA determined by the branched DNA assay (Quantiplex HCV-RNA 2.0 assay, Chiron Corporation, Calif., USA), HCV genotypes determined by line probe assay (Versant HCV Genotype Assay, Bayer, Tarrytown, N.Y., USA), persistently elevated levels of ALT on at least three occasions and lasting at least 6 months, as well as histological features of chronic inflammation on the pretreatment liver biopsy. The exclusion criteria included advanced liver cirrhosis, hemolytic anemia, depression, autoimmune disease, infection with hepatitis B virus or human immunodeficiency virus type 1, previous IFN-α therapy and pregnancy.

All eligible patients received IFN-α_{2b} (Intron A, Schering-Plough, Kenilworth, N.J., USA) 5 million units three times per week and ribavirin 1,200 or 1,000 mg daily for patients with a body weight >75 or ≤75 kg for 52 weeks. Protocol liver biopsy was performed at 1 month before and 6 months after the treatment. All patients were followed every 4 weeks during the treatment period and at a 3-month interval after treatment. The end of treatment response was defined as HCV RNA undetectable by the branched DNA method at the end of treatment. Sustained virological response (SVR) was defined as HCV RNA undetectable by the branched DNA assay 6 months after the completion of treatment.

During 2 years, from 1999 to 2000, 196 patients with chronic hepatitis C attended our clinic. The prevalence of HCV genotypes was as follows: 1a, 8.1%; 1b, 54.7%; 2a, 2.6%; 2b, 0.5%; 3a, 1.5%; 6a, 21.9%; 6b, 5.1%, and mixed/indeterminate, 5.6%. Among these 196 patients, 176 possessed either HCV genotype 1 (n = 123) or 6 (n = 53). Of those, 103 patients were not eligible for the study because of one or more of the following reasons: normal ALT levels, previous IFN-α treatment, liver cirrhosis, receiving liver transplantation or renal transplantation, Graves' disease and depression. Of the remaining 73 patients, 40 agreed to participate in the study, including 24 with genotype 1 and 16 with genotype 6 infection.

There were no differences in the age, sex ratio and biochemical parameters of the liver between patients with genotype 1 and 6 infections. The median baseline ALT levels were 90 and 120 IU/l for patients with genotypes 1 and 6 (p = 0.17). The median baseline HCV RNA levels were 1.0×10^6 and 6.1×10^6 genome equivalents/ml for patients with genotypes 1 and 6 (p = 0.22). According to the criteria for histological assessment by Desmet et al. [8], high inflammatory activity (grade 2–3) was found in 25 and 18.8% of patients with genotypes 1 and 6 (p = 0.72). Advanced fibrosis (grade 3) was found in 45.8 and 37.5% of patients with genotypes 1 and 6 (p = 0.6). Therefore, all the baseline characteristics were comparable between patients with genotypes 1 and 6.

Treatment responses (SVRs) at week 24, at the end of treatment and at 6 months after completion of treatment are listed in table 1. Patients with genotype 6 showed consistently higher rates of treatment response compared with patients with genotype 1 at these three different time points.

Patients with genotype 6 had a higher chance of improvement in the liver histology (defined by a reduction of ≥ 1 score at posttreatment from the baseline). Of these patients, 25% gained improvement in inflammatory activity and 25% in fibrosis, in comparison with 12.5 and 8.3% of patients with genotype 1; the differences were not statistically significant (p = 0.41 and p = 0.2, respectively).

Five patients (13%) experienced a reduction of hemoglobin level by more than 2 g/dl, and 2 patients had a hemoglobin level less than 10 g/dl and required a reduction of the ribavirin dose. Two patients developed thyrotoxicosis and 1 patient had depression.

Discussion

Patients infected with HCV genotype 6 have a better response to IFN-α (5 million units three times per week) and ribavirin (1,000–1,200 mg daily) for 52 weeks than those with HCV genotype 1 during, at the end and 6 months after treatment. According to two registration trials using IFN-α and ribavirin [9, 10], the SVRs for genotype 1 and genotype 2 or 3 are approximately 30 and 65%, respectively. Therefore, the SVR of genotype 6 as shown in the study from Hong Kong (63%) is comparable with that of genotype 2 or 3. Since the SVRs for genotype 2 or 3 are maintained even after shortening the duration of treatment with IFN-α and ribavirin to 6 months, it is likely that the duration of treatment for genotype 6 may also be shortened to 6 months without jeopardizing the efficacy. Future studies are required to evaluate the treatment efficacy of pegylated IFN combined with ribavirin in patients with HCV genotype 6 and determine the optimal treatment duration (6 or 12 months) as well as the optimal dose of ribavirin (800 or 1,000/1,200 mg).

References

1 Davidson F, Simmonds P, Ferguson JC, Jarvis LM, Dow BC, Follett EA, Seed CR, Krusius T, Lin C, Medgyesi GA: Survey of major genotypes and subtypes of hepatitis C virus using RFLP of sequences amplified from the 5′ noncoding region. J Gen Virol 1995;76:1197–1204.

2 McOmish F, Yap PL, Dow BC, Follett EA, Seed C, Keller AJ, Cobain TJ, Krusius T, Kolho E, Naukkarinen R: Geographical distribution of hepatitis C virus genotypes in blood donors: An international collaborative survey. J Clin Microbiol 1994;32:884–892.

3 Zhang YY, Lok AS, Chan DT, Widell A: Greater diversity of hepatitis C virus genotypes found in Hong Kong than in mainland China. J Clin Microbiol 1995;33:2931–2934.

4 Prescott LE, Simmonds P, Lai CL, Chan NK, Pike I, Yap PL, Lin CK: Detection and clinical features of hepatitis C virus type 6 infections in blood donors from Hong Kong. J Med Virol 1996;50:168–175.

5 Wong DA, Tong LK, Lim W: High prevalence of hepatitis C virus genotype 6 among certain risk groups in Hong Kong. Eur J Epidemiol 1998;14:421–426.

6 Mellor J, Walsh EA, Prescott LE, Jarvis LM, Davidson F, Yap PL, Simmonds P: Survey of type 6 group variants of hepatitis C virus in Southeast Asia by using a core-based genotyping assay. J Clin Microbiol 1996;34:417–423.

7 Hui CK, Yuen MF, Sablon E, Chan AO, Wong BC, Lai CL: Interferon and ribavirin therapy for chronic hepatitis C virus genotype 6: A comparison with genotype 1. J Infect Dis 2003;187:1071–1074.

8 Desmet VJ, Gerber M, Hoofnagle JH, Manns M, Scheuer PJ: Classification of chronic hepatitis: Diagnosis, grading and staging. Hepatology 1994;19:1513–1520.

9 McHutchison JG, Gordon SC, Schiff ER, Shiffman ML, Lee WM, Rustgi VK, Goodman ZD, Ling MH, Cort S, Albrecht JK: Interferon alfa-2b alone or in combination with ribavirin as initial treatment for chronic hepatitis C. N Engl J Med 1998;339:1485–1492.

10 Poynard T, Marcellin P, Lee SS, Niederau C, Minuk GS, Ideo G, Bain V, Heathcote J, Zeuzem S, Trepo C, Albrecht J: Randomised trial of interferon alpha2b plus ribavirin for 48 weeks or for 24 weeks versus interferon alpha2b plus placebo for 48 weeks for treatment of chronic infection with hepatitis C virus. Lancet 1998;352:1426–1432.

Intervirology

Intervirology 2006;49:99–106
DOI: 10.1159/000087271

Treatment of Chronic Hepatitis C in Southern Taiwan

Wang-Long Chuang Ming-Lung Yu Chia-Yen Dai Wen-Yu Chang

Hepatobiliary Division, Department of Internal Medicine, Kaohsiung Medical University, Kaohsiung, Taiwan, ROC

Key Words
Chronic hepatitis C · Genotypes · Hepatitis C virus · Interferon · Ribavirin

Abstract
Chronic hepatitis C virus (HCV) infection may lead to cirrhosis and hepatocellular carcinoma. Interferon (IFN)-α is effective in the treatment of chronic hepatitis C. The rate of response to IFN is enhanced by increasing the IFN dose. Extending the treatment duration can reduce the relapse rate. Addition of ribavirin to IFN increases the sustained virological response (SVR). Thus, combination therapy with IFN and ribavirin was adopted for the treatment of chronic hepatitis C in Kaohsiung Medical University Hospital in 1998. Approximately 60% of patients receiving IFN/ribavirin therapy gained SVR. IFN 6 million units three times per week combined with daily ribavirin for 6 months achieved SVR more frequently than combination therapy with 3 million units. Factors for SVR in these combination regimens were HCV genotype, viral load and early virological response. Long-term follow-up of patients treated with IFN has shown that SVR might reduce the risk of progression to cirrhosis and hepatocellular carcinoma. Pegylated (peg)-IFN has a longer half-life and better efficacy. Combination therapy with peg-IFN and ribavirin accomplished higher SVR than conventional IFN and ribavirin. A multicenter clinical trial was conducted in Taiwan to compare the efficacy of combination therapy between peg-IFN/ribavirin and conventional IFN/ribavirin for 6 months. SVR was higher in patients receiving peg-IFN and ribavirin, especially in those infected with HCV genotype 1b. Based on the results obtained, the national health insurance started to sponsor the combination therapy in October 2003, with a suggested duration for 6 months. Some small-scale studies in Taiwan have postulated higher SVR for treatment duration of 12 than of 6 months in patients with genotype 1b. Further investigation should be conducted in the near future.

Introduction

Hepatitis C virus (HCV) infection is a major health problem throughout the world. There are more than 170 million people chronically infected with HCV [1, 2], and approximately 280,000 deaths per year are related to HCV infection [2, 3]. HCV is a single-stranded RNA virus of the Flaviviridae family. It is mainly transmitted through parenteral exposure to blood and blood products. Although transmission through blood products and organ transplants has been eliminated by the introduction of tests for anti-HCV since 1992, HCV infection may exist in patients with injection drug use, blood transfusion before 1992, solid organ transplantation from infected donors, unsafe medical practices, occupational exposure to

KARGER
Fax +41 61 306 12 34
E-Mail karger@karger.ch
www.karger.com

0300–5526/06/0492–0099$23.50/0

Accessible online at:
www.karger.com/int

Wen-Yu Chang, MD
Hepatobiliary Division, Department of Internal Medicine
Kaohsiung Medical University, No. 100 Shih-Chuan 1st Road
Kaohsiung 807, Taiwan (ROC)
Tel. +886 7 3121101, ext. 7475, Fax +886 7 3123955, E-Mail waloch@kmu.edu.tw

infected blood, sex with an infected person, high-risk sexual practices and possibly intranasal cocaine use, and in children of infected mothers [4].

Prospective studies have shown that 60–85% of HCV-infected subjects develop chronic infection [4, 5]. The most important sequelae of chronic HCV infection are progressive liver fibrosis leading to cirrhosis, end-stage liver disease and hepatocellular carcinoma (HCC) [2, 4–8]. The estimated proportion of chronically infected people who develop cirrhosis 20 years after the initial infection varies widely. The actual risk is estimated at around 10–15% [4]. The risk whether a person with chronic hepatitis C will develop HCC appears to be 1–5% after 20 years. Once cirrhosis is established, the rate of developing HCC increases to 1–4% per year [5]. Thus, effective management of chronic HCV infection is very important. The goal of treatment for chronic HCV infection is sustained virological response (SVR) accompanied by improvement of liver damage. SVR was defined by the absence of HCV RNA in serum detectable by qualitative HCV RNA assays with a lower limit of detection at 50 IU/ml or less than 24 weeks after the end of treatment [4]. Potential benefits of SVR would be decreased infectivity, prevention of liver damage and improvement of the necroinflammatory process. In the long run, SVR may decrease the risk of developing cirrhosis, decompensation and HCC, along with prolonged survival and improved quality of life [2, 4].

Seroepidemiology of HCV Infection in Southern Taiwan

There is considerable geographic variation in the incidence and prevalence of HCV infection. The estimated prevalence of HCV infection is 1–3% in Western countries [4, 9, 10]. However, anti-HCV prevalence in the general population of Egypt is much higher at 15–20% [11]. A similar situation might be present in different areas of the same country. For example, although the prevalence of anti-HCV in Taiwan was 1–3% [12–15], there were several HCV hyperendemic townships in southern Taiwan where anti-HCV prevailed in more than 15% of inhabitants [16–19]. To investigate the actual prevalence of HCV infection, we conducted a large-scale community-based survey in southern parts of Taiwan including some HCV hyperendemic townships from 2000 to 2003. Surprisingly, the prevalence of anti-HCV around Kaohsiung, the second largest city in Taiwan, was quite high at 5.4% (877/16,320) in comparison with that reported in northern Taiwan (table 1). Furthermore, the prevalence of HCV infection in the adults of two villages in Masago was over 60% (table 1). Age-specific prevalence of anti-HCV has demonstrated that HCV infection increases in parallel with age both in northern and southern Taiwan (table 2). The prevalence of anti-HCV was not significantly different between men and women in southern Taiwan (data not shown).

Table 1. The prevalence (%) of anti-HCV in the general population of Taiwan

Area and study	Subjects examined	Anti-HCV	Prevalence
Northern Taiwan			
Chen et al. [12], 1990	420	4	0.95
Lee et al. [13], 1991	1,419	4	0.28
Sheu et al. [14], 1993	1,500	37	2.5
Southern Taiwan			
Chuang et al. [15], 1993	275	8	2.9
Chuang et al. [39], 2004			
Kaohsiung	16,320	877	5.4
A-Lien	407	32	7.9
Tzukuan	5,881	120	20.4
Masago	600	417	69.5

Taiwan is a country hyperendemic for hepatitis B virus (HBV). Besides HBV, HCV is also a major cause of chronic liver disease including HCC in Taiwan. The prevalence of anti-HCV in patients with chronic liver disease without hepatitis B surface antigen (HBsAg) in serum was between 60 and 80% in Taiwan [12, 20]; however, HCV also plays an important role in patients with HBsAg. The frequency of anti-HCV in HBsAg-positive patients was 10–20% [12, 15, 20]. In addition, concurrent HCV infection in patients with chronic HBV infection may accelerate the progression of liver damage and contribute to the development of HCC [6, 15].

Distribution of HCV Genotypes in Southern Taiwan

Several HCV strains have been identified on the basis of nucleotide and amino acid diversities. Although these strains can be classified into six major types [21, 22], predominant geographical distribution of a few particular genotypes has been reported [22–24]. Genotypes help predict SVR and plan treatment duration [2, 4, 5]. HCV genotype 1b was most prevalent in Taiwan [25–27], but

Table 2. The age-specific prevalence (%) of anti-HCV in Taiwan

Area	Anti-HCV	Age group						
		6–10	11–20	21–40		>40		
Northern Taiwan								
Lee et al. [13], 1991 (n = 1,419)	0.28	0	0	0.6		2.5		
				21–30	31–40	41–50	51–60	>60
Sheu et al. [14], 1993 (n = 1,500)	2.5			2.0	1.5	2.1	4.5	6.7
			<20	21–40		41–60		>60
Southern Taiwan								
Chuang et al. [39], 2004 (n = 16,320)	5.4		2.3	2.5		5.1		7.2

Table 3. Distribution of HCV genotypes in Taiwan

Area and study	Genotypes							
	n	1a	1b	2a	2b	3a	mixed	unclassified
Northern Taiwan								
Wu et al. [25], 1994	122		89 (73)	16 (13)	13 (11)			4 (3)
Chen et al. [26], 1994	81		47 (58)	6 (7)	4 (5)		11 (14)	13 (16)
Kao et al. [27], 1995	175	1 (0.6)	125 (71)	21 (12)	6 (3)		18 (10)	4 (2)
Southern Taiwan								
Yu et al. [28], 1996	56		25 (45)	23 (41)	2 (4)		4 (7)	2 (4)
Yu et al. [29], 2001								
Kaohsiung	690	2 (0.3)	324 (47)	236 (34)	56 (8.1)	2 (0.3)	39 (5.7)	31 (4.5)
Taoyuan	169		130 (77)	6 (3.6)	14 (8.3)	1 (0.6)	6 (3.6)	12 (7.1)
Tzukuan	113	2 (1.8)	70 (62)	17 (15)	12 (11)		2 (1.8)	10 (8.8)
Masago	192	1 (0.5)	43 (22)	122 (64)	3 (1.6)	1 (0.5)	11 (5.7)	11 (5.7)

Figures in parentheses are percentages.

genotype 2a also contributed to the pathogenesis of HCV-related chronic liver disease in southern Taiwan in previous studies [25, 28]. This indicates that regional differences of genotype distribution might exist between northern and southern Taiwan. In addition, several areas hyperendemic for HCV have been discovered in southern Taiwan [16–19]; the molecular epidemiology of HCV may differ in these areas. In 1,164 subjects positive for anti-HCV and HCV RNA in serum from three HCV hyperendemic areas (community-based; Masago, Tzukuan and Taoyuan) and a tertiary referral center (hospital-based) in southern Taiwan, we determined genotype distribution to evaluate the age-specific prevalence of HCV genotypes and clarify the relationship between genotype and pathogenesis of HCV infection [29]; HCV genotypes were examined by the method of Okamoto et al. [30].

HCV genotypes were able to be determined in 1,100 of 1,164 (94.5%) subjects. Overall, genotype 1b (48.7%, n = 567) was the most prevalent, followed by genotype 2a (32.7%, n = 381), 2b (7.3%, n = 85), mixed genotypes (5.0%, n = 58), 1a (4%, n = 5) and 3a (0.3%, n = 4). In particular, genotype 1b prevailed in Tzukuan (61.9%), Taoyuan (76.9%) and the referral center (47.0%). By contrast, 2a was the major HCV genotype in Masago (63.5%) (table 3). Since genotypes 1b and 2a were most prevalent in study populations, the age-specific prevalence of these

Table 4. SVR to IFN therapy in chronic hepatitis C patients with respect to two different virological risks (genotype 1b and HCV RNA levels >5.8 log/ml)[a]

Regimen	SVR			
	total	two risks	one risk	no risks
Fixed	36/123 (29)	3/36 (8)[b]	17/64 (27)[c]	16/23 (70)
Tailored	42/90 (47)	6/23 (26)[b]	22/45 (49)[c]	14/22 (64)

Figures in parentheses are percentages.
[a] Adapted from Yu et al. [35], 2004.
[b] p = 0.06.
[c] p = 0.02.

two major genotypes was analyzed. HCV genotypes 1b and 2a inversely correlated with age ($p < 0.01$, χ^2 test with the linear trend). Based on multivariate analysis, factors significantly associated with cirrhosis, with or without HCC, in patients with chronic hepatitis C were genotype 1b and age. Our study suggested that independent HCV outbreaks continue in hyperendemic areas in Taiwan, and that the HCV infection keeps changing along with the relative prevalence of HCV genotypes in relation to age. Both the correlation of genotype 1b with age (cohort effect) and intrinsic properties of HCV genotypes are probably responsible for the association between genotype and pathogenesis of HCV infection [29].

Interferon Monotherapy for Chronic Hepatitis C in Southern Taiwan

Interferon (IFN)-α was the therapy first approved for chronic HCV infection in the 1980s. With the standard regimen of IFN-α monotherapy, 3 million units (MU) 3 times in a week (tiw) for 24–48 weeks, SVR could be achieved in 8–20% of patients with chronic hepatitis C [31, 32]. To evaluate the efficacy and safety of IFN treatment in Taiwanese patients with chronic hepatitis C and to find out the potential predictor(s) of SVR, we have conducted serial studies since 1992.

In an initial small-scale pilot study, we found that 30% (8/27) of patients can gain SVR [33]. Patients who received a higher dose of IFN and a longer duration of treatment had higher SVR. Patients with non-1 genotypes achieved higher SVR (40%, 8/20) than those with genotype 1 (0%, 0/7) [33]. Based on these preliminary results, we treated a further 200 patients. Again, the end of treatment response was greater in patients receiving a higher- (6 MU 3 tiw) than a lower-dose regimen (3 MU 3 tiw) for 6 months, 83% (103/124) versus 47% (36/76) ($p < 0.001$). Nevertheless, the relapse rates were quite high at 55 and 50%. SVR in patients with 6-MU and 3-MU regimens were 37 and 24%, respectively. Multivariate analysis demonstrated that viral load, HCV genotype, cirrhosis and IFN dose were independent predictors of SVR in Taiwanese patients with chronic hepatitis C (unpublished data).

Further analysis was performed with reference to virologically unfavorable risks, i.e. HCV genotype (genotype 1b) and viral load (>5.8 log/ml) [34]. Patients with no virological risks had a high SVR (68% for the 3-MU regimen and 75% for the 6-MU regimen), while those with two virological risks had a low SVR (11 and 13% for 3-MU and 6-MU regimens for 24 weeks, respectively). Higher-dose IFN (6 MU 3 tiw for 6 months) was superior to the standard IFN dose (3 MU 3 tiw) only among patients with one virological risk. The SVR for the 6-MU regimen was 30% (18/61) compared with 8% (3/39) for the 3-MU regimen ($p < 0.01$).

Therefore, a tailored 9- to 12-month regimen was instituted in 1997 with a higher IFN dose and longer duration for patients with higher virological risks (table 4) [35]. Again, the tailored regimen improved treatment in comparison with the fixed-dose regimen. SVR of tailored and fixed-dose regimens were 47% (42/90) and 29% (36/123), respectively. SVR was significantly increased both in patients with one and two virological risks. SVR were 49 and 27% in patients with only one virological risk treated with tailored and fixed-dose regimens, respectively ($p = 0.02$). Likewise, SVR were 26 and 8% in patients with two virological risks treated with tailored and fixed-dose regimens, respectively ($p = 0.06$).

IFN Combined with Ribavirin for Higher SVR than IFN Alone

Addition of ribavirin increased SVR of IFN monotherapy in treatment of chronic hepatitis C [36]. IFN/ribavirin combination therapy for 24 or 48 weeks elevated SVR to 31–43% [37, 38]. Thus, combined IFN and ribavirin therapy was adopted for treatment of chronic hepatitis C in the Kaohsiung Medical University Hospital in 1998. A total of 145 treatment-naive patients with chronic hepatitis C received IFN 6 MU 3 tiw plus daily ribavirin 1,000–1,200 mg for 6 months. End of treatment response (70%, 101/145) was similar to that of IFN monotherapy. Nonetheless, SVR of IFN/ribavirin reached 58% (84/145), which is much higher than that of IFN monotherapy ($p < 0.001$). Thus, addition of ribavirin may decrease the risk of relapse after treatment. Further analysis with the logistic regression method showed that HCV genotype, viral load, early virological response (EVR) with a minimum decrease of 2 logs in viral load, during the first 12 weeks of treatment, and addition of ribavirin were independent predictive factors of SVR. Our limited study has revealed that prolonging the duration of combination therapy may increase SVR, especially in patients with HCV genotype 1b and a viral load >0.8 mega international units/ml. SVR for 6-month and 12-month regimens were 28% (13/47) and 63% (12/19), respectively (unpublished data).

Retreatment of patients with a failure in IFN monotherapy is another important issue. Patients who failed to respond to previous IFN-α monotherapy may still benefit from retreatment with the combination regimen. To elucidate the efficacy and safety of IFN/ribavirin and to determine the possible predictors of SVR on retreatment, 120 patients who had failed to respond to the initial IFN monotherapy were treated [39]. They were randomly assigned (with a ratio of 1:1:2) to receive one of the three regimens for retreatment during 24 weeks: group A, IFN 6-MU monotherapy; group B, IFN 3 MU 3 tiw combined with ribavirin, and group C, combination therapy with ribavirin and IFN 6 MU 3 tiw (table 5). The overall SVR was 38% based on the intent-to-treat analysis, and SVR in group C (53%) was significantly higher than those of group A (17%, $p < 0.005$) and group B (30%, $p < 0.05$). Patients achieving SVR had significant improvement of liver damage. The logistic regression analysis revealed that non-1b genotype of HCV, lower pretreatment HCV RNA level, combination with ribavirin, higher IFN dose and relapse were independent predictors of SVR. Thus, more than one third of Taiwanese patients with chronic hepatitis C achieved SVR by combination therapy for 24 weeks. The results of our study also suggested that combination therapy with a higher dose of IFN can gain a higher efficacy [39].

Table 5. SVR to IFN combined with ribavirin in patients with chronic hepatitis C who failed to respond to previous IFN-α monotherapy[a]

Regimen for 6 months		SVR	p value
Group A	IFN 6 MU 3 tiw	5/30 (17)	<0.005[b]
Group B	IFN 3 MU 3 tiw plus ribavirin 1,000–1,200 mg/day	9/30 (30)	<0.05[b]
Group C	IFN 6 MU 3 tiw plus ribavirin 1,000–1,200 mg/day	32/60 (53)	

Figures in parentheses are percentages.
[a] Adapted from Chuang et al. [39], 2004.
[b] Compared with group C.

Effect of IFN on the Occurrence of Cirrhosis and HCC

Potential benefits of SVR include decrease in infectivity, prevention of liver damage and improvement in the necroinflammatory process. Long-term benefits may be decrease in the risk of cirrhosis, decompensation and HCC, as well as prolonged patient survival and improved quality of life [2, 4]. Although there is an obvious ethical problem in performing large-scale randomized trials with placebos to prove the reduction in morbidity and mortality, several studies have shown a decrease in morbidity and mortality among patients given IFN, especially in the development of cirrhosis and HCC [2, 40, 41]. We have followed 427 patients with chronic hepatitis C who were treated with IFN (214 patients received IFN monotherapy and 213 IFN/ribavirin) for 10–117 months (median 60 months). Clinical evaluation, liver biochemistry, α-fetoprotein and abdominal ultrasonography were performed every 3–6 months on patients without cirrhosis at the baseline, and every 2–3 months on those with baseline cirrhosis. For the 367 patients noncirrhotic at the baseline, 17 of 166 (10.2%) nonresponders and 6 of 201 (3.0%) sustained responders progressed to cirrhosis ($p < 0.01$ by the Kaplan-Meier survival analysis). In 427 patients without HCC at the baseline, 16 of 204 (7.8%) nonresponders and 3 of 223 (1.4%) sustained responders developed HCC ($p < 0.01$ by the Kaplan-Meier survival analysis). These results have confirmed that treatment with IFN monotherapy or IFN/ribavirin combination therapy can decrease the development of liver cirrhosis and HCC in Taiwanese patients with chronic hepatitis C.

Pegylated IFN Combined with Ribavirin for Chronic Hepatitis C

Pegylation or addition of polyethylene glycol to IFN prolongs half-life in plasma, reduces clearance and decreases immunogenicity. Hence, pegylated (peg)-IFN

Table 6. SVR to peg-IFN combined with ribavirin in patients with chronic hepatitis C

Patient group	n	SVR	p value
Genotype 1	23	13 (56)	
Genotype non-1	38	36 (95)	<0.001[a]
Total	61	49 (80)	

Figures in parentheses are percentages.
[a] Compared with genotype 1 group.

have a longer half-life and better efficacy. Combination therapy with peg-IFN and ribavirin accomplished higher SVR than the conventional IFN/ribavirin [2, 4, 42–44]. To evaluate the safety and efficacy of peg-INF/ribavirin compared with the conventional IFN/ribavirin, a multicenter randomized clinical trial was conducted in five clinical centers in Taiwan on 153 treatment-naive patients with chronic hepatitis C [45]. Patients received peg-IFN-α_{2b}/ribavirin for 6 months or the conventional IFN-α_{2b}/ribavirin for 6 months. Patients treated with peg-IFN/ribavirin gained higher SVR than those with the conventional IFN/ribavirin. Per-protocol analysis revealed an overall significant difference in SVR between peg-IFN/ribavirin and the conventional IFN/ribavirin regimens, especially in patients infected with HCV genotype 1 (74 vs. 44% on peg-IFN and conventional IFN regimens, respectively). For patients with genotype non-1 infection, SVR was above 90% with either regimen [45]. In our study, peg-IFN/ribavirin gained higher SVR than the conventional IFN/ribavirin regimen. Of patients treated with peg-IFN/ribavirin for 6 months, SVR in those with genotype 1 and non-1 reached 56 and 95%, even in the intent-to-treat analysis (table 6).

Based on encouraging results of the multicenter clinical trial [45], the national health insurance started to sponsor the treatment of chronic hepatitis C in October 2003, with a suggested duration of 6 months. Fried et al. [43] demonstrated that hepatitis C patients without an EVR after peg-IFN/ribavirin had a small chance of achieving SVR. The NIH consensus statement also suggests that IFN does not need to be extended beyond 12 weeks in patients without EVR [4]. Nonetheless, the Taiwanese patients without EVR have been observed to achieve an SVR in up to 33% [45]. Therefore, it is suggested that patients with chronic hepatitis C in Taiwan should be treated for 6 months even if EVR is not accomplished. In addition, patients with HCV genotype 1 responded well to the 6-month regimen in Taiwan [45]. Hence, the Bureau of National Health Insurance in Taiwan is now supporting HCV treatment with 6-month combination therapy regardless of genotypes.

Longer duration of IFN treatment leads to higher SVR, both in IFN monotherapy and combined with ribavirin [31, 32, 35, 37, 38]. Hadziyannis et al. [44] postulated that in patients infected with HCV genotype 1, 48-week treatment with peg-IFN/ribavirin is statistically superior to 24-week treatment. In a small-scale multicenter clinical trial conducted by Professor M.-Y. Lai of the National Taiwan University Hospital, SVR with the 48-week regimen of peg-IFN/ribavirin was higher than that of the 24-week regimen in patients with HCV genotype 1b who had failed to respond to previous IFN-α monotherapy (85 vs. 36%) [pers. commun.]. We have treated 6 treatment-naive patients infected with HCV genotype 1b with peg-IFN/ribavirin for 48 weeks. Five of them (83%) gained SVR at a frequency much higher than that of 24-week peg-IFN/ribavirin. Further investigation should be conducted in the near future in Taiwan to confirm the advantage of extending the duration of therapy.

Conclusion

HCV infection is a major health problem throughout the world. The estimated prevalence of HCV infection is 1–3% in Taiwan. However, there were several townships hyperendemic for HCV in southern Taiwan with an anti-HCV prevalence at 15%, which is much higher than the overall prevalence of anti-HCV around 5%. The distribution of HCV genotypes differs between northern and southern Taiwan. HCV genotype 1b is most prevalent in Taiwan, but genotype 2a plays an important role in HCV-associated chronic liver disease of southern Taiwan. Thus, effective management of chronic HCV infection is very important in southern Taiwan. Treatment of chronic hepatitis C patients with IFN/ribavirin can achieve SVR in 50–60%. Retreatment of patients who have failed to respond to previous IFN monotherapy can achieve satisfactory results. Therefore, combination therapy should be considered as the first-line treatment of patients with chronic hepatitis C. The long-term benefits of IFN monotherapy or IFN/ribavirin combination therapy in patients with chronic hepatitis C may decrease the risk of cirrhosis and HCC. The peg-IFN has a longer half-life and better efficacy. Combination therapy with peg-IFN and ribavirin has achieved higher SVR than the conventional IFN/ribavirin therapy. Based on these results, the national health insurance in Taiwan has sponsored the treatment of chronic hepatitis C since October 2003, for a suggested duration of 6 months. Nevertheless, some small-scale studies in Taiwan have postulated that SVR with a 12-month regimen is higher than that with a 6-month regimen in patients infected with HCV genotype 1b. Further investigation should be conducted in the near future to find out the most efficient treatment of patients with chronic hepatitis C.

References

1 Lauer GM, Walker BD: Hepatitis C virus infection. N Engl J Med 2001;345:41–52.
2 Poynard T, Yuen MF, Ratziu V, Lai CL: Viral hepatitis C. Lancet 2003;362:2095–2100.
3 El-Serag HB: Hepatocellular carcinoma: An epidemiologic view. J Clin Gastroenterol 2002; 35:S72–S78.
4 Anonymous: NIH Consensus Statement on Management of Hepatitis C, 2002. NIH Consens State Sci Statements 2002;19:1–46.
5 Anonymous: Management of hepatitis C. NIH Consens Statement 1997;15:1–41.
6 Chuang WL, Chang WY, Lu SN, Su WP, Lin ZY, Chen SC, Hsieh MY, Wang LY, You SL, Chen CJ: The role of hepatitis B and C viruses in hepatocellular carcinoma in a hepatitis B endemic area. A case-control study. Cancer 1992; 69:2052–2054.
7 Poynard T, Bedossa P, Opolon P: Natural history of liver fibrosis progression in patients with chronic hepatitis C. Lancet 1997;349: 825–832.
8 Seeff LB: Natural history of hepatitis C. Am J Med 1999;107:S10–S15.
9 Wasley A, Alter MJ: Epidemiology of hepatitis C: Geographic differences and temporal trends. Semin Liver Dis 2000;20:1–16.
10 Touzet S, Kraemer L, Colin C, Pradat P, Lanoir D, Bailly F, Coppola RC, Sauleda S, Thursz MR, Tillmann H, Alberti A, Braconier JH, Esteban JI, Hadziyannis SJ, Manns MP, Saracco G, Thomas HC, Trepo C: Epidemiology of hepatitis C virus infection in seven European Union countries: A critical analysis of the literature. Eur J Gastroenterol Hepatol 2000;12:667–678.
11 Frank C, Mohamed MK, Strickland GT, Lavanchy D, Arthur RR, Magder LS, El Khoby T, Abdel-Wahab Y, Aly Ohn ES, Anwar W, Sallam I: The role of parenteral antischistosomal therapy in the spread of hepatitis C virus in Egypt. Lancet 2000;355:887–891.
12 Chen DS, Kuo GC, Sung JL, Lai MY, Sheu JC, Chen PJ, Yang PM, Hsu HM, Chang MH, Chen CJ: Hepatitis C virus infection in an area hyperendemic for hepatitis B and chronic liver disease: The Taiwan experience. J Infect Dis 1990;162:817–822.
13 Lee SD, Chan CY, Wang YJ, Wu JC, Lai KH, Tsai YT, Lo KJ: Seroepidemiology of hepatitis C virus infection in Taiwan. Hepatology 1991; 13:830–833.
14 Sheu JC, Wang JT, Wang TH, Wang CY, Yang PM, Huang GT, Shih LN, Lee HS, Chen DS: Prevalence of hepatitis C viral infection in a community in Taiwan. Detection by synthetic peptide-based assay and polymerase chain reaction. J Hepatol 1993;17:192–198.
15 Chuang WL, Chang WY, Lu SN, Lin ZY, Chen SC, Hsieh MY, Wang LY, You SL, Chen CJ: The role of hepatitis C virus in chronic hepatitis B virus infection. Gastroenterol Jpn 1993; 28:S23–S27.
16 Wu JS, Lu CF, Chou WH, Chen HY, Lee HF, Wu YC, Lin SY: High prevalence of hepatitis C virus infection in aborigines in Taiwan. Jpn J Med Sci Bio 1992;45:165–171.
17 Lu SN, Chue PY, Chen HC, Wu MH, Chen IL, Huang JF, Wang JH, Peng CF, Shih CH, You SL, Lu CF, Chen CJ, Chang WY: Different viral aetiology of hepatocellular carcinoma between two hepatitis B and C endemic townships in Taiwan. J Gastroenterol Hepatol 1997;12:547–550.
18 Wang JH, Lu SN, Wu JC, Huang JF, Yu ML, Chen SC, Chuang WL: A hyperendemic community of hepatitis B virus and hepatitis C virus infection in Taiwan. Trans R Soc Trop Med Hyg 1999;93:253–254.
19 Wang CS, Chang TT, Yao WJ, Chou P: Comparison of hepatitis B virus and hepatitis C virus prevalence and risk factors in a community-based study. Am J Trop Med Hyg 2002;66: 389–393.
20 Liaw YF, Chien RN, Sheen IS, Lin DY, Lin HH, Chu CM: Hepatitis C virus infection in patients with chronic liver diseases in an endemic area for hepatitis B virus infection. Gastroenterol Jpn 1991;26:S167–S169.
21 Simmonds P, Holmes EC, Cha TA, Chan SW, McOmish F, Irvine B, Beall E, Yap PL, Kolberg J, Urdea MS: Classification of hepatitis C virus into six major genotypes and a series of subtypes by phylogenetic analysis of the NS-5 region. J Gen Virol 1993;74:2391–2399.
22 Simmonds P, Smith DB: Investigation of the pattern of diversity of hepatitis C virus in relation to times of transmission. J Viral Hepat 1997;4:S69–S74.
23 Dusheiko G, Schmilovitz-Weiss H, Brown D, McOmish F, Yap PL, Sherlock S, McIntyre N, Simmonds P: Hepatitis C virus genotypes: An investigation of type-specific differences in geographic origin and disease. Hepatology 1994;19:13–18.
24 McOmish F, Yap PL, Dow BC, Follett EA, Seed C, Keller AJ, Cobain TJ, Krusius T, Kolho E, Naukkarinen R: Geographical distribution of hepatitis C virus genotypes in blood donors: An international collaborative survey. J Clin Microbiol 1994;32:884–892.
25 Wu JS, Lee HF, Hsiau HL, Lu HY, Chou WH, Lu CF, Chen HY, Lee FN, Chen PY, Tam KM: Genotype distribution of hepatitis C virus infection in Taiwan. J Med Virol 1994;44:74–79.
26 Chen CH, Sheu JC, Wang JT, Huang GT, Yang PM, Lee HS, Lee CZ, Chen DS: Genotypes of hepatitis C virus in chronic liver disease in Taiwan. J Med Virol 1994;44:234–236.
27 Kao JH, Chen PJ, Lai MY, Yang PM, Sheu JC, Wang TH, Chen DS: Genotypes of hepatitis C virus in Taiwan and the progression of liver disease. J Clin Gastroenterol 1995;21:233–237.
28 Yu ML, Chuang WL, Lu SN, Chen SC, Wang JH, Lin ZY, Hsieh MY, Wang LY, Chang WY: The genotypes of hepatitis C virus in patients with chronic hepatitis C virus infection in southern Taiwan. Kaohsiung J Med Sci 1996; 12:605–612.
29 Yu ML, Chuang WL, Chen SC, Dai CY, Hou C, Wang JH, Lu SN, Huang JF, Lin ZY, Hsieh MY, Tsai JF, Wang LY, Chang WY: Changing prevalence of hepatitis C virus genotypes: Molecular epidemiology and clinical implications in the hepatitis C virus hyperendemic areas and a tertiary referral center in Taiwan. J Med Virol 2001;65:58–65.
30 Okamoto H, Tokita H, Sakamoto M, Horikita M, Kojima M, Iizuka H, Mishiro S: Characterization of the genomic sequence of type V (or 3a) hepatitis C virus isolates and PCR primers for specific detection. J Gen Virol 1993;74: 2385–2390.
31 Poynard T, Leroy V, Cohard M, Thevenot T, Mathurin P, Opolon P, Zarski JP: Meta-analysis of interferon randomized trials in the treatment of viral hepatitis C: Effects of dose and duration. Hepatology 1996;24:778–789.
32 Thevenot T, Regimbeau C, Ratziu V, Leroy V, Opolon P, Poynard T: Meta-analysis of interferon randomized trials in the treatment of viral hepatitis C in naive patients: 1999 update. J Viral Hepat 2001;8:48–62.

33 Yu ML, Chuang WL, Chen SC, Lu SN, Wang JH, Lin ZY, Hsieh MY, Wang LY, Chang WY: Treatment of chronic hepatitis C with interferon-alpha: A preliminary report. Kaohsiung J Med Sci 1996;12:581–589.

34 Yu ML, Chuang WL, Chen SC, Lin ZY, Hsieh MY, Wang LY, Chang WY: Clinical application of the Quantiplex HCV RNA 2.0 and Amplicor HCV Monitor assays for quantifying serum hepatitis C virus RNA. J Clin Pathol 1999; 52:807–811.

35 Yu ML, Dai CY, Chen SC, Lee LP, Huang JF, Lin ZY, Hsieh MY, Wang LY, Chuang WL, Chang WY: A prospective study on treatment of chronic hepatitis C with tailored and extended interferon-alpha regimens according to pretreatment virological factors. Antiviral Res 2004;63:25–32.

36 Lai MY, Kao JH, Yang PM, Wang JT, Chen PJ, Chan KW, Chu JS, Chen DS: Long-term efficacy of ribavirin plus interferon alfa in the treatment of chronic hepatitis C. Gastroenterology 1996;111:1307–1312.

37 McHutchison JG, Gordon SC, Schiff ER, Shiffman ML, Lee WM, Rustgi VK, Goodman ZD, Ling MH, Cort S, Albrecht JK: Interferon alfa-2b alone or in combination with ribavirin as initial treatment for chronic hepatitis C. N Engl J Med 1998;339:1485–1492.

38 Poynard T, Marcellin P, Lee SS, Niederau C, Minuk GS, Ideo G, Bain V, Heathcote J, Zeuzem S, Trepo C, Albrecht J: Randomised trial of interferon alpha2b plus ribavirin for 48 weeks or for 24 weeks versus interferon alpha2b plus placebo for 48 weeks for treatment of chronic infection with hepatitis C virus. Lancet 1998;352:1426–1432.

39 Chuang WL, Dai CY, Chen SC, Lee LP, Lin ZY, Hsieh MY, Wang LY, Yu ML, Chang WY: Randomized trial of three different regimens for 24 weeks for re-treatment of chronic hepatitis C patients who failed to respond to interferon-alpha monotherapy in Taiwan. Liver Int 2004;24:595–602.

40 Shiratori Y, Imazeki F, Moriyama M, Yano M, Arakawa Y, Yokosuka O, Kuroki T, Nishiguchi S, Sata M, Yamada G, Fujiyama S, Yoshida H, Omata M: Histologic improvement of fibrosis in patients with hepatitis C who have sustained response to interferon therapy. Ann Intern Med 2000;132:517–524.

41 Nishiguchi S, Shiomi S, Nakatani S, Takeda T, Fukuda K, Tamori A, Habu D, Tanaka T: Prevention of hepatocellular carcinoma in patients with chronic active hepatitis C and cirrhosis. Lancet 2001;357:196–197.

42 Manns MP, McHutchison JG, Gordon SC, Rustgi VK, Shiffman M, Reindollar R, Goodman ZD, Koury K, Ling M, Albrecht JK: Peginterferon alfa-2b plus ribavirin compared with interferon alfa-2b plus ribavirin for initial treatment of chronic hepatitis C: A randomised trial. Lancet 2001;358:958–965.

43 Fried MW, Shiffman ML, Reddy KR, Smith C, Marinos G, Goncales FL Jr, Haussinger D, Diago M, Carosi G, Dhumeaux D, Craxi A, Lin A, Hoffman J, Yu J: Peginterferon alfa-2a plus ribavirin for chronic hepatitis C virus infection. N Engl J Med 2002;347:975–982.

44 Hadziyannis SJ, Sette H Jr, Morgan TR, Balan V, Diago M, Marcellin P, Ramadori G, Bodenheimer H Jr, Bernstein D, Rizzetto M, Zeuzem S, Pockros PJ, Lin A, Ackrill AM: Peginterferon-alpha2a and ribavirin combination therapy in chronic hepatitis C: A randomized study of treatment duration and ribavirin dose. Ann Intern Med 2004;140:346–355.

45 Lee SD, Yu ML, Lai MY, Chao YC, Cheng PN, Hwang SJ, Chang WY, Chang TT, Hsieh TY, Liu CJ, Chen DS: Comparison of peginterferon-α_{2b} plus ribavirin and interferon-α_{2b} plus ribavirin in treating Chinese patients with chronic hepatitis C in Taiwan. J Viral Hepat, in press.

Intervirology

Intervirology 2006;49:107–111
DOI: 10.1159/000087272

Treatment of Chronic Hepatitis C in Patients with End-Stage Renal Disease and Hemophilia – The Singapore Experience

Wan-Cheng Chow[a] Sim-Leng Tien[b] Chee-Kiat Tan[a] Hock-Foong Lui[a] Anantharaman Vathsala[c] Han-Seong Ng[a]

Departments of [a]Gastroenterology, [b]Haematology and [c]Renal Medicine, Singapore General Hospital, Singapore, Singapore

Key Words
Hemophilia · Hepatitis C virus · Interferon · Renal failure · Thyroid dysfunction

Abstract
Objective: The aim of this study was to determine the response to treatment with interferon-alpha (IFN-α) in patients with chronic hepatitis C who had end-stage renal disease (ESRD) or hemophilia in Singapore. ***Methods:*** Treatment-naive hepatitis patients with ESRD or hemophilia were given IFN-α_{2a} 3 million units three times per week for 12 months in an open-label study. Hepatitis C virus RNA was determined before treatment, at the end of treatment and 6 months thereafter. Regular clinical examinations including blood counts and biochemistry were carried out during and after the treatment. ***Results:*** Nine consecutive patients with ESRD (8 men and 1 woman) and 6 consecutive male patients with hemophilia, with a mean age of 43 and 40 years, received treatment. Patients in both groups were predominantly infected with hepatitis C virus genotype 1 and had significant cytopenia affecting all three cell lines during the treatment; only 1 patient developed serious neutropenia, temporarily demanding a reduction of his IFN dose. Biochemical and virological responses at the end of treatment were accomplished by 8 of the 9 (89%) patients with ESRD and 4 of the 6 (67%) patients with hemophilia; however, 1 patient with ESRD and 2 with hemophilia relapsed after the treatment. Four of the 7 patients with ESRD who had sustained virological response underwent successful kidney transplantation later on. ***Conclusion:*** Monotherapy with IFN-α for 12 months is safe for treatment of the patients with chronic hepatitis C who had ESRD or those with hemophilia. A higher sustained virological response rate was observed in patients with ESRD than in those with hemophilia (78 vs. 33%).

Introduction

The prevalence of infection with chronic hepatitis C virus (HCV) is low in the general population of Singapore, with merely 0.37% of blood donors seropositive for anti-HCV [1]. In remarkable contrast, the prevalence of HCV infection is high in populations at risk, such as patients with end-stage renal disease (ESRD) and hematologic disorders. The prevalence of anti-HCV among Singaporean patients with ESRD undergoing peritoneal dialysis and hemodialysis was 5 and 28% [2], and that in patients with hemophilia was 46% [3]. The majority of these patients were infected with genotype 1 [3, 4]. Therefore, taking clinical and virological profiles of our patients into consideration, treatment of chronic hepatitis C, albeit in small numbers of patients, is a potential challenge for us.

KARGER

Fax +41 61 306 12 34
E-Mail karger@karger.ch
www.karger.com

0300–5526/06/0492–0107$23.50/0

Accessible online at:
www.karger.com/int

Wan-Cheng Chow, MD
Department of Gastroenterology
Singapore General Hospital
Outram Road, 169608 (Singapore)
Tel. +65 63214684, Fax +65 62273623, E-Mail gm2cwc@sgh.com.sg

Toward this goal, we examined the outcome of treatment of chronic hepatitis C in some patients with ESRD or hemophilia.

Patients and Methods

Treatment-naive patients with chronic hepatitis C who had ESRD or hemophilia were offered to receive monotherapy with interferon (IFN)-α for treatment of their liver disease. Independently, 9 consecutive ESRD patients were enrolled by their attending hepatologists and 6 consecutive hemophilia patients were enrolled by their managing hematologist from June 1997 to March 2002 and from June 1998 to May 1999, respectively. An open-label study for treatment with IFN-α_{2a} 3 million units subcutaneously three times per week was planned for these patients.

All patients were confirmed to be positive for anti-HCV by recombinant immunoblot assay (RIBA, Chiron, Emeryville, Calif., USA) with detectable HCV RNA in serum at baseline. Treatment was offered to all hemophilia patients whose serum levels of alanine aminotranasferase (ALT) were greater than 1.5 × upper limit of the normal. However, there was no exclusion limit of serum ALT for treatment of ESRD patients, because they needed to clear HCV RNA from serum to be logged in the waiting list for kidney transplantation.

At the beginning of treatment, the baseline physical examination was carried out along with tests for various laboratory parameters, including blood counts, liver and thyroid functions. Genotypes of HCV RNA were determined by the line-probe assay (InnoLiPA, Innogenetics, Ghent, Belgium). Pretreatment liver biopsies were performed on all patients with ESRD. During treatment, regular clinical check-ups were carried out at week 1, 2 and 4 of treatment and monthly thereafter till the end of treatment. After the treatment, patients were examined every 3 months for the first 6 months and every 6 months thereafter. Their blood counts, liver as well as thyroid function, and blood glucose levels were monitored during these visits up to 6 months after the treatment. HCV RNA was determined by the reverse transcription polymerase chain reaction (Amplicor, Roche, N.J., USA) before treatment, at 6 months of treatment, at the end of treatment and 6 months after the treatment.

Patients with ESRD

We treated 1 female and 8 male patients with ESRD, whose mean age was 43 years. They were all on regular hemodialysis, which was continued throughout their treatment of chronic hepatitis C. Genotyping was performed on 5 patients which were all infected with HCV genotype 1; 4 had infections with HCV genotype 1b, including 1 with a mixed infection with genotype 3a, and the remaining subject had an infection with HCV genotype 1a (table 1). Their mean serum levels of ALT and aspartate aminotransferase (AST) at the baseline were 88 and 54 U/l, respectively. Two of the 9 patients had a Knodell score for hepatic fibrosis ≥ 3 at the baseline. Clinically, all patients were in Child's class A.

Treatment Outcome

Treatment was discontinued in 1 patient at 6 months, because his HCV RNA stayed positive and serum ALT remained elevated at the same time point; therefore, he was considered a nonresponder to IFN. All the other 8 patients completed the course of treatment during a mean period of 53 weeks and achieved virological and biochemical responses at the end of treatment; they were negative for HCV RNA in serum, and their mean serum levels of ALT and AST at the end of treatment were 19 and 22 U/l, respectively. Unfortunately, 1 of the 8 patients developed a virological relapse and HCV RNA turned positive at 6 months after treatment. This patient was the only one who required transient attenuation in the dose of IFN due to significant neutropenia. However, he resumed the standard dose of IFN 1 week later. Thus, sustained virological and biochemical responses were accomplished in 7 of the 9 (78%) patients with ESRD. Up to the present, these 7 sustained responders to IFN remain well and aviremic through a mean follow-up period of 32 months after the treatment, and 4 of them have successfully undergone kidney transplantation. The incidence of allograft rejection did not increase in these patients.

Table 1. Baseline characteristics and treatment response to 1-year IFN monotherapy in patients with chronic hepatitis C who had ESRD or hemophilia

Features	ESRD	Hemophilia
Number of patients (men:women)	9 (8:1)	6 (6:0)
Mean age, years	43	40
HCV genotypes		
1a	1	1
1b	3	2
3a	0	1
Mixed with 1b	1 (plus 3a)	1 (plus 4a)
Mixed with 3	0	1 (plus 4)
Mean ALT level, U/l		
Pretreatment	88	190
Posttreatment	19	101
Mean AST level, U/l		
Pretreatment	54	117
Posttreatment	22	90
Response to IFN, number of patients (%)		
Sustained response	7 (78)	2 (33)
End-of-treatment response with relapse	1 (11)	2 (33)
No response	1 (11)	2 (33)
Mean treatment duration, weeks	53[a]	53
Mean follow-up period in sustained responders, months	32	41

Figures in parentheses are percentages, unless otherwise indicated.

[a] Not including treatment of a nonresponder to IFN that was discontinued at 24 weeks after the treatment.

Adverse Reactions

Overall, the ESRD patients tolerated well the IFN monotherapy at the conventional standard dose for treatment of hepatitis C. Seven of the 9 patients experienced some flu-like symptoms, with fever, myalgia and easy fatigability being the most persistent symptoms that lasted for 3–4 months. While the baseline blood counts of all

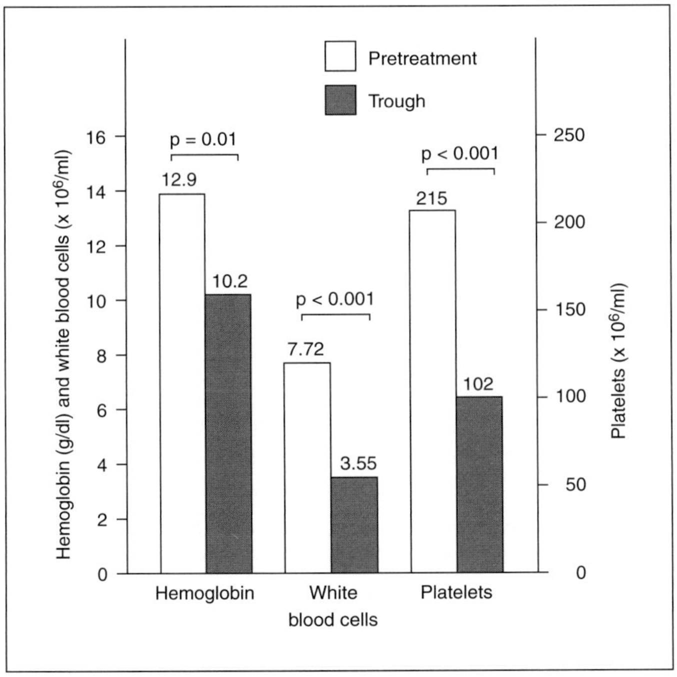

Fig. 1. Influence of IFN treatment on peripheral blood counts in patients with chronic hepatitis C who had ESRD.

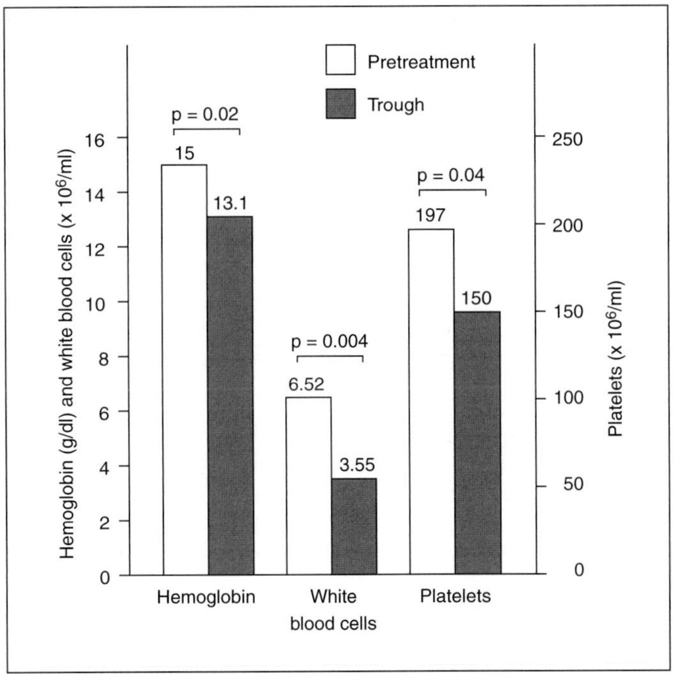

Fig. 2. Influence of IFN treatment on peripheral blood counts in patients with chronic hepatitis C who had hemophilia.

three cell lines were normal (table 1), there were statistically significant decreases in cell counts affecting all lineages during the treatment (fig. 1). However, transient attenuation of the IFN dose was required in only 1 patient. None developed sepsis related to neutropenia. All patients were on routine subcutaneous erythropoietin before and throughout the course of IFN treatment. Subclinical and reversible thyroid dysfunction was found in scheduled blood tests in 3 of the 9 patients. Two patients developed elevated levels of thyroid-stimulating hormone on and off, while their free thyroxine (T_4) levels remained normal throughout treatment. The other patient already had hypothyroidism before the treatment and required an increased dose of *L*-thyroxine replacement towards the end of the course of IFN treatment, as thyroid-stimulating hormone levels increased despite the usual maintenance treatment. However, the patient was asymptomatic of his hypothyroid state even before he had received an increased dose of *L*-thyroxine.

Patients with Hemophilia

Six patients with hemophilia, all men, with a mean age of 40 years, received IFN during a mean period of 53 weeks. Three patients were infected with HCV genotype 1b (including 1 having a mixed infection with HCV genotype 4a), 1 with HCV genotype 1a and 2 others with HCV genotype 3 (1 with genotype 3a infection and the other having a mixed infection with genotypes 3 and 4) (table 1). All of them were negative for antibody to human immunodeficiency virus type 1. Their mean serum levels of ALT and AST at the baseline were 190 and 117 U/l, respectively. No liver biopsy was performed on any of the 6 patients treated. None had clinical evidence of liver cirrhosis or hepatic decompensation.

Treatment Outcome

Of the 6 patients treated with IFN, 2 did not respond to it, with HCV RNA persisting in serum despite treatment. The other 4 patients gained virological and biochemical responses at the end of treatment and accomplished normalization of ALT levels and clearance of HCV RNA from serum. Unfortunately, 2 patients relapsed 4 and 6 weeks after the end of treatment. Therefore, sustained response was achieved in only 2 of the 6 (33%) patients who were followed up for 38 and 44 months after the treatment, respectively.

Adverse Reactions

All 6 patients treated with IFN complained of fever that lasted 6 weeks at the longest. The other two most common complaints were myalgia and easy fatigability, each affecting 4 of the 6 (67%) patients. In addition, there was a statistically significant drop in the mean hemoglobin level and a decrease in white cell and platelet counts during treatment, although they did not incur any clinical consequences (fig. 2). There was no increase in the bleeding diathesis during the treatment. No serious adverse events were documented in this cohort of patients.

Discussion

It is well known that chronic hepatitis C in patients with ESRD, if left untreated, increases their mortality and morbidity, with [5–7] or without kidney transplantation [8, 9]. However, as there is a substantial risk of allograft failure during IFN treatment of chronic hepatitis C in patients with kidney transplantation [10, 11], it makes sense to treat chronic hepatitis C before transplantation, with the aim of achieving sustained virological response (SVR) in patients with ESRD.

Earlier studies suggested poor SVR and high incidence of adverse events associated with IFN treatment of chronic hepatitis C in patients with ESRD [12, 13]. However, recently reported clinical data seem more encouraging [14, 15], and our findings are in agreement with these reports. Longer duration (12 instead of 6 months) and the use of the full dose, rather than attenuated doses, of IFN would contribute to an improved therapeutic outcome. Fortunately, our patients tolerated the full course of IFN treatment fairly well. None, with the exception of 1 patient, required temporary attenuation of the IFN dose. It is likely that the motivation of patients to receive kidney transplantation determines the tolerability for adverse symptoms. In Singapore, in view of a shortage of organ donors and a less favorable outcome associated with liver diseases after kidney transplantation, the absence of viremia with HCV has determined chances of patients on the waiting list for transplantation for receiving an allograft. This background may have been an important motivating factor and incentive for the treatment compliance. In addition, provision with adequate moral supports along with effective treatments, such as erythropoietin, during the course of treatment is probably just as important as the active treatment with IFN itself.

Unfortunately, we did not gain the same success in treatment of chronic hepatitis C in patients with hemophilia as we did in those with ESRD. However, the limited response accomplished was consistent with that reported in other published series in the Western populations, even with combined IFN and ribavirin [16–18].

Following the therapeutic success with the advent of pegylated (peg)-IFN, taken together with the established efficacy of combination therapy with ribavirin and IFN in the treatment of chronic hepatitis C in adult patients without high risks, we should explore possible benefits of these newer modalities of treatment on our subgroups of patients with ESRD or hemophilia. While ribavirin is generally not recommended for patients with ESRD, its use has been attempted by some investigators. These studies involving a small number of patients have proven the feasibility of ribavirin usage, but with limited therapeutic success [19, 20]. As for the usage of peg-IFN in patients with ESRD, it seems that we need to take into consideration the molecular sizes of various available peg-IFN, in relation to diverse ranges of permeability and the pore size of dialysers [21], in planning therapies with it. Given the current contradictory data [22, 23], not only the safety of the use of peg-IFN in patients with ESRD is required to be established, we also need to ascertain if SVR is influenced by different pharmacokinetics of various peg-IFN preparations in patients who are on maintenance hemodialysis.

Conclusion

Treatment with subcutaneous IFN-α_{2a} at a dose of 3 million units three times per week for 12 months gained SVR in 78% of patients with chronic hepatitis C and ESRD. The treatment was well tolerated and patients remained well after they received renal transplantation later on. However, a similar therapeutic regimen yielded poorer response, with only 33% accomplishing SVR in patients with chronic hepatitis C and hemophilia. Large-scale, randomized, controlled studies with newer agents, such as peg-IFN used singly or in combination, need to be conducted to evaluate the potential of various therapeutic regimens in these subgroups of patients for the purpose of establishing treatment guidelines.

References

1 Wang JE: A study on the epidemiology of hepatitis C infection among blood donors in Singapore. J Public Health Med 1995;17:387–391.
2 Choong HL: Hepatitis C in end-stage renal failure (abstract); in Oon CJ, Aw SE and Goh KT (eds): Selected Papers from the International Symposia on Viral Hepatitis and Hepatocellular Carcinoma Research. Singapore, Department of Clinical Research (Ministry of Health), 1992, p 105.
3 Tien SL, Ho LP, Lee ASG, Teng SW, Oon CJ: Hepatitis C infection in haemophilia patients at Singapore General Hospital (abstract). APASL Commemorative International Congress on Viral Hepatitis, Prevention and Control, Singapore, 2000, p 241.
4 Lee AS, Ng KY, Chee MK, Vathsala A, Choong HL, Ng HS, Oon CJ: Partial sequence analysis of the hepatitis C viral genome in Singapore patients. Biochem Biophys Res Commun 1994;199:37–40.
5 Pereira BJ, Levey AS: Hepatitis C virus infection in dialysis and renal transplantation. Kidney Int 1997;51:981–999.
6 Huang CC, Liaw YF, Lai MK, Chu SH, Chuang CK, Huang JY: The clinical outcome of hepatitis C virus antibody-positive renal allograft recipients. Transplantation 1992;53:763–765.
7 Chan TM, Wu PC, Lok AS, Lai CL, Cheng IK: Clinicopathological features of hepatitis C virus antibody negative fatal chronic hepatitis C after renal transplantation. Nephron 1995;71:213–217.
8 Nakayama E, Akiba T, Marumo F, Sato C: Prognosis of anti-hepatitis C virus antibody-positive patients on regular hemodialysis therapy. J Am Soc Nephrol 2000;11:1896–1902.
9 Stehman-Breen CO, Emerson S, Gretch D, Johnson RJ: Risk of death among chronic dialysis patients infected with hepatitis C virus. Am J Kidney Dis 1998;32:629–634.
10 Rostaing L, Modesto A, Baron E, Cisterne JM, Chabannier MH, Durand D: Acute renal failure in kidney transplant patients treated with interferon alpha 2b for chronic hepatitis C. Nephron 1996;74:512–516.
11 Kakimoto K, Takahara S, Kokado Y, Kameoka H, Ishibashi M, Okuyama A, Kyo M, Nagano S: A case of allograft rejection induced by the interferon-alpha therapy to hepatitis type C after renal transplantation. Hinyokika Kiyo 1994;40:529–532.
12 Duarte R, Huraib S, Said R, Abdel-Khadir A, Sullivan S, Chaballout A, Sbeih F, Mughal T: Interferon-alpha facilitates renal transplantation in hemodialysis patients with chronic viral hepatitis. Am J Kidney Dis 1995;25:40–45.
13 Koenig P, Vogel W, Umlauft F, Weyrer K, Prommegger R, Lhotta K, Neyer U, Stummvoll HK, Gruenewald K: Interferon treatment for chronic hepatitis C virus infection in uremic patients. Kidney Int 1994;45:1507–1509.
14 Fabrizi F, Dulai G, Dixit V, Bunnapradist S, Martin P: Meta-analysis: Interferon for the treatment of chronic hepatitis C in dialysis patients. Aliment Pharmacol Ther 2003;18:1071–1081.
15 Russo MW, Goldsweig CD, Jacobson IM, Brown RS Jr: Interferon monotherapy for dialysis patients with chronic hepatitis C: An analysis of the literature on efficacy and safety. Am J Gastroenterol 2003;98:1610–1615.
16 Makris M, Preston FE, Triger DR, Underwood JC, Westlake L, Adelman MI: A randomized controlled trial of recombinant interferon-alpha in chronic hepatitis C in hemophiliacs. Blood 1991;78:1672–1677.
17 Rumi MG, Santagostino E, Morfini M, Gringeri A, Tagariello G, Chistolini A, Pontisso P, Tagger A, Colombo M, Mannucci PM: A multicenter controlled, randomized, open trial of interferon alpha2b treatment of anti-human immunodeficiency virus-negative hemophilic patients with chronic hepatitis C. Hepatitis Study Group of the Association of Italian Hemophilia Centers. Blood 1997;89:3529–3533.
18 Dasani H, Loran CM, Collines PW: Treatment of chronic HCV with alpha-interferon and ribavirin in 28 patients with inherited bleeding disorders (abstract). Haemophilia 2000;6:326.
19 Bruchfeld A, Stahle L, Andersson J, Schvarcz R: Interferon and ribavirin therapy in dialysis patients with chronic hepatitis C. Nephrol Dial Transplant 2001;16:1729–1730.
20 Tan AC, Brouwer JT, Glue P, van Leusen R, Kauffmann RH, Schalm SW, de Vries RA, Vroom B: Safety of interferon and ribavirin therapy in haemodialysis patients with chronic hepatitis C: Results of a pilot study. Nephrol Dial Transplant 2001;16:193–195.
21 Barril G, Quiroga JA, Sanz P, Rodriguez-Salvanes F, Selgas R, Carreno V: Pegylated interferon-alpha2a kinetics during experimental haemodialysis: Impact of permeability and pore size of dialysers. Aliment Pharmacol Ther 2004;20:37–44.
22 Lamb MW, Marks IM, Wynohradnyk L, Modi MW, Preston RA, Pappas SC: 40 KDa peginterferon alfa-2a (Pegasys) can be administered safely in patients with end-sage renal disease (abstract). Hepatology 2001;34:326A.
23 Annicchiarico BE, Siciliano M: Pegylated interferon-alpha 2b monotherapy for haemodialysis patients with chronic hepatitis C. Aliment Pharmacol Ther 2004;20:123–124.

Treatment

Intervirology

Intervirology 2006;49:112–118
DOI: 10.1159/000087273

Treatment of Chronic Hepatitis C with Interferon Alone or Combined with Ribavirin in Japan

Takashi Kumada[a] Hidenori Toyoda[a] Takashi Honda[b] Teiji Kuzuya[a]
Yosiaki Katano[b] Isao Nakano[b] Hidemi Goto[b]

[a]Department of Gastroenterology, Ogaki Municipal Hospital, Ogaki, and [b]Department of Gastroenterology, Nagoya University School of Medicine, Nagoya, Japan

Key Words

Body mass index · Chronic hepatitis · Hepatitis C virus · Interferon · Ribavirin

Abstract

We treated 665 patients with chronic hepatitis C with interferon (IFN) monotherapy and 288 with combined IFN and ribavirin. At the baseline, age (53.8 ± 11.1 vs. 49.7 ± 10.5 years, p < 0.0001) and activity (p = 0.0207) as well as fibrosis (p = 0.0270) were higher in patients who received combination therapy than in those receiving monotherapy. Compliance to treatment (64.2 vs. 62.1%, p < 0.0001) and discontinuation were more frequent (18.1 vs. 14.5%, p < 0.0001) in patients with combination therapy than in those with monotherapy. Patients with combination therapy with genotype 2 infection achieved sustained viral response (SVR) at a rate of 77.0%, regardless of viral loads, in contrast to those with genotype 1 infection, of whom only 24.4% gained SVR. Of patients with combination therapy, reduction (42.6 vs. 29.0%, p = 0.0453) and discontinuation (34.0 vs. 21.6%, p = 0.0414) of ribavirin were more frequently required in the 47 patients ≥65 years than in the 241 patients <65 years. Although a trend for higher SVR to combination therapy was observed in patients aged <65 than in those aged ≥65 years (39.4 vs. 25.2%), the difference was not significant (p = 0.0819). In patients with genotype 1 infection, IFN monotherapy in addition to the 24-week combination therapy increased the SVR rate (18.3 vs. 42.6%, p = 0.0003). A decrease in SVR was observed with an increased body mass index in patients who received combination therapy.

Introduction

Hepatitis C virus (HCV) is a major cause of chronic hepatitis, cirrhosis and hepatocellular carcinoma (HCC). In Japan, annual deaths due to HCC have increased and exceeded 30,000, 75–80% of which are related to HCV infection [1, 2]. Since the approval of interferon (IFN) therapy for the treatment of chronic hepatitis C in 1992 in Japan, more than 300,000 patients have been treated with it. However, sustained virological response (SVR), which is defined by the absence of serum HCV RNA detectable by qualitative methods at the end of treatment and 6 months after the end of treatment, has been achieved in about one third of patients. The reasons for such a low SVR is attributed, at least partly, to restrictions on IFN therapy, such as the limitation of treatment duration within 6 months and prohibition of retreatment with IFN in Japan. Since April 2004, retreatment without any restriction on the duration of therapy has been approved in Japan. However, more than 70% of patients in Japan are

KARGER

Fax +41 61 306 12 34
E-Mail karger@karger.ch
www.karger.com

0300–5526/06/0492–0112$23.50/0

Accessible online at:
www.karger.com/int

Takashi Kumada, MD
Ogaki Municipal Hospital
4-86 Minaminokawa
Ogaki, Gifu, 503-8502 (Japan)
Tel. +81 584 81 3341, Fax +81 584 75 5715, E-Mail hosp3@omh.ogaki.gifu.jp

infected with HCV genotype 1b, for which the efficacy of IFN monotherapy is limited [3–5]. Most recently, combination therapy with ribavirin and IFN-α for 6 months, as well as monotherapy with consensus IFN or pegylated (peg)-IFN, was also approved. With these new regimens of IFN treatment, the efficacy in patients infected with HCV genotype 1b in high viral titers has slightly improved. However, with the 6-month limitation on the duration of combined IFN and ribavirin, the SVR rate has not been markedly improved and remains low at around 20%. The aim of this study is to provide an overview of the current status of treatment of hepatitis C in Japan.

Materials and Methods

Patients with Chronic Hepatitis C

During August 1989 to September 2003, 943 patients were treated with IFN and evaluated for therapeutic efficacy at the Ogaki Municipal Hospital, the Nagoya University School of Medicine and affiliated hospitals. The diagnosis of chronic hepatitis C was based on detection of HCV RNA by reverse transcription polymerase chain reaction with nested primers and histological confirmation of chronic hepatitis by liver biopsy. Patients received IFN therapies and were followed for clinical course and virological markers in serum. The protocol was approved by the ethics committees of each hospital and a written informed consent was obtained from each patient before therapy.

IFN Monotherapy and Combination Therapy

Patients received IFN monotherapy or combination therapy with IFN and ribavirin. From August 1989 to September 2003, 665 patients received IFN monotherapy. All patients were naive to IFN. Natural IFN-α (Otsuka Pharmaceutical Co., Ltd., Osaka, Japan, or Sumitomo Pharmaceutical Co., Ltd., Tokyo, Japan) was given to 272 patients, recombinant IFN-α_{2a} (Takeda Pharmaceutical Co., Ltd., Osaka, Japan) to 128 patients, recombinant IFN-α_{2b} (Schering-Plough, N.J., USA) to 110 patients, natural IFN-β (Daiichi Pharmaceutical Co., Ltd., Tokyo, Japan) to 99 patients, consensus IFN (IFN alfacon-1, Infergen, Amgen Inc., Calif., USA) to 18 patients, natural IFN-α and natural IFN-β to 17 patients and peg-IFN-α_{2a} (F. Hoffmann-La Roche, Basel, Switzerland) to 11 patients. The standard course of up to 30 weeks was administered to 560 patients and an extended course of more than 40 weeks to 95 patients. Between December 1999 and September 2003, 288 patients received combination therapy, 161 of whom were IFN naive and 127 retreated. IFN-naive patients received combination therapy, because they all presented with high viral loads in serum. Among retreated patients, 59 had transient viral response and 45 had no response to initial treatment, while response was unknown in the remaining 23 patients. The standard course therapy of 6 months was given to 222 patients and the long course therapy was given to 66 patients.

SVR was defined as HCV RNA in the serum undetectable by qualitative methods at the end and 6 months after the completion of treatment, along with normalized serum levels of alanine aminotransferase. Transient viral response was diagnosed when serum HCV RNA reappeared within 24 weeks after the end of treatment, usually accompanied by reelevation of serum alanine aminotransferase levels. No response was defined as the presence of HCV RNA during the treatment period.

Genotypes of HCV

HCV genotypes were determined by polymerase chain reaction with genotype-specific primers in 928 patients [6, 7]. HCV RNA was quantified by the target amplification technique using Amplicor HCV Monitor assay (Roche Molecular Systems, Calif., USA) in 943 patients [8]. Nucleotide sequences of the IFN sensitivity-determining region (ISDR) were determined by the method similar to those described by Enomoto et al. [9, 10]. The mutant type was defined as four or more substitutions of amino acids in the ISDR, the intermediate type as one to three substitutions, and the wild type as the complete identity with the prototype strain of genotype 1b (HCV-J).

Histology in the Liver

Fibrosis stage and activity grade were determined on biopsied liver specimens according to the Metavir criteria [11], and fibrosis was staged on a scale of F0–F4 (F0, no fibrosis; F1, portal fibrosis without septa; F2, few septa; F3, numerous septa without cirrhosis, and F4, cirrhosis) in 775 patients. Necroinflammatory activity was graded on a scale of A0–A3 (A0, no histological activity; A1, mild activity; A2, moderate activity, and A3, severe activity) in 744 patients.

Statistical Analyses

Variables having normal distribution were expressed by the mean ± standard deviation (SD) or by the median with the range in parentheses, and differences were evaluated by Student's t test and the Mann-Whitney U test. Differences in proportions were tested by the χ^2 test. For multivariate analysis, the multiple logistic regression analysis was used to predict the SVR. All p values were two-tailed, and those less than 0.05 were considered statistically significant.

Results

Comparison between IFN Monotherapy and Combination Therapies

Characteristics of patients who received IFN monotherapy or combination treatment are compared in table 1. The patients with combination therapy were older, more frequently infected with HCV genotype 2, with higher viral load and a higher grade of histological activity, as well as with an advanced stage of fibrosis. After treatment, patients receiving combination treatment gained a higher SVR rate for those with non-genotype 1 infection and had lower compliance to treatment, more frequent treatment discontinuation and shorter treatment duration than those with IFN monotherapy.

Among patients with genotype 1 infection in low viral load (<100 × 10^3 IU/ml), no differences were observed

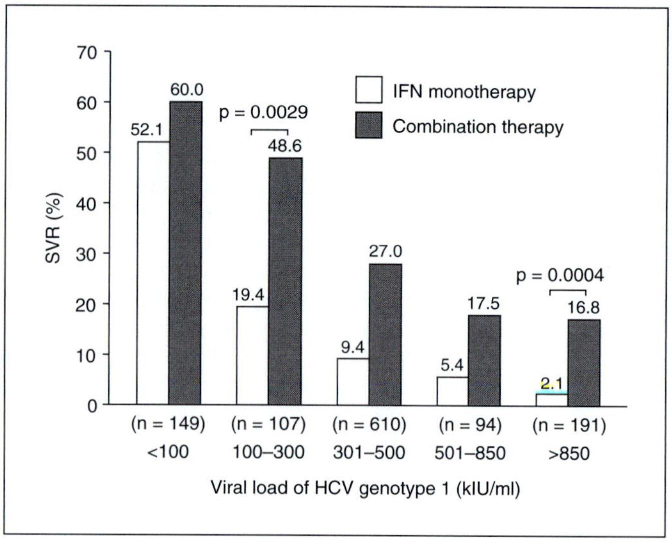

Fig. 1. SVR to IFN monotherapy or combination therapy in patients infected with HCV genotype 1 in various viral loads.

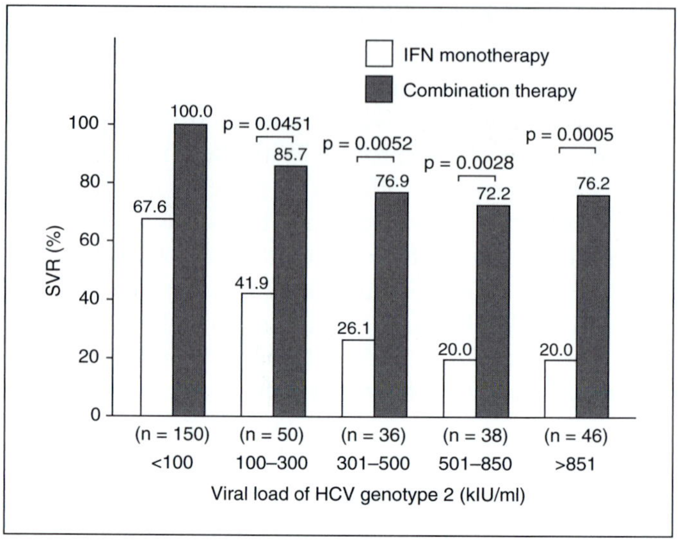

Fig. 2. SVR to IFN monotherapy or combination therapy in patients infected with HCV genotype 2 in various viral loads.

Table 1. Comparison between patients with IFN monotherapy and patients with combination therapy

Features	IFN monotherapy (n = 655)	Combination therapy (n = 288)	p value
Age, years[a]	49.7 ± 10.5	53.8 ± 11.1	<0.0001
Male	426 (65.0)	190 (66.0)	NS
BMI[a]	23.1 ± 2.9	23.3 ± 2.3	NS
ALT[b], IU/l	73 (8–1,450)	73 (15–1,111)	NS
Genotype (1/2/others)	382/255/9	219/55/2	0.0409
Viral load[b], kIU/ml	220 (0.5–2,800)	720 (20–2,500)	<0.0001
Activity (A0/A1/A/A3)	41/307/180/12	7/103/87/24	0.0207
Fibrosis (F0/F1/F2/F3/F4)	113/261/145/50/4	10/99/60/35/14	0.0270
SVR	234 (35.7)	105 (36.5)	NS
Compliance to treatment ≥80%	408 (62.3)	185 (64.2)	<0.0001
Discontinuation of treatment	95 (14.5)	54 (18.8)	<0.0001
Duration of treatment (standard/long)[c]	560/95	222/66	0.0019

Figures in parentheses are percentages, unless otherwise indicated. NS = Not significant.
[a] Mean ± SD.
[b] Median values are shown with ranges in parentheses.
[c] Standard duration was 30 weeks and long duration exceeded 40 weeks.

between those receiving IFN monotherapy and those with combination therapy. However, in patients with a high viral load (>850 kIU/ml) and in those with a lower viral load (100–300 kIU/ml), the SVR rate was significantly higher in patients with combination therapy than in those with IFN monotherapy (fig. 1). In contrast, among patients with genotype 2 infection, a significantly higher SVR rate was gained by the combination therapy than by the IFN monotherapy, except in those with a low viral load (<100 kIU/ml), while no reduction in the SVR rate was observed with increase in viral load (fig. 2).

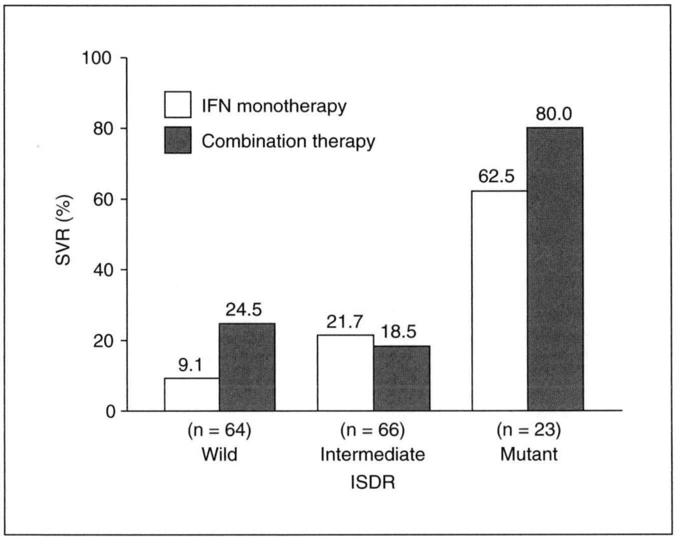

Fig. 3. SVR to IFN monotherapy or combination therapy in patients infected with HCV with or without mutations in ISDR.

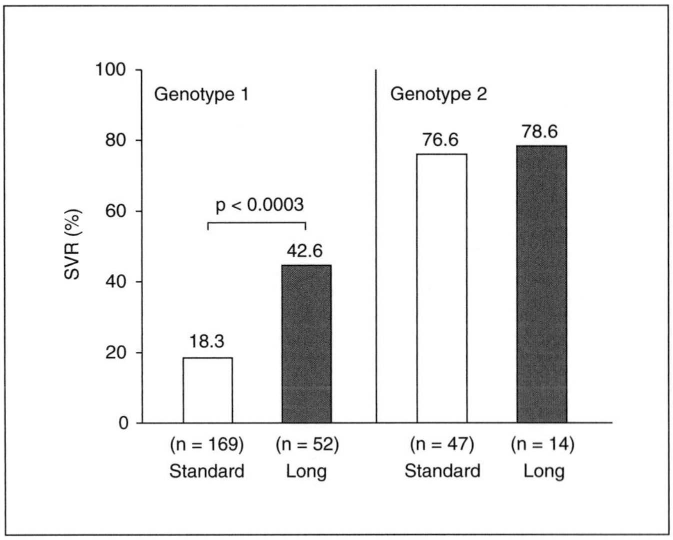

Fig. 4. SVR to the standard (up to 30 weeks) or a long (more than 40 weeks) course of IFN therapy.

Table 2. Factors associated with SVR to IFN monotherapy and combination therapy in multivariate analysis

Factors	Odds ratio (95% CI)	p value
Non-1 genotypes	3.85 (2.66–5.61)	<0.0001
Viral load <100 kIU/ml	7.12 (4.59–11.22)	<0.0001
Ribavirin combined with IFN	3.99 (2.53–6.36)	<0.0001
Compliance to treatment ≥80%	3.13 (1.93–5.20)	<0.0001
Age ≤65 years	5.20 (1.96–13.90)	0.0009
BMI <24	3.27 (1.09–10.05)	0.0363

The relationship between ISDR and the SVR rate was examined in patients infected with HCV genotype 1. A trend for a higher SVR rate was observed with the wild type in the combination therapy group, but differences were not significant (fig. 3).

The factors associated with SVR were examined in all patients by multivariate analysis (table 2). Non-1 genotypes, low viral load, combined ribavirin, good compliance to treatment, age <65 years and low body mass index (BMI) were factors significantly associated with SVR.

Factors Influencing SVR to Combination Therapy

SVR was achieved by 105 of the 288 (37.5%) patients who received combined IFN and ribavirin. Of those, 47 aged ≥65 and 241 aged <65 years were compared (table 3). Of the patients aged ≥65, the proportion of men was significantly lower and many had advanced fibrosis, and they required the reduction or discontinuation of the ribavirin dose more often than those <65 years old. Although a trend for a higher SVR rate was observed in patients aged <65 than in those ≥65 years, the difference fell just short of being significant (p = 0.0819).

The influence of treatment duration on the SVR rate was evaluated in patients infected with HCV of different genotypes (fig. 4). The SVR rate was high in patients with genotype 2 infection, regardless of the duration of treatment: 76.6% for the standard course (up to 30 weeks) and 78.6% for a long course (≥40 weeks). However, in patients with genotype 1, a longer duration of treatment resulted in a higher SVR rate (18.3% for the standard course vs. 42.6% for a long course, p = 0.0003).

Figure 5 compares the SVR among patients with different BMI levels who were infected with HCV genotype 1 or 2. In patients with either genotype, the SVR rate decreased with an increase in BMI, and the decrease was greater in patients infected with genotype 2 than in those infected with genotype 1 (p = 0.0212).

The factors associated with SVR in combination therapy were examined by multivariate analysis (table 4). Non-1 genotypes, serum HCV RNA negative at 4 weeks after the start of therapy, treatment course ≥40 weeks and low BMI were factors significantly associated with SVR.

Table 3. Comparison of patients treated with combined IFN and ribavirin who were aged ≥65 years and <65 years

Features	≥65 years (n = 47)	<65 years (n = 241)	p value
Male	24 (51.1)	166 (68.9)	0.0278
BMI[a]	23.6 ± 2.2	23.2 ± 2.9	NS
ALT[b], IU/l	75 (22–1,110)	73 (15–592)	NS
Genotype (1/2/others)	40/4/0	179/57/3	NS
Viral load[b], kIU/ml	780 (37–2,300)	706 (21–2,500)	NS
Activity (A0/A1/A/A3)	0/14/12/5	7/80/68/18	NS
Fibrosis (F0/F1/F2/F3/F4)	0/9/8/9/4	10/80/49/24/9	0.0332
SVR	12 (25.2)	93 (38.6)	NS
Compliance to treatment (≥80%)	37 (78.7)	207 (85.9)	NS
The standard duration of treatment[c]	35 (74.5)	184 (76.3)	NS
Dose reduction of IFN	8 (17.0)	35 (14.5)	NS
Discontinuation of IFN	11 (23.4)	43 (17.8)	NS
Dose reduction of ribavirin	20/44 (45.5)	70/233 (30.0)	0.0453
Discontinuation of ribavirin	16/44 (36.4)	51/232 (22.0)	0.0414

Figures in parentheses are percentages, unless otherwise indicated. NS = Not significant.
[a] Mean ± SD.
[b] Median values are shown with ranges in parentheses.
[c] Standard duration was 30 weeks and long duration exceeded 40 weeks.

Table 4. Factors influencing SVR to combination therapy in multivariate analysis

Factors	Odds ratio (95% CI)	p value
Non-1 genotypes	21.24 (6.54–82.78)	<0.0001
HBV RNA negative at 4 weeks	18.35 (7.72–48.68)	<0.0001
Treatment duration longer than 40 weeks	7.35 (2.55–23.26)	0.0004
BMI <24	77.21 (5.27–1,404.42)	0.0021

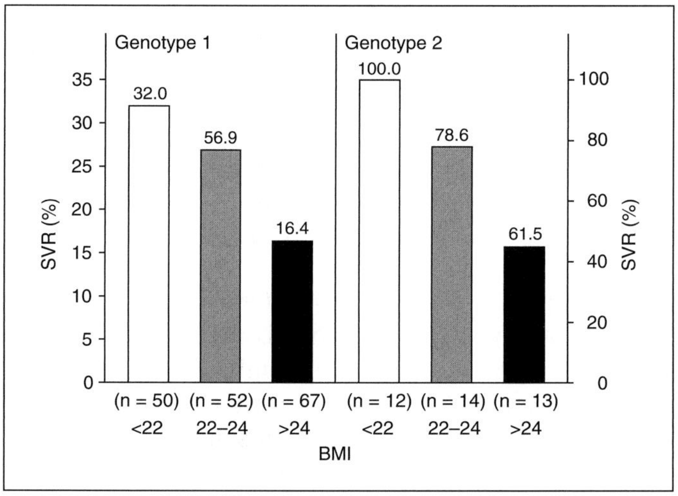

Fig. 5. SVR to combination therapy in patients with different BMI levels.

Discussion

The current status of treatment of chronic hepatitis C in Japan is presented based on our experiences at several major hospitals in the Tokai area. With IFN monotherapy, an overall SVR rate of 35.7% (234/655) has been obtained. The SVR rate in patients infected with non-1 genotypes in low viral loads was high, as has been reported [3–5, 12, 13]. However, in Japan, the patients with hardly treatable viral characteristics (genotype 1b infection in high viral loads) account for 70%. Combination therapy with ribavirin became possible in Japan in December 2001. Although the approved duration of treatment remains 24 weeks, combination therapy is currently the main treatment in Japan; it is focused on patients with a high viral load, particularly of HCV genotype 1b.

Although the SVR rate remains low in patients with genotype 1b infection in high viral loads, it has improved with combination therapy. A trend for increased SVR rates with combination therapy was also observed with genotype 1b infection of the wild type, although the difference was not significant (fig. 3). In remarkable contrast, the SVR rate in genotype 2 infection with combination therapy was high at 70–80%, regardless of the viral load (fig. 5).

The age was significantly higher in patients with combination therapy than with IFN monotherapy. This is inevitable, because new HCV infection has become rare in Japan, and the age of patients with chronic hepatitis is much higher than in other countries [14, 15]. It is well known that there are more side effects with combination therapy than with monotherapy. In this study, compliance to treatment was clearly lower and the rate of treatment discontinuation higher with the combination therapy than with IFN monotherapy. The proportion of male patients was significantly lower, and liver disease was more advanced in 45 patients aged ≥65 years than in the 241 aged <65 years who received the combination therapy. The requirement for reduction of ribavirin dose and treatment discontinuation was more frequent in older patients. Although the SVR rate was somewhat higher in patients aged <65 than in those aged ≥65 years, 38.6% (93/241) versus 25.5% (12/47), the difference was not significant. Few studies have compared side effects and complications in the elderly with IFN monotherapy and combination therapy [16, 17]. A good SVR rate would be achievable in the elderly by avoiding early treatment discontinuation by careful monitoring for instituting treatment modification including dose reduction as required.

Since the duration of ribavirin treatment is limited to 24 weeks in Japan, IFN alone was continued in 66 patients after they had completed combination therapy for 24 weeks. Although no benefits were observed with extended IFN monotherapy in patients infected with genotype 2, a clear advantage of additional IFN monotherapy was observed in those with genotype 1. In the very near future, 48-week treatment with combined peg-IFN and ribavirin is expected to be approved; until then, the type of therapy we used will be given to patients. Extended IFN monotherapy will also be useful in patients for whom long-term treatment with ribavirin is not indicated.

Obesity starting in the middle age is a growing problem in Japan, as elsewhere in the world. Recently, reports on the association of the BMI as well as the body weight with the SVR rate are accumulating [18–23]. An association between the BMI and SVR was also observed in our study, with the SVR rate decreasing in parallel with an increased BMI. Furthermore, this tendency was particularly clear in patients with genotype 2 infection. Several mechanisms for treatment responses reduced by obesity and hepatic steatosis have been proposed. They include a decrease in IFN-α available in the liver and impaired immune responses to HCV associated with obesity. Actually, weight reduction in obese patients improves histological changes in the liver, which may reflect an increased efficacy of IFN-α [24, 25].

Acknowlegements

We thank the following institutions for their participation in this study: Anjo Kosei Hospital, Department of Internal Medicine; Inazawa City Hospital, Department of Internal Medicine; Kakegawa City General Hospital, Department of Internal Medicine; Toyota Medical Corporation Kariya General Hospital, Department of Internal Medicine; Gamagori City Hospital, Department of Internal Medicine; Aihoku Hospital, Department of Internal Medicine; Kamo Hospital, Department of Internal Medicine; Yokkaichi City Hospital, Department of Internal Medicine; Seirei Hospital, Department of Internal Medicine; Chubu-Rosai Hospital, Department of Gastroenterology; Toyohashi Municipal Hospital, Department of Gastroenterology; Japanese Red Cross Nagoya First Hospital, Department of Gastroenterology.

References

1 Kiyosawa K, Sodeyama T, Tanaka E, Gibo Y, Yoshizawa K, Nakano Y, Furuta S, Akahane Y, Nishioka K, Purcell RH: Interrelationship of blood transfusion, non-A, non-B hepatitis and hepatocellular carcinoma: Analysis by detection of antibody to hepatitis C virus. Hepatology 1990;12:671–675.
2 Takano S, Yokosuka O, Imazeki F, Tagawa M, Omata M: Incidence of hepatocellular carcinoma in chronic hepatitis B and C: A prospective study of 251 patients. Hepatology 1995; 21:650–655.
3 Tsubota A, Chayama K, Ikeda K, Yasuji A, Koida I, Saitoh S, Hashimoto M, Iwasaki S, Kobayashi M, Hiromitsu K: Factors predictive of response to interferon-alpha therapy in hepatitis C virus infection. Hepatology 1994;19: 1088–1094.
4 Kanai K, Kako M, Okamoto H: HCV genotypes in chronic hepatitis C and response to interferon (letter). Lancet 1992;339:1543.
5 Kumada T, Nakano S, Takeda I, Sugiyama K, Osada T, Kiriyama S, Toyoda H, Sasa T, Shibata M, Morishima T, Nakano I, Fukuda Y, Kosaka Y, Tameda Y, Nakashima M: Long-term administration of natural interferon-alpha in patients with chronic hepatitis C: Relationship to serum RNA concentration, HCV-RNA genotypes, histological changes and hepatitis C virus. J Gastroenterol Hepatol 1996;11:159–165.
6 Okamoto H, Mishiro S, Tokita H, Tsuda F, Miyakawa Y, Mayumi M: Superinfection of chimpanzees carrying hepatitis C virus of genotype II/1b with that of genotype III/2a or I/1a. Hepatology 1994;20:1131–1136.
7 Simmonds P, Alberti A, Alter HJ, Bonino F, Bradley DW, Brechot C, Brouwer JT, Chan SW, Chayama K, Chen DS: A proposed system for the nomenclature of hepatitis C viral genotypes. Hepatology 1994;19:1321–1324.
8 Pawlotsky JM: Use and interpretation of virological tests for hepatitis C. Hepatology 2002; 36:S65–S73.
9 Enomoto N, Sakuma I, Asahina Y, Kurosaki M, Murakami T, Yamamoto C, Izumi N, Marumo F, Sato C: Comparison of full-length sequences of interferon-sensitive and resistant hepatitis C virus 1b. Sensitivity to interferon is conferred by amino acid substitutions in the NS5A region. J Clin Invest 1995;96:224–230.
10 Enomoto N, Sakuma I, Asahina Y, Kurosaki M, Murakami T, Yamamoto C, Ogura Y, Izumi N, Marumo F, Sato C: Mutations in the nonstructural protein 5A gene and response to interferon in patients with chronic hepatitis C virus 1b infection. N Engl J Med 1996;334: 77–81.
11 Bedossa P, Poynard T: An algorithm for the grading of activity in chronic hepatitis C. Hepatology 1996;24:289–293.
12 Yoshioka K, Kakumu S, Wakita T, Ishikawa T, Itoh Y, Takayanagi M, Higashi Y, Shibata M, Morishima T: Detection of hepatitis C virus by polymerase chain reaction and response to interferon-alpha therapy: Relationship to genotypes of hepatitis C virus. Hepatology 1992;16:293–299.
13 Tsubota A, Chayama K, Arase Y, Koida I, Saitoh S, Ikeda K, Iwasaki S, Matsumoto T, Kobayashi M, Kumada H: Factors useful in predicting the response to interferon therapy in chronic hepatitis C. J Gastroenterol Hepatol 1993;8:535–539.
14 Sasaki F, Tanaka J, Moriya T, Katayama K, Hiraoka M, Ohishi K, Nagakami H, Mishiro S, Yoshizawa H: Very low incidence rates of community-acquired hepatitis C virus infection in company employees, long-term inpatients, and blood donors in Japan. J Epidemiol 1996;6:198–203.
15 Tanaka J, Kumagai J, Katayama K, Komiya Y, Mizui M, Yamanaka R, Suzuki K, Miyakawa Y, Yoshizawa H: Sex- and age-specific carriers of hepatitis B and C viruses in Japan estimated by the prevalence in the 3,485,648 first-time blood donors during 1995–2000. Intervirology 2004;47:32–40.
16 Alessi N, Freni MA, Spadaro A, Ajello A, Turiano S, Migliorato D, Ferrau O: Efficacy of interferon treatment (IFN) in elderly patients with chronic hepatitis C. Infez Med 2003;11: 208–212.
17 Terranova R, Luca S: Preliminary results of beta-interferon treatment in the elderly. Control Clin Trials 1996;17:123–129.
18 Zeuzem S, Feinman SV, Rasenack J, Heathcote EJ, Lai MY, Gane E, O'Grady J, Reichen J, Diago M, Lin A, Hoffman J, Brunda MJ: Peginterferon alfa-2a in patients with chronic hepatitis C. N Engl J Med 2000;343:1666–1672.
19 Akuta N, Suzuki F, Tsubota A, Suzuki Y, Someya T, Kobayashi M, Saitoh S, Arase Y, Ikeda K, Kumada H: Efficacy of interferon monotherapy to 394 consecutive naive cases infected with hepatitis C virus genotype 2a in Japan: Therapy efficacy as consequence of tripartite interaction of viral, host and interferon treatment-related factors. J Hepatol 2002;37: 831–836.
20 Camma C, Di Bona D, Schepis F, Heathcote EJ, Zeuzem S, Pockros PJ, Marcellin P, Balart L, Alberti A, Craxi A: Effect of peginterferon alfa-2a on liver histology in chronic hepatitis C: A meta-analysis of individual patient data. Hepatology 2004;39:333–342.
21 Bressler BL, Guindi M, Tomlinson G, Heathcote J: High body mass index is an independent risk factor for nonresponse to antiviral treatment in chronic hepatitis C. Hepatology 2003; 38:639–644.
22 Fried MW, Shiffman ML, Reddy KR, Smith C, Marinos G, Goncales FL Jr, Haussinger D, Diago M, Carosi G, Dhumeaux D, Craxi A, Lin A, Hoffman J, Yu J: Peginterferon alfa-2a plus ribavirin for chronic hepatitis C virus infection. N Engl J Med 2002;347:975–982.
23 Lee SS, Heathcote EJ, Reddy KR, Zeuzem S, Fried MW, Wright TL, Pockros PJ, Haussinger D, Smith CI, Lin A, Pappas SC: Prognostic factors and early predictability of sustained viral response with peginterferon alfa-2a (40KD). J Hepatol 2002;37:500–506.
24 Giannini E, Ceppa P, Testa R: Steatosis in chronic hepatitis C: Can weight reduction improve therapeutic efficacy? J Hepatol 2001;35: 432–433.
25 Gao B, Hong F, Radaeva S: Host factors and failure of interferon-alpha treatment in hepatitis C virus. Hepatology 2004;39:880–890.

Intervirology

Author Index Vol. 49, No. 1–2, 2006

Fax +41 61 306 12 34
E-Mail karger@karger.ch
www.karger.com

Accessible online at:
www.karger.com/int

Intervirology

Subject Index Vol. 49, No. 1–2, 2006

KARGER

Fax +41 61 306 12 34
E-Mail karger@karger.ch
www.karger.com

Accessible online at:
www.karger.com/int